METABOLIC MEMORY

METABOLIC MEMORY

Past, Present and Future Implications

JEENA GUPTA
Lovely Professional University, Phagwara, Punjab, India

ELSEVIER
ACADEMIC PRESS
An imprint of Elsevier

Academic Press is an imprint of Elsevier
125 London Wall, London EC2Y 5AS, United Kingdom
50 Hampshire Street, 5th Floor, Cambridge, MA 02139, United States

ISBN: 978-0-443-44591-0

For information on all Academic Press publications visit our website at
https://www.elsevier.com/books-and-journals

Publisher: Megan Ball
Acquisitions Editor: Patricia Osborn
Editorial Project Manager: Apoorva Shrivastava
Production Project Manager: M. Balakrishnan
Cover Designer: Mark Rogers

Typeset by TNQ Tech

Contents

Preface

The concept of metabolic memory, the persistent impact of past metabolic states on future physiological outcomes, has transformed our understanding of chronic metabolic diseases such as diabetes, obesity, and cardiovascular disorders. Once regarded merely as an epiphenomenon of poor glycemic control, metabolic memory is now recognized as a complex interplay of molecular, cellular, and epigenetic mechanisms that imprint lasting effects long after metabolic normalization has been achieved.

This book, *Metabolic Memory: Past, Present and Future Implications*, offers a comprehensive exploration of this evolving field, tracing its origins, current scientific insights, and emerging therapeutic frontiers. The book delve into the historical development of the concept, from early clinical trials like the DCCT and UKPDS, which first hinted at the long-term consequences of transient hyperglycemia, to the discovery of oxidative stress, advanced glycation end-products (AGEs), and mitochondrial dysfunction as central mediators of metabolic memory.

The subsequent sections illuminate the molecular underpinnings of metabolic memory, including the pivotal roles of epigenetic remodeling, and persistent inflammatory signaling. Together, these insights reveal how "metabolic scars" become embedded within the genome and proteome, perpetuating cellular dysfunction and disease progression even after metabolic correction.

Equally vital are the discussions on contemporary and future perspectives, showing how understanding metabolic memory paves the way for precision medicine, personalized nutrition, and targeted epigenetic therapies. The book emphasizes the translational potential of this knowledge, exploring how interventions that reverse or reprogram metabolic memory may hold the key to mitigating long-term complications in metabolic disorders.

This volume is intended for researchers, clinicians, and students across disciplines like biochemistry, molecular biology, pharmacology, endocrinology, and systems medicine, who seek a holistic view of how our metabolic past continues to shape our biological future.

It is my hope that this book serves not only as a scholarly reference but also as an inspiration for new hypotheses, innovative research, and collaborative efforts aimed at deciphering metabolic memory and its role in governing human health and disease.

Dr. Jeena Gupta

1

Introduction to metabolic memory

1. Definition and historical background

1.1 Definition

Metabolic memory is a concept that has gained traction in recent years, referring to the phenomenon where prior metabolic states, particularly those involving glucose levels, leave a lasting imprint on the body's physiology. This imprint influences future responses to metabolic changes and can significantly affect the progression and management of chronic diseases such as diabetes, cardiovascular diseases, and obesity. Essentially, it means that the body "remembers" past metabolic conditions and this memory influences current and future health outcomes.

Metabolic diseases, such as diabetes, obesity, and metabolism-associated fatty liver disease (MAFLD), are growing public health concerns globally (Wu et al., 2023). According to (He et al., 2021) Diabetes Atlas, diabetes affects 10.5% of adults worldwide, and this number is projected to increase by 46% by 2045 (Sun et al., 2022). Obesity and overweight rates are similarly rising (Afshin et al., 2017), having nearly doubled since 1975, with over 1.9 billion people classified as overweight or obese by 2016 (Koenen et al., 2021). MAFLD affects 25%–30% of the global population and is the most common liver disease, with rates increasing alongside obesity and type 2 diabetes mellitus (T2DM) (Eslam et al., 2020) These diseases and their complications pose significant health challenges, highlighting the need to investigate their mechanisms and develop effective treatments.

The development of metabolic diseases involves complex mechanisms, requiring comprehensive therapeutic approaches (Pillai et al., 2023). Recent studies show that cells retain harmful effects even after returning to a normal metabolic environment, a phenomenon known as metabolic memory (Lachin and Nathan, 2021). Metabolic memory refers to the lasting cellular changes and characteristics from an earlier abnormal metabolic

Metabolic Memory. https://doi.org/10.1016/B978-0-443-44591-0.00013-8

state. Traditional treatments for metabolic diseases, like glycemic control in T2DM, are challenged by metabolic memory (Smith and Adams, 2011). Despite good glycemic control, inflammation and complications can persist due to metabolic memory (Holman, 2013; Writing Team for the Diabetes Control and Complications Trial, 2003). This calls for deeper research into the molecular mechanisms of metabolic memory and developing treatments that address its adverse effects, potentially improving disease management (Singh et al., 2020). Evidence suggests that mechanisms such as epigenetic regulation, glycosylation end products, and oxidative stress play roles in metabolic memory. These mechanisms form a complex network that could be targeted for detecting and treating metabolic diseases (Vasishta et al., 2022).

This chapter outlines the research history and features of metabolic memory, summarizing its molecular and cellular mechanisms. We highlight its impact on metabolic diseases and connections to disease progression, focusing on links between metabolic memory and cancer risk. Finally, we explore metabolic memory as a target for detecting and treating metabolic diseases.

1.2 Historical background

The concept of "metabolic memory" originated from studies on diabetes, specifically the Diabetes Control and Complications Trial (DCCT) that began in 1983. This trial investigated how hyperglycemia affects long-term complications in diabetes, involving 1441 individuals with type 1 diabetes mellitus (T1DM) (Nathan, 1996). Participants were divided into intensive therapy and conventional therapy groups, with the former receiving at least three daily insulin injections or continuous infusion to achieve tight glycemic control, while the latter received one or two daily injections for asymptomatic glucose control (The Diabetes Control and Complications Trial (DCCT), 1986; Diabetes Control and Complications Trial (DCCT), 1987). By 1993, after an average follow-up of 6.5 years, results showed that intensive therapy significantly reduced diabetic complications like retinopathy, nephropathy, and neuropathy compared to conventional therapy, primarily due to differences in mean glycosylated hemoglobin A1c (HbA1c) levels (The Relationship of Glycemic Exposure (HbA1c), 1995; The Absence of a Glycemic Threshold, 1996). These findings supported the "glucose hypothesis," emphasizing the critical role of blood glucose levels in diabetic complications (Nathan, 2014).

After the DCCT, the Epidemiology of Diabetes Interventions and Complications (EDIC) study began in 1994, continuing to observe 1394 surviving participants (Epidemiology of Diabetes Interventions and Complications (EDIC), 1999). Initially, conventional therapy participants were switched to intensive treatment. Although HbA1c levels between groups converged, the first 4-year EDIC follow-up revealed widening disparities in complication rates. The intensively treated group showed reduced progression of retinopathy and nephropathy (Lachin et al., 2000). These outcomes highlighted that early HbA1c levels significantly impact long-term complications, even after hyperglycemia normalization, a phenomenon termed "metabolic memory" (Lachin and Nathan, 2021).

Similar findings emerged from the UK Prospective Diabetes Study (UKPDS) and the Steno-2 trial, where early intensive glycemic control offered prolonged benefits (Chalmers and Cooper, 2008; Intensive blood-glucose control, 1998). The UKPDS, which involved newly diagnosed diabetic patients, showed a 25% risk reduction in microvascular lesions and a 16% reduction in myocardial infarction with intensive therapy (Intensive blood-glucose control, 1998). In the Steno-2 trial, intensive therapy reduced cardiovascular risks and mortality over 13.3 years, despite eventual glycemic control convergence (Gæde et al., 2008).

Recent research has expanded the concept of metabolic memory to include hyperlipidemia and hypoxia. Abnormal fat and cholesterol levels can cause lasting cellular changes (Lu et al., 2021; Duan et al., 2022). Crisóstomo et al. found that an early high-fat diet can cause irreversible changes in testicular lipid content and metabolism, affecting sperm quality for generations (Crisóstomo et al., 2022a, 2022b). This "inherited metabolic memory" is linked to sperm small non-coding RNAs (sncRNAs) and epigenetic changes in chromatin accessibility and histone modifications (Leung et al., 2016). Similarly, a study on medaka fish demonstrated that early high-fat diets induced lasting epigenetic changes in liver genes associated with fibrosis and cancer, even after returning to a normal diet (Inoue et al., 2023).

Hypoxia-induced metabolic reprogramming also contributes to metabolic memory. Hypoxic fibroblasts exhibit persistent metabolic changes, shifting toward aerobic glycolysis and increasing inflammation, even after returning to normoxia (Li et al., 2016a; Watson et al., 2014). In tumors, hypoxia and hypoxia-inducible factor-1α (HIF-1α) trigger transcriptional reprogramming and epigenetic modifications, promoting cancer progression and resistance (Tian et al., 2020; Fan et al., 2023). Additionally, high uric acid levels can cause persistent immune changes through epigenetic modifications. In gout patients, differential DNA methylation of immune-related genes persists even after uric acid levels normalize (Wang et al., 2020b). Histone methyltransferase and histone deacetylase inhibitors can reverse some of these changes (Cleophas et al., 2019). Further research is needed to understand hyperuricemia's long-term effects and potential interventions.

In summary, metabolic memory, initially focused on diabetes, describes how short-term metabolic abnormalities can have long-term health effects. Recent studies have expanded this concept to include lipid, oxygen, and uric acid metabolism, emphasizing the importance of early and strict metabolic control to mitigate these long-lasting effects (Fig. 1.1).

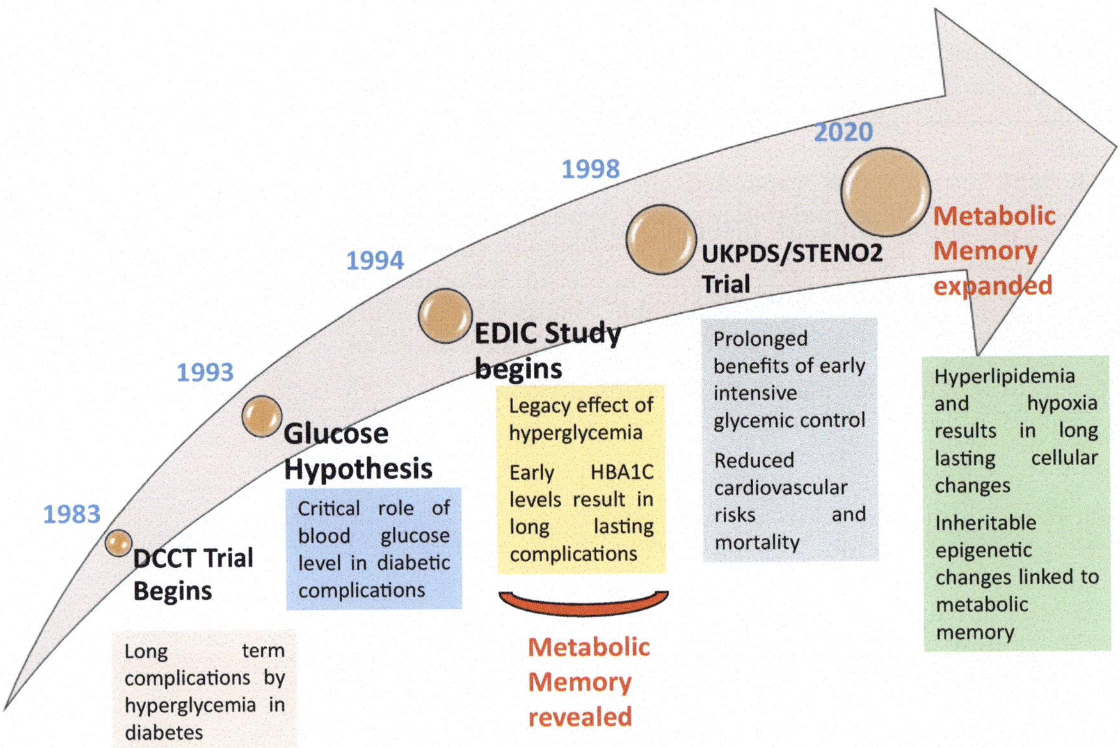

Figure 1.1 History of metabolic memory.

2. The scientific basis of metabolic memory

The concept of metabolic memory encompasses several complex biological mechanisms, explaining how early metabolic states, even if transient, can have long-lasting effects on health. The scientific basis of metabolic memory involves the interplay of epigenetic modifications, persistent inflammatory responses, oxidative stress, and structural changes in tissues. Understanding these mechanisms provides insights into how early metabolic experiences influence long-term health outcomes.

2.1 Epigenetic modifications

Epigenetics refers to changes in gene expression that do not involve alterations to the underlying DNA sequence. These changes can be influenced by environmental factors, including metabolic states such as hyperglycemia. Epigenetic modifications include DNA methylation, histone modification, and noncoding RNA expression.

Recent studies have demonstrated a strong link between epigenetic modifications and metabolic memory. Epigenetic changes are observed in various cell types exposed to abnormal metabolic conditions, and these changes often persist even after normal metabolic levels are restored. This suggests that epigenetic modifications are a fundamental mechanism underlying metabolic memory (Li et al., 2023; Alvarez and DiStefano, 2013). Chromosomes are made up of DNA-protein complexes called chromatin, with nucleosomes as their basic units. Each nucleosome consists of an octamer of histone proteins, including H2A, H2B, H3, and H4, wrapped by 147 base pairs of DNA. Epigenetic modifications regulate gene expression without altering the DNA sequence (Bošković and Rando, 2018). These modifications occur at the level of DNA and histones and include DNA methylation, histone modifications, and non-coding RNAs (ncRNAs), which work together to control gene function (Kato and Natarajan, 2019; Aranyi and Susztak, 2019). Disrupted metabolic conditions can trigger cellular metabolic reprogramming, leading to changes in metabolites that affect enzymes involved in modifying the epigenome. These epigenetic changes allow cells to quickly respond to environmental changes and maintain long-term responsiveness even after the original stimulus is gone (Whitelaw and Whitelaw, 2008; Breton et al., 2021).

DNA Methylation: One of the most studied epigenetic mechanisms in metabolic memory is DNA methylation. DNA methylation is a key biochemical process where methyl groups are added to DNA molecules, primarily at CpG dinucleotides, forming 5-methylcytosines. This process often suppresses gene expression by preventing transcription factor binding or recruiting chromatin inactivation complexes. Methylation in gene bodies can affect transcription elongation and alternative splicing (Moore et al., 2013). DNA methylation is primarily maintained by DNA methyltransferases (DNMTs), where DNMT1 ensures methylation during DNA replication, and DNMT3a and DNMT3b initiate de novo methylation (Portela and Esteller, 2010; Chen and Riggs, 2011). Demethylation can occur through the inhibition of DNMT1 and activation of TET enzymes, which remove methyl groups.

Research indicates a link between DNA methylation and metabolic memory, influenced by environmental factors and diet, contributing to metabolic disease susceptibility (Jirtle and Skinner, 2007; Wang et al., 2012). For instance, the Diabetes Control and Complications Trial/Epidemiology of Diabetes Interventions and Complications (DCCT/EDIC) study found correlations between long-term glycemic history and changes in DNA methylation at 186 CpGs associated with HbA1c levels (Wang, Tar and Davies, 2020a). These CpGs are often enriched in enhancer regions, particularly at CCAAT/enhancer binding protein (C/EBP) sites, which are crucial for hematopoiesis and linked to oxidative stress and inflammation (Avellino and Delwel, 2017; Zhuo et al., 2016).

Specific methylation patterns have been identified in diabetes-related genes. For example, differences in methylation levels at CpG loci near the insulin gene are associated with type 1 diabetes mellitus (T1DM) susceptibility (Fradin et al., 2012). Similarly, DNA methylation changes are observed in complications like diabetic nephropathy and retinopathy, where altered methylation patterns contribute to disease progression (Maghbooli et al., 2014). Notably, DNA methylation changes induced by early metabolic abnormalities often persist even after normalization of metabolic conditions. For instance, hypermethylation in the POLG1 promoter region in diabetic rats remains despite normal glucose levels. This persistence is also seen in other diabetic models, suggesting a lasting impact on gene expression (Olsen et al., 2012; Wang et al., 2020b).

Short-term high-fat diets can cause long-lasting DNA methylation changes, affecting genes involved in lipid metabolism (Gomez-Arango et al., 2016; Peng et al., 2023). These changes persist even after returning to a normal diet, as demonstrated by altered methylation patterns in genes like Apoa4, affecting triglyceride transport. Offspring of mothers on high-fat diets show increased susceptibility to liver disease and inflammation due to sustained methylation changes in key metabolic genes (Wankhade et al., 2017). Overall, these findings suggest that abnormal metabolic stimuli can induce persistent promoter methylation changes, affecting gene expression related to oxidative stress and apoptosis, thus contributing to metabolic memory.

Histone Modification: Histones are proteins around which DNA is wrapped, and their modification can influence gene expression by altering chromatin structure. Histone modifications are post-translational changes that occur on the N-terminal amino acids of histones, including acetylation, methylation, phosphorylation, and ubiquitination (Bannister and Kouzarides, 2011). These modifications regulate the interaction between histones, DNA, and nuclear proteins, thus influencing gene transcription. The impact on gene expression depends on the type, degree, and location of the modification, which affects cellular metabolism through various mechanisms (Tessarz and Kouzarides, 2014).

Histone acetylation, mediated by histone acetyltransferases (HATs) like p300 and CREB-binding protein, and histone deacetylases (HDACs) including HDAC1-11 and sirtuins, is a dynamic process that reduces the positive charge on histone tails, decreasing their binding to negatively charged DNA (Alvarez and DiStefano, 2013). This opens chromatin and promotes gene transcription. Acetylation at promoters (e.g., H3K9ac, H3K14ac, and H3K56ac) typically activates transcription, while deacetylation represses it (Li, Li and Sun, 2016b). Hyperglycemia activates HATs, leading to increased acetylation of pro-inflammatory gene promoters and amplifying inflammatory responses (Yun et al., 2011). In hyperglycemic conditions, the expression and function of Class III HDAC sirtuin 1 (SIRT1) are reduced, linking metabolic memory to histone acetylation (Zheng et al., 2012). High glucose inhibits SIRT1, increasing acetylation of genes like Foxo1 and NF-κB, leading to oxidative stress and inflammation (Tu et al., 2021). Additionally, HDAC3 and HDAC4 are upregulated in high glucose, worsening inflammation and fibrosis (Chen et al., 2021; Wang et al., 2014). Histone acetylation also affects DNA methylation by modifying DNMT proteins (Allis and Jenuwein, 2016). For example, H3K9 acetylation at the DNMT1 promoter can activate DNMT1 by downregulating SIRT1 (Mishra et al., 2018).

Histone methylation can either activate or repress transcription depending on the modified residues and methylation level. Activation is associated with methylation at H3K4me1/2/3, H3K36me2/3, H3K48me3, and H3K79me3, while H3K9me3, H3K27me3, and H4K20me3 are linked to repression (Brooks et al., 2010). Histone methyltransferases (HMTs) add methyl groups to lysine or arginine residues, which can be removed by histone demethylases (HDMs) (Klose and Zhang, 2007). Diabetic rat studies show reduced H3K9me3 and H3K27me3, lifting repression of genes related to fibrosis and inflammation, like Il-6 and Mcp-1 (Villeneuve et al., 2008; Komers et al., 2013; Jia et al., 2019). Markers like H3K4me1 are upregulated at p65 promoters in high glucose and persist after glucose normalization (El-Osta et al., 2008). Mice on a high-fat diet followed by a normal diet show persistent lipid accumulation, with FAIRE-seq analysis indicating chromatin changes affecting transcription factors such as HNF4α, linked to repressive histone modifications like H3K9me2 (Inoue et al., 2023). Histone methylation also influences DNA methylation by modulating DNMT proteins (Cedar and Bergman, 2009). H3K4 methylation can activate transcription by initiating de novo DNA methylation, while interaction with DNMTs at H3K9 leads to transcriptional repression (Hashimoto et al., 2010; Gowher and Jeltsch, 2018).

Histone phosphorylation affects histone-DNA interactions by altering histone charge, primarily occurring on serine, threonine, and tyrosine residues. Elevated H3Ser10 phosphorylation in diabetic patients' glomerular endothelial cells increases VCAM-1 expression, promoting leukocyte adhesion and advancing diabetic nephropathy (Alghamdi et al., 2018; Liu et al., 2015). Histone ubiquitination typically occurs at lysine residues in histone H2A and H2B's C-terminal tail (Svikle et al., 2022). High glucose induces H2A ubiquitination and reduces H2B ubiquitination, activating the TGF-β pathway and accelerating disease progression (Gao et al., 2013). Recently, histone lactylation has gained interest for its role in gene transcription and metabolic regulation, highlighting the need for further study in its link to metabolic disorders (Zhang et al., 2019).

Non-Coding RNAs: Non-coding RNAs, including microRNAs (miRNAs) and long non-coding RNAs (lncRNAs), play significant roles in regulating gene expression. Non-coding RNAs (ncRNAs) are RNA molecules that do not code for proteins but regulate gene expression at post-transcriptional and translational levels (Taft et al., 2010). They are classified into structural RNAs, like rRNAs and tRNAs, and regulatory RNAs. Regulatory RNAs include small ncRNAs (sncRNAs) under 200 nucleotides (nt) and long ncRNAs (lncRNAs) over 200 nt (Palazzo and Lee, 2015). sncRNAs include microRNAs (miRNAs), small interfering RNAs (siRNAs), PIWI-interacting RNAs (piRNAs), and other sncRNAs. lncRNAs are categorized based on their origin, such as intergenic, bidirectional, sense/antisense, intronic, and enhancer lncRNAs (Wang et al., 2015; Nojima and Proudfoot, 2022). Recent studies indicate that both miRNAs and lncRNAs influence gene expression and modulate growth and inflammatory factors related to metabolic diseases.

miRNAs are short, endogenous non-coding RNAs, usually 17 to 25 bases long, that bind to mRNA to cause degradation or inhibition after transcription (Shantikumar et al., 2012). They can regulate multiple target genes involved in metabolic memory pathways, and a single target gene can be regulated by multiple miRNAs (Hartig et al., 2015). Dysregulated miRNA expression contributes to metabolic complications by affecting angiogenesis, apoptosis, inflammation, and oxidative stress (Agbu and Carthew, 2021; Macvanin et al., 2023). For example, miRNA-21 (miR-21) is upregulated in hyperglycemic conditions, activating TGF-β and NF-κB signaling pathways and leading to inflammation and apoptosis (Zhong et al., 2013). Thus, miRNAs have potential as diagnostic and prognostic biomarkers and therapeutic targets for metabolic diseases and their complications (Kato and Natarajan, 2014).

LncRNAs are transcribed by RNA polymerase II or III and resemble protein-coding mRNAs but do not translate into proteins (Guttman and Rinn, 2012; Cabili et al., 2011). Typically expressed at low levels under normal conditions, lncRNAs play key roles in cell proliferation, differentiation, and senescence (Zhao and Lin, 2015; Schmitz et al., 2016). Aberrant expression of lncRNAs is linked to certain diseases (Forrest and Khalil, 2017; Yang et al., 2022; Thomas et al., 2017). Recent research shows that lncRNAs regulate metabolic disorders through epigenetic modifications, transcriptional regulation, and post-transcriptional modulation (Goyal et al., 2018). For example, the lncRNA maternally expressed gene 3 (MEG3) is downregulated in the retina of mice with STZ-induced diabetes, worsening retinal microvascular dysfunction by activating the PI3K/Akt signaling pathway (Qiu et al., 2016). The decrease in MEG3 expression is controlled by DNMT1-mediated methylation at the MEG3 promoter, promoting endothelial-mesenchymal transition (endMT) in diabetic retinopathy patients (He et al., 2021) (Table 1.1).

2.2 Inflammatory responses

Chronic inflammation is a hallmark of many metabolic diseases, and metabolic memory can perpetuate inflammatory responses initiated during periods of poor metabolic control. Hyperglycemia induces the production of pro-inflammatory

Table 1.1 Influences of different epigenetic modifications on metabolic memory.

Epigenetic mechanism	Description	Impact on metabolic disorders	Examples	References
DNA methylation	Addition of methyl groups to DNA, primarily at CpG dinucleotides, forming 5-methylcytosines. Suppresses gene expression by preventing transcription factor binding or recruiting chromatin inactivation complexes.	Contributes to metabolic disease susceptibility through persistent promoter methylation changes induced by abnormal metabolic stimuli.	- Methylation in gene bodies affecting transcription elongation and alternative splicing. - Hyperglycemia causes hypermethylation in diabetic models. - Long-term glycemic history linked to changes in DNA methylation at 186 CpGs associated with HbA1c levels.	Moore et al. (2013), Portela and Esteller (2010), Chen and Riggs (2011), Jirtle and Skinner (2007), Wang et al. (2012, 2020b), Avellino and Delwel (2017), Zhuo et al. (2016), Fradin et al. (2012), Maghbooli et al. (2014), Olsen et al. (2012), Gomez-Arango et al. (2016), Peng et al. (2023), Wankhade et al. (2017)
Histone modification	Post-translational changes to histone proteins, including acetylation, methylation, phosphorylation, and ubiquitination. These modifications alter chromatin structure and influence gene transcription.	Dysregulated histone modifications contribute to the persistence of metabolic memory, promoting inflammation, fibrosis, and oxidative stress in metabolic diseases.	- Hyperglycemia activates HATs, increasing acetylation of pro-inflammatory gene promoters. - High glucose inhibits SIRT1, linking metabolic memory to histone acetylation. - Histone phosphorylation increases VCAM-1 expression, advancing diabetic nephropathy.	Bannister and Kouzarides (2011), Alvarez and DiStefano (2013), Tessarz and Kouzarides (2014), Yun et al. (2011), Zheng et al. (2012), Tu et al. (2021), Chen et al. (2021), Gao et al. (2013), Zhang et al. (2019)

Table 1.1 Influences of different epigenetic modifications on metabolic memory.—*continued*

Epigenetic mechanism	Description	Impact on metabolic disorders	Examples	References
Non-coding RNAs	RNA molecules that do not code for proteins but regulate gene expression at post-transcriptional and translational levels, including miRNAs and lncRNAs.	Dysregulated expression of ncRNAs contributes to metabolic complications by affecting processes like angiogenesis, apoptosis, inflammation, and oxidative stress.	- miRNA-21 upregulation in hyperglycemia activates TGF-β and NF-κB pathways. - Downregulation of lncRNA MEG3 in diabetic retina worsens retinal microvascular dysfunction.	Taft et al. (2010), Shantikumar et al. (2012), Kato and Natarajan (2014), Guttman and Rinn (2012), Cabili et al. (2011), He et al. (2021)

cytokines such as interleukin-6 (IL-6), tumor necrosis factor-alpha (TNF-α), and C-reactive protein (CRP). These cytokines activate inflammatory pathways that can lead to endothelial dysfunction, a key factor in the development of vascular complications. The activation of NF-κB is key to increasing pro-inflammatory gene expression, which, in diabetes, results in elevated inflammatory cytokines associated with vascular inflammation. This promotes the synthesis of endothelial adhesion molecules and proteases, recruiting monocytes that adhere to endothelial and vascular smooth muscle cells and differentiate into macrophages (Guarner and Rubio-Ruiz, 2014). Toll-like receptors also play a significant role in linking inflammation and oxidative stress, contributing to obesity and insulin resistance (Thompson and Webb, 2013).

Even after glycemic control is achieved, the inflammatory response can remain elevated due to the persistence of activated immune cells and sustained production of inflammatory mediators. This ongoing inflammation contributes to the progression of complications such as atherosclerosis, nephropathy, and retinopathy in diabetic patients.

Immune cells play a critical role in the development and maintenance of metabolic memory. Hyperglycemia causes innate immune cells like monocytes and macrophages to acquire metabolic memory, leading to sustained pro-inflammatory responses (Mossel et al., 2020). This metabolic reprogramming in response to high blood sugar contributes to atherosclerosis (van Diepen et al., 2016). In diabetic mice, hyperglycemia increases H3K4me3 and H3K27ac marks on inflammation-related gene promoters in macrophages through a glycolysis-dependent mechanism, enhancing pro-inflammatory gene expression (Edgar et al., 2021). These changes persist even when cells are switched to normal glucose levels, and normoglycemic mice receiving bone marrow transplants from diabetic mice show increased atherosclerosis, indicating a lasting impact of hyperglycemia through metabolic memory (Chen et al., 2020).

Histone-modifying enzymes upregulate MCP-1 expression, activate inflammatory monocyte differentiation, and promote macrophage M1 polarization, which contributes to diabetic wound healing (Cabanel et al., 2015; Davis et al., 2020). Additionally, hyperglycemia increases DNMT1 expression, stimulating the mTOR pathway and activating peripheral blood mononuclear cells (Chen et al., 2019). High lipid levels can also lead to insulin resistance in monocytes, which persists due to metabolic memory. THP-1 monocytes treated with palmitate, a saturated fatty acid, for 6–12 h show resistance to insulin-mediated glucose uptake, lasting at least 60 h after palmitate removal (Gao et al., 2009).

Prolonged inflammation may drive metabolic memory through enhanced reactive oxygen species (ROS) production, which links epigenetic changes to environmental factors and increases the expression of inflammatory factors. This creates a positive feedback loop involving ROS, metabolic byproducts, inflammation, and epigenetic changes, leading to metabolic disorders (Reddy and Natarajan, 2011; Schroen and Heymans, 2012). Increasing evidence shows that excessive ROS-mediated metabolic memory leads to a pro-inflammatory environment and endothelial dysfunction in the aorta (Cai and Harrison, 2000). This process involves NADPH oxidase 4 (Nox4) and endothelial nitric oxide synthase (eNOS), which are regulated by altered histone methylation (Liao et al., 2018). In hyperglycemia, endothelial cells show increased H3K4me1 at Nox4 and eNOS promoters, opposing H3K9me2 and H3K9me3. Transient high blood sugar recruits the methyltransferase SET7 and demethylase LSD1 to the NF-κB-p65 promoter. SET7 upregulates H3K4me1, while LSD1 downregulates H3K9me2 and H3K9me3, activating the NF-κB pathway and increasing inflammatory factors like MCP-1 and VCAM-1, leading to vascular dysfunction (Rana et al., 2012).

Studies also show that hyperglycemia-induced NF-κB pathway enhancement, increased miR-27a-3p, decreased NRF2 expression, and ROS overproduction in endothelial cells persist even after normalizing glucose levels, causing perivascular fibrosis and heart dysfunction (Yao et al., 2022). This confirms metabolic memory in endothelial cells, where insulin alone does not improve cardiac function, but miR-27a-3p inhibitors can reverse adverse effects. Additionally, research on retinal endothelial cells indicates hyperglycemia upregulates miR-23b-3p via NF-κB signaling, targeting SIRT1 to mediate NF-κB acetylation, creating a feedback loop to maintain metabolic memory (Zhao et al., 2016). Studies have shown that early intervention to reduce inflammation during hyperglycemic episodes can mitigate the long-term inflammatory response, highlighting the importance of timely and effective management of metabolic states to prevent chronic complications.

2.3 Oxidative stress

Oxidative stress, characterized by the excessive production of reactive oxygen species (ROS), is a critical factor in the development of metabolic memory. Hyperglycemia increases the production of ROS through several mechanisms, including the activation of the mitochondrial electron transport chain, increased flux through the polyol pathway, and the formation of advanced glycation end-products (AGEs).

Brownlee et al. discovered that hyperglycemia significantly increases reactive oxygen species (ROS) production, a key factor in various pathological conditions (Brownlee, 2001). Under hyperglycemic conditions, excess electron donors like NADH and FADH2 increase the voltage gradient across the mitochondrial membrane, promoting superoxide (O2−) and ROS generation (Trumpower, 1990; Creager et al., 2003). High blood sugar also raises diglycerides (DAG), activating protein kinase C (PKC) and NADPH oxidase, further increasing O2− production. ROS, such as peroxynitrite (ONOO−), disrupts cellular structures and damages nuclear and mitochondrial DNA (Geraldes and King, 2010). Mitochondrial DNA is particularly sensitive to oxidative stress, causing structural and functional impairments, leading to a cycle of ROS production (Foury et al., 2004).

Excessive ROS production explains hyperglycemic metabolic memory, even after blood sugar levels normalize. Although free ROS have a short half-life, their effects persist, contributing to metabolic memory and cell damage (Kowluru et al., 2004). Broad-spectrum antioxidants can counteract ROS effects at the mitochondrial level (Savitha et al., 2005). Excessive ROS also drives pathological cellular mechanisms, including increased polyol and hexosamine fluxes, AGEs, and NF-κB-induced vascular inflammation (Giacco et al., 2010). Interventions aimed at reducing oxidative stress, such as antioxidant supplementation and lifestyle modifications, have shown promise in mitigating the effects of metabolic memory and improving long-term outcomes in patients with metabolic diseases.

2.4 Advanced glycation end products (AGEs)

AGEs are glycosylated adducts produced internally and externally via the "Maillard reaction" (Garay-Sevilla et al., 2021). They form when sugars react with amino groups of proteins, lipids, and nucleic acids through non-enzymatic reactions (Henning and Glomb, 2016). While AGEs naturally accumulate with age, insulin resistance, inflammation, and oxidative stress accelerate their formation, causing cytopathic changes like inflammation, fibrosis, and thrombosis (Yamagishi, 2011). AGEs levels are higher in patients with MAFLD, diabetes, and complications, linked to disease progression and mortality (De Vos et al., 2014; Genuth et al., 2015). Resistant to degradation, AGEs-modified proteins persist in diabetic patients' blood vessels, kidneys, and heart, contributing to metabolic memory (Flier et al., 1988).

AGEs harm the body through three main mechanisms: modifying extracellular and intracellular proteins, and activating signaling cascades via the RAGE receptor. Extracellular protein modification leads to abnormal crosslinks in proteins like collagen and laminin, thickening blood vessel walls, and affecting factors like fibrinogen and LDL, which enhance blood clot formation and cause diabetic cataracts (Fishman et al., 2018; Bahmani et al., 2016). Intracellularly, AGEs disrupt cellular homeostasis by modifying proteins, causing improperly folded proteins to accumulate in the ER, leading to ER stress and apoptosis. They also bind to mitochondrial complexes, decreasing ATP and increasing ROS, leading to mitochondrial dysfunction and diminishing antioxidant enzymes (Ramasamy et al., 2005). The AGE-RAGE interaction is a major pathogenic mechanism, triggering signaling cascades that produce pro-inflammatory factors and ROS, leading to tissue damage and inflammation (Hudson and Lippman, 2018). This interaction activates pathways like MAPK and NF-κB, overexpressing cytokines and adhesion molecules, enhancing oxidative stress, and contributing to fibrosis, apoptosis, vascular inflammation, and diabetic complications (Stitt et al., 2002).

2.5 Structural changes in tissues

Metabolic memory encompasses the long-term structural changes in tissues due to prolonged hyperglycemia and metabolic dysregulation, contributing to complications like diabetic nephropathy (DN) (Zheng et al., 2012). These structural alterations include the accumulation of extracellular matrix (ECM) components, basement membrane thickening, and fibrosis, all of which can persist even after blood glucose levels are controlled, emphasizing the importance of early and sustained metabolic management to prevent long-term damage.

2.5.1 Extracellular matrix (ECM) accumulation

Hyperglycemia stimulates the production of ECM components such as collagen and fibronectin, resulting in tissue fibrosis and stiffness (Hu et al., 2025). This is particularly evident in diabetic kidney disease (DKD), where excessive ECM deposition in the glomeruli leads to glomerular sclerosis and impaired kidney function (Qian et al., 2008). In the early stages of DKD, ECM protein buildup in the mesangial space is driven by continuous ECM protein synthesis and deposition, decreased degradation, and post-translational modifications, leading to significant collagen deposition in advanced stages (Stokes et al., 2000).

2.5.2 Basement membrane thickening

In diabetes, the basement membrane of capillaries becomes thickened due to the accumulation of glycosylated proteins and increased production of ECM components. This thickening impairs nutrient and oxygen exchange, contributing to tissue hypoxia and further damage (Harlan et al., 2018).

2.5.3 Fibrosis

Chronic inflammation and oxidative stress promote the activation of fibroblasts and the deposition of fibrotic tissue in organs such as the heart, kidneys, and liver (Barnes et al., 2011). Fibrosis reduces tissue elasticity and function, contributing to the progression of chronic complications. The TGF-β signaling pathway plays a key role in renal fibrosis by enhancing ECM protein and plasminogen activator inhibitor-1 expression via Smad2-4 transcription factors. Connective tissue growth factor (CTGF) enhances fibrotic activity by boosting fibronectin and collagen expression, facilitating ECM deposition (Kok et al., 2014).

Epigenetic modifications, including DNA methylation and histone modifications, are crucial in regulating fibrosis in diabetic kidney disease (DKD), especially in type 2 diabetic nephropathy (T2DN). DNA methylation changes, such as the hypomethylation of TIMP-2 and AKR1B1, are linked to increased extracellular matrix (ECM) accumulation and proteinuria in early DKD (Aldemir et al., 2017). In db/db mice, the pregnane X receptor (PXR) activates Rgc32, contributing to fibrosis (Watanabe et al., 2019). Transforming growth factor-beta 1 (TGF-β1) influences renal fibrosis through DNA methylation, leading to DNMT1-mediated hypermethylation of RASAL1, which increases fibroblast activation and fibrosis. However, TET3-mediated demethylation of the RASAL1 promoter can reverse fibrosis in STZ-induced DKD models (Tao et al., 2018).

Histone modifications also play a significant role in regulating ECM-related gene expression in both type 1 and type 2 diabetic nephropathy (T1DN and T2DN). In STZ-induced diabetic mice, MRTF-A recruits p300 and WDR5 to the collagen I promoter, enhancing renal fibrosis by increasing H3K18/27ac and H3K4me3 transcription (Xu et al., 2015). TGF-β increases SET7/9 recruitment to gene promoters, enhancing active chromatin markers and reducing repressive markers (Li et al., 2016a). Elevated H3K9/14ac and H3K18ac levels in high-glucose-induced mesangial cells boost the expression of profibrotic factors like CTGF and TGF-β1 (Gaikwad et al., 2010) (Fig. 1.2).

MicroRNAs (miRNAs) are significant regulators in the progression of diabetic nephropathy by controlling gene expression related to inflammation and fibrosis (Chung and Lan, 2015). In T1DN, miR-192 promotes ECM and collagen expression. Elevated miR-214 and miR-22 contribute to renal fibrogenesis by inhibiting PTEN expression, while miR-455-3p overexpression in STZ-induced DN rats improves renal fibrosis by targeting ROCK2 (Zhang et al., 2019; Wu et al., 2018). In T2DN, miR-146a has an anti-inflammatory role, and miR-29b reduces inflammation and fibrogenesis by inhibiting TGF-β/Smad3-dependent fibrosis and NF-κB-driven inflammation (Bhatt et al., 2016). MiR-133b and miR-199b facilitate TGF-β1-induced EMT and renal fibrosis by inhibiting sirt1 expression, while miR-199a upregulation activates pathways leading to fibrosis and inflammation (Sun et al., 2018; Wu et al., 2016).

These hyperglycemia-induced epigenetic changes can persist even after glucose control, highlighting the need for early metabolic management to prevent long-term damage.

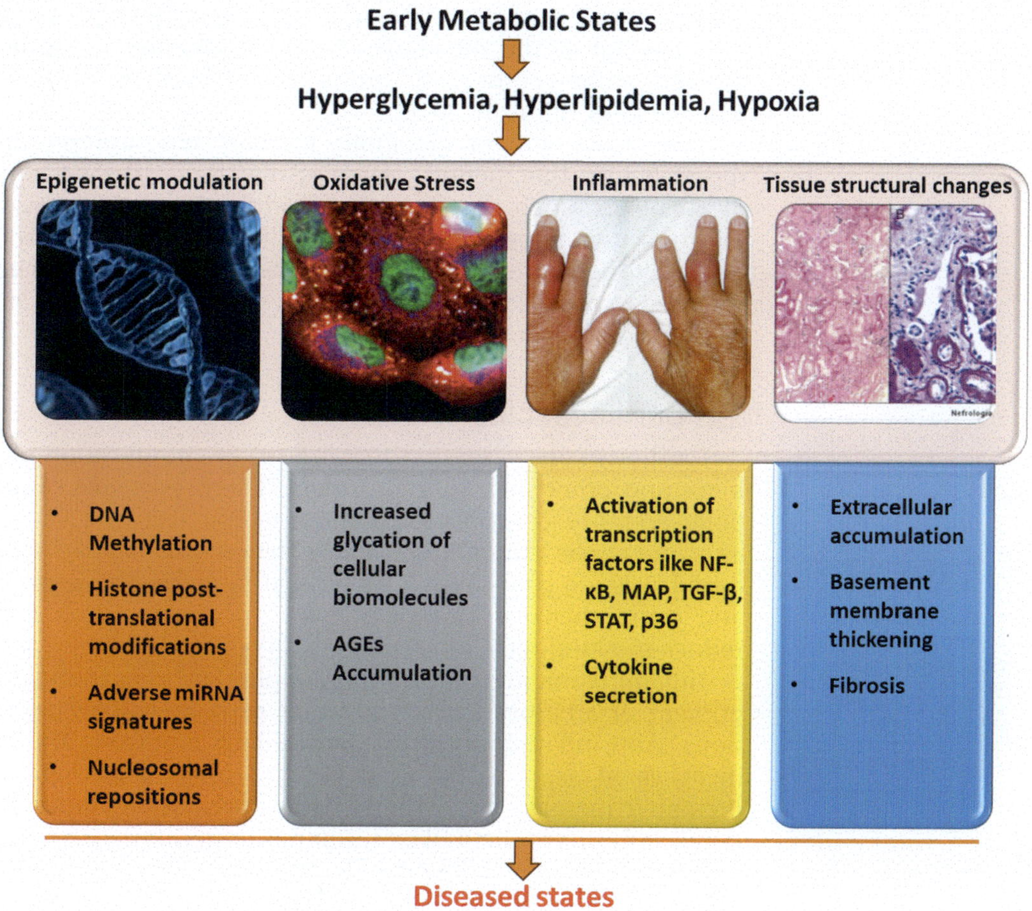

Figure 1.2 Scientific basis of metabolic memory.

3. Clinical implications of metabolic memory

The concept of metabolic memory has significant clinical implications, particularly in the management of chronic diseases such as diabetes, cardiovascular diseases, and obesity. Understanding the mechanisms underlying metabolic memory can inform treatment strategies and improve patient outcomes.

3.1 Diabetes management

In diabetes, the concept of metabolic memory underscores the importance of early and intensive glycemic control. Both the DCCT and UKPDS highlighted that tight glucose control in the early stages of diabetes could reduce the risk of complications even after transitioning to less intensive therapy. This has led to the recommendation of maintaining stringent glycemic targets, especially during the initial phase of diabetes management (Berezin, 2016).

The recognition of metabolic memory has also prompted research into therapeutic strategies that target the underlying mechanisms, such as epigenetic modifications, inflammation, and oxidative stress. Drugs that modulate these pathways, as well as lifestyle interventions such as diet and exercise, are being explored as means to mitigate the long-term effects of metabolic memory (Zhang et al., 2026).

3.2 Cardiovascular disease

Cardiovascular disease (CVD) is a major complication of diabetes and other metabolic disorders. The persistence of metabolic memory contributes to the ongoing risk of CVD, even after metabolic parameters such as blood glucose and cholesterol levels are controlled. This has led to an emphasis on early and comprehensive management of metabolic risk factors to reduce the long-term burden of CVD (Yao et al., 2022).

Inflammation and oxidative stress play key roles in the development of atherosclerosis and other cardiovascular complications. Anti-inflammatory and antioxidant therapies are being investigated as potential strategies to mitigate the effects of metabolic memory and improve cardiovascular outcomes in patients with metabolic diseases (Phillips, 2022).

3.3 Obesity and weight management

Obesity is another condition where metabolic memory plays a critical role. Early life metabolic states, such as childhood obesity and maternal diet during pregnancy, can imprint lasting effects on an individual's metabolism and predispose them to obesity and related complications later in life. Understanding these early influences is crucial for developing effective prevention and intervention strategies (Mobbs, 2018).

Interventions that target metabolic memory in obesity include lifestyle modifications, such as diet and exercise, as well as pharmacological approaches that address underlying mechanisms such as inflammation and insulin resistance. Early intervention and sustained management are key to preventing the long-term consequences of obesity (Fruh, 2017).

4. Future directions in metabolic memory research

The field of metabolic memory is rapidly evolving, with ongoing research aimed at elucidating the underlying mechanisms and developing targeted interventions. Future directions in metabolic memory research include.

4.1 Epigenetic therapies

Advancements in epigenetic research are opening new avenues for therapeutic interventions that target DNA methylation, histone modification, and non-coding RNA expression. Epigenetic therapies have the potential to reverse aberrant gene expression patterns induced by early metabolic states, offering a promising approach to mitigate the effects of metabolic memory (Kushwaha et al., 2024).

4.2 Precision medicine

The concept of metabolic memory underscores the importance of personalized approaches to disease management. Precision medicine, which tailors treatment strategies based on an individual's genetic, epigenetic, and metabolic profile, holds promise for improving outcomes in patients with chronic diseases influenced by metabolic memory.

4.3 Biomarkers of metabolic memory

Identifying biomarkers that reflect the presence and extent of metabolic memory is a critical area of research. These biomarkers could provide valuable insights into an individual's long-term risk of complications and inform targeted interventions to mitigate the effects of metabolic memory.

4.4 Integrative approaches

Integrative approaches that combine lifestyle modifications, pharmacological interventions, and novel therapies targeting epigenetic and inflammatory pathways are being explored to address the multifaceted nature of metabolic memory. These approaches aim to provide comprehensive and sustained management of chronic diseases influenced by metabolic memory.

5. Conclusion

Metabolic memory is a profound concept that has reshaped our understanding of chronic disease management and prevention. From its origins in diabetes research to its broader implications for cardiovascular disease and obesity, metabolic memory highlights the lasting impact of early metabolic states on long-term health. The scientific basis of metabolic memory encompasses epigenetic modifications, persistent inflammatory responses, oxidative stress, and structural changes in tissues. Understanding these mechanisms is crucial for developing effective strategies to mitigate the long-term effects of metabolic memory and improve patient outcomes.

As research in this field continues to evolve, it holds the promise of novel therapeutic interventions and personalized approaches that can transform the management of chronic diseases. By recognizing and addressing the enduring legacy of our biochemical past, we can pave the way for a healthier future.

References

Afshin, A., Forouzanfar, M.H., Reitsma, M.B., Sur, P., Estep, K., Lee, A., Marczak, L., Mokdad, A.H., Moradi-Lakeh, M., Naghavi, M., Salama, J.S., Vos, T., Abate, K.H., Abbafati, C., Ahmed, M.B., Al-Aly, Z., Alkerwi, A., Al-Raddadi, R., Amare, A.T., Amberbir, A., Amegah, A.K., Amini, E., Amrock, S. M., Anjana, R.M., Ärnlöv, J., Asayesh, H., Banerjee, A., Barac, A., Baye, E., Bennett, D.A., Beyene, A.S., Biadgilign, S., Biryukov, S., Bjertness, E., Boneya, D.J., Campos-Nonato, I., Carrero, J.J., Cecilio, P., Cercy, K., Ciobanu, L.G., Cornaby, L., Damtew, S.A., Dandona, L., Dandona, R., Dharmaratne, S.D., Duncan, B.B., Eshrati, B., Esteghamati, A., Feigin, V.L., Fernandes, J.C., Fürst, T., Gebrehiwot, T.T., Gold, A., Gona, P.N., Goto, A., Habtewold, T.D., Hadush, K.T., Hafezi-Nejad, N., Hay, S.I., Horino, M., Islami, F., Kamal, R., Kasaeian, A., Katikireddi, S.V., Kengne, A.P., Kesavachandran, C.N., Khader, Y.S., Khang, Y.H., Khubchandani, J., Kim, D., Kim, Y.J., Kinfu, Y., Kosen, S., Ku, T., Defo, B.K., Kumar, G.A., Larson, H.J., Leinsalu, M., Liang, X., Lim, S.S., Liu, P., Lopez, A.D., Lozano, R., Majeed, A., Malekzadeh, R., Malta, D.C., Mazidi, M., McAlinden, C., McGarvey, S.T., Mengistu, D.T., Mensah, G.A., Mensink, G.B.M., Mezgebe, H.B., Mirrakhimov, E.M., Mueller, U.O., Noubiap, J.J., Obermeyer, C.M., Ogbo, F. A., Owolabi, M.O., Patton, G.C., Pourmalek, F., Qorbani, M., Rafay, A., Rai, R.K., Ranabhat, C.L., Reinig, N., Safiri, S., Salomon, J.A., Sanabria, J.R., Santos, I.S., Sartorius, B., Sawhney, M., Schmidhuber, J., Schutte, A.E., Schmidt, M.I., Sepanlou, S.G., Shamsizadeh, M., Sheikhbahaei, S., Shin, M. J., Shiri, R., Shiue, I., Roba, H.S., Silva, D.A.S., Silverberg, J.I., Singh, J.A., Stranges, S., Swaminathan, S., Tabarés-Seisdedos, R., Tadese, F., Tedla, B.A., Tegegne, B.S., Terkawi, A.S., Thakur, J.S., Tonelli, M., Topor-Madry, R., Tyrovolas, S., Ukwaja, K.N., Uthman, O.A., Vaezghasemi, M., Vasankari, T., Vlassov, V.V., Vollset, S.E., Weiderpass, E., Werdecker, A., Wesana, J., Westerman, R., Yano, Y., Yonemoto, N., Yonga, G., Zaidi, Z., Zenebe, Z.M.,

Zipkin, B., Murray, C.J.L., 2017. Health effects of overweight and obesity in 195 countries over 25 years. N. Engl. J. Med. 377 (1), 13–27. https://doi.org/10.1056/NEJMoa1614362. Available from: http://www.nejm.org/doi/pdf/10.1056/NEJMoa1614362.

Agbu, P., Carthew, R.W., 2021. MicroRNA-mediated regulation of glucose and lipid metabolism. Nat. Rev. Mol. Cell Biol. 22 (6), 425–438. https://doi.org/10.1038/s41580-021-00354-w.

Aldemir, O., Turgut, F., Gokce, C., 2017. The association between methylation levels of targeted genes and albuminuria in patients with early diabetic kidney disease. Renal Failure 39 (1), 597–601.

Alghamdi, T.A., Batchu, S.N., Hadden, M.J., Yerra, V.G., Liu, Y., Bowskill, B.B., Advani, S.L., Geldenhuys, L., Siddiqi, F.S., Majumder, S., Advani, A., 2018. Histone H3 serine 10 phosphorylation facilitates endothelial activation in diabetic kidney disease. Diabetes 67 (12), 2668–2681. https://doi.org/10.2337/db18-0124.

Allis, C.D., Jenuwein, T., 2016. The molecular hallmarks of epigenetic control. Nat. Rev. Genet. 17 (8), 487–500. https://doi.org/10.1038/nrg.2016.59.

Alvarez, M.L., DiStefano, J.K., 2013. The role of non-coding RNAs in diabetic nephropathy: potential applications as biomarkers for disease development and progression. Diabetes Res. Clin. Pract. 99 (1), 1–11. https://doi.org/10.1016/j.diabres.2012.10.010.

Aranyi, T., Susztak, K., 2019. Cytosine methylation studies in patients with diabetic kidney disease. Curr. Diabetes Rep. 19, 91.

Avellino, R., Delwel, R., 2017. Expression and regulation of C/EBPα in normal myelopoiesis and in malignant transformation. Blood 129 (15), 2083–2091. https://doi.org/10.1182/blood-2016-09-687822.

Bahmani, F., Bathaie, S.Z., Aldavood, S.J., Ghahghaei, A., 2016. Inhibitory effect of crocin(s) on lens α-crystallin glycation and aggregation, results in the decrease of the risk of diabetic cataract. Molecules 21 (2). https://doi.org/10.3390/molecules21020143. Available from: http://www.mdpi.com/1420-3049/21/2/143/pdf.

Bannister, A.J., Kouzarides, T., 2011. Regulation of chromatin by histone modifications. Cell Res. 21 (3), 381–395. https://doi.org/10.1038/cr.2011.22.

Barnes, T.C., Anderson, M.E., Moots, R.J., 2011. The many faces of interleukin-6: the role of IL-6 in inflammation, vasculopathy, and fibrosis in systemic sclerosis. Int. J. Rheumatol. 2011 (1), 721608.

Berezin, A., 2016. Metabolic memory phenomenon in diabetes mellitus: achieving and perspectives. Diabetes Metab. Syndr.: Clin. Res. Rev. 10 (2), S176–S183.

Bhatt, K., Kato, M., Natarajan, R. 2016. Mini-review: emerging roles of microRNAs in the pathophysiology of renal diseases. Am. J. Physiol. Renal Physiol. 310 (2), F109–F118.

Bošković, A., Rando, O.J., 2018. Transgenerational epigenetic inheritance. Ann. Rev. Genet. 52, 21–41. https://doi.org/10.1146/annurev-genet-120417-031404.

Breton, C.V., Landon, R., Kahn, L.G., Enlow, M.B., Peterson, A.K., Bastain, T., Braun, J., Comstock, S.S., Duarte, C.S., Hipwell, A., Ji, H., LaSalle, J.M., Miller, R.L., Musci, R., Posner, J., Schmidt, R., Suglia, S.F., Tung, I., Weisenberger, D., Zhu, Y., Fry, R., 2021. Exploring the evidence for epigenetic regulation of environmental influences on child health across generations. Commun. Biol. 4 (1). https://doi.org/10.1038/s42003-021-02316-6. Available from: https://www.springer.com/journal/11852.

Brooks, W.H., Le Dantec, C., Pers, J.O., Youinou, P., Renaudineau, Y., 2010. Epigenetics and autoimmunity. J. Autoimmun. 34 (3), J207. https://doi.org/10.1016/j.jaut.2009.12.006.

Brownlee, M., 2001. Biochemistry and molecular cell biology of diabetic complications. Nature 414 (6865), 813–820. https://doi.org/10.1038/414813a.
Cabanel, M., Brand, C., Oliveira-Nunes, M.C., Cabral-Piccin, M.P., Freitas Lopes, M., Brito, J.M., Oliveira, F.L.de, El-Cheikh, M.C., Carneiro, K., Cotterill, S., 2015. Epigenetic control of macrophage shape transition towards an atypical elongated phenotype by histone deacetylase activity. PLoS One 10 (7), e0132984. https://doi.org/10.1371/journal.pone.0132984.
Cabili, M., Trapnell, C., Goff, L., Koziol, M., Tazon-Vega, B., Regev, A., Rinn, J.L., 2011. Integrative annotation of human large intergenic noncoding RNAs reveals global properties and specific subclasses. Genes Dev. 25 (18), 1915–1927. https://doi.org/10.1101/gad.17446611.
Cai, H., Harrison, D.G., 2000. Endothelial dysfunction in cardiovascular diseases: the role of oxidant stress. Circ. Res. 87 (10), 840–844. https://doi.org/10.1161/01.RES.87.10.840.
Cedar, H., Bergman, Y., 2009. Linking DNA methylation and histone modification: patterns and paradigms. Nat. Rev. Genet. 10 (5), 295–304. https://doi.org/10.1038/nrg2540.
Chalmers, J., Cooper, M.E., 2008. UKPDS and the legacy effect. New Engl. J. Med. 359 (15), 1618–1620. https://doi.org/10.1056/NEJMe0807625.
Chen, Z.X., Riggs, A.D., 2011. DNA methylation and demethylation in mammal. J. Biol. Chem. 286 (21), 18347–18353. https://doi.org/10.1074/jbc.R110.205286.
Chen, G., Chen, H., Ren, S., Xia, M., Zhu, J., Liu, Y., Zhang, L., Tang, L., Sun, L., Liu, H., Dong, Z., 2019. Aberrant DNA methylation of mTOR pathway genes promotes inflammatory activation of immune cells in diabetic kidney disease. Kidney Int. 96 (2), 409–420. https://doi.org/10.1016/j.kint.2019.02.020.
Chen, Z., Miao, F., Braffett, B.H., Lachin, J.M., Zhang, L., Wu, X., Roshandel, D., Carless, M., Li, X.A., Tompkins, J.D., Kaddis, J.S., Riggs, A.D., Paterson, A.D., Braffet, B.H., Lachin, J.M., Chen, Z., Miao, F., Zhang, L., Natarajan, R., Paterson, A.D., Natarajan, R., 2020. DNA methylation mediates development of HbA1c-associated complications in type 1 diabetes. Nat. Metab. 2 (8), 744–762. https://doi.org/10.1038/s42255-020-0231-8.
Chen, F., Qi, G., Wei, A., Chen, X., Shi, Y., Wang, H., Cao, W., 2021. Histone deacetylase 3 aberration inhibits Klotho transcription and promotes renal fibrosis. Cell Death Differ. 28 (3), 1001–1012. https://doi.org/10.1038/s41418-020-00631-9.
Chung, A.C.K., Lan, H.Y., 2015. MicroRNAs in renal fibrosis. Front. Physiol. 6, 50.
Cleophas, M.C.P., Crisan, T.O., Klück, V., Hoogerbrugge, N., Netea-Maier, R.T., Dinarello, C.A., Netea, M.G., Joosten, L.A.B., 2019. Romidepsin suppresses monosodium urate crystal-induced cytokine production through upregulation of suppressor of cytokine signaling 1 expression. Arthritis Res. Ther. 21 (1). https://doi.org/10.1186/s13075-019-1834-x.
Creager, M.A., Lüscher, T.F., Cosentino, F., Beckman, J.A., 2003. Diabetes and vascular disease. Pathophysiology, clinical consequences, and medical therapy: Part I. Circulation 108 (12), 1527–1532. https://doi.org/10.1161/01.CIR.0000091257.27563.32.
Crisóstomo, L., et al., 2022a. Inherited metabolic memory of high-fat diet impairs testicular fatty acid content and sperm parameters. Mol. Nutr. Food Res. 66, e2100680.
Crisóstomo, L., Bourgery, M., Rato, L., Raposo, J.F., Batterham, R.L., Kotaja, N., Alves, M.G., 2022b. Testicular "inherited metabolic memory" of ancestral

high-fat diet is associated with sperm sncRNA content. Biomedicines 10 (4), 909. https://doi.org/10.3390/biomedicines10040909.

Davis, F.M., denDekker, A., Joshi, A.D., Wolf, S.J., Audu, C., Melvin, W.J., Mangum, K., Riordan, M.O., Kunkel, S.L., Gallagher, K.A., 2020. Palmitate-TLR4 signaling regulates the histone demethylase, JMJD3, in macrophages and impairs diabetic wound healing. Eur. J. Immunol. 50 (12), 1929–1940. https://doi.org/10.1002/eji.202048651. Available from: http://onlinelibrary.wiley.com/journal/10.1002/(ISSN)1521-4141.

De Vos, L.C., Mulder, D.J., Smit, A.J., Dullaart, R.P.F., Kleefstra, N., Lijfering, W. M., Kamphuisen, P.W., Zeebregts, C.J., Lefrandt, J.D., 2014. Skin autofluorescence is associated with 5-year mortality and cardiovascular events in patients with peripheral artery disease. Arterioscler. Thromb. Vasc. Biol. 34 (4), 933–938. https://doi.org/10.1161/ATVBAHA.113.302731.

Diabetes control and complications trial (DCCT): results of feasibility study. The DCCT research group. Diabetes Care 10, 1987, 1–19.

Duan, Y., Gong, K., Xu, S., Zhang, F., Meng, X., Han, J., 2022. Regulation of cholesterol homeostasis in health and diseases: from mechanisms to targeted therapeutics. Signal Transduct. Targeted Ther. 7 (1). https://doi.org/10.1038/s41392-022-01125-5.

Edgar, L., Akbar, N., Braithwaite, A.T., Krausgruber, T., Gallart-Ayala, H., Bailey, J., Corbin, A.L., Khoyratty, T.E., Chai, J.T., Alkhalil, M., Rendeiro, A.F., Ziberna, K., Arya, R., Cahill, T.J., Bock, C., Laurencikiene, J., Crabtree, M.J., Lemieux, M.E., Riksen, N.P., Netea, M.G., Wheelock, C.E., Channon, K.M., Rydén, M., Udalova, I.A., Carnicer, R., Choudhury, R.P., 2021. Hyperglycemia induces trained immunity in macrophages and their precursors and promotes atherosclerosis. Circulation 144 (12), 961–982. https://doi.org/10.1161/circulationaha.120.046464.

El-Osta, A., Brasacchio, D., Yao, D., Pocai, A., Jones, P.L., Roeder, R.G., Cooper, M.E., Brownlee, M., 2008. Transient high glucose causes persistent epigenetic changes and altered gene expression during subsequent normoglycemia. J. Exp. Med. 205 (10), 2409–2417. https://doi.org/10.1084/jem.20081188.

Epidemiology of diabetes interventions and complications (EDIC). Design, implementation, and preliminary results of a long-term follow-up of the diabetes control and complications trial cohort. Diabetes Care 22, 1999, 99–111.

Eslam, M., Sanyal, A.J., George, J., Sanyal, A., Neuschwander-Tetri, B., Tiribelli, C., Kleiner, D.E., Brunt, E., Bugianesi, E., Yki-Järvinen, H., Grønbæk, H., Cortez-Pinto, H., Fan, J., Valenti, L., Abdelmalek, M., Romero-Gomez, M., Rinella, M., Arrese, M., Bedossa, P., Newsome, P.N., Anstee, Q. M., Jalan, R., Bataller, R., Loomba, R., Sookoian, S., Sarin, S.K., Harrison, S., Kawaguchi, T., Wong, V.W.S., Ratziu, V., Yilmaz, Y., Younossi, Z., 2020. MAFLD: a consensus-driven proposed nomenclature for metabolic associated fatty liver disease. Gastroenterology 158 (7), 1999. https://doi.org/10.1053/j.gastro.2019.11.312.

Fan, P., Zhang, N., Candi, E., Agostini, M., Piacentini, M., Francesca, B., Pierluigi, B., Alessandro, M., Giuseppe, N., Valentina, R., Manuel, S., Giuseppe, S., Sun, Q., Giuseppe, T., Wang, Y., Shi, Y., Huang, Y., Melino, G., 2023. Alleviating hypoxia to improve cancer immunotherapy. Oncogene 42 (49), 3591–3604. https://doi.org/10.1038/s41388-023-02869-2.

Fishman, S.L., Sonmez, H., Basman, C., Singh, V., Poretsky, L., 2018. The role of advanced glycation end-products in the development of coronary artery disease in patients with and without diabetes mellitus: a review. Molecular Medicine 24 (1). https://doi.org/10.1186/s10020-018-0060-3.

Flier, J.S., Underhill, L.H., Brownlee, M., Cerami, A., Vlassara, H., 1988. Advanced glycosylation end products in tissue and the biochemical basis of diabetic complications. N. Engl. J. Med. 318 (20), 1315–1321. https://doi.org/10.1056/nejm198805193182007.

Forrest, M.E., Khalil, A.M., 2017. Review: regulation of the cancer epigenome by long non-coding RNAs. Cancer Lett. 407, 106–112. https://doi.org/10.1016/j.canlet.2017.03.040.

Foury, F., Hu, J., Vanderstraeten, S., 2004. Mitochondrial DNA mutators. Cell. Mol. Life Sci. 61 (22), 2799–2811. https://doi.org/10.1007/s00018-004-4220-y.

Fradin, D., Le Fur, S., Mille, C., Naoui, N., Groves, C., Zelenika, D., McCarthy, M.I., Lathrop, M., Bougnères, P., Lynn, F.C., 2012. Association of the CpG methylation pattern of the proximal insulin gene promoter with type 1 diabetes. PLoS One 7 (5), e36278. https://doi.org/10.1371/journal.pone.0036278.

Fruh, S.M., 2017. Obesity: Risk factors, complications, and strategies for sustainable long-term weight management. J. Am. Assoc. Nurse Pract. 29 (S1), S3–S14.

Gæde, P., Lund-Andersen, H., Parving, H.H., Pedersen, O., 2008. Effect of a multifactorial intervention on mortality in type 2 diabetes. New Engl. J. Med. 358 (6), 580–591. https://doi.org/10.1056/NEJMoa0706245.

Gaikwad, A.B., Gupta, J., Tikoo, K., 2010. Epigenetic changes and alteration of Fbn1 and Col3A1 gene expression under hyperglycaemic and hyperinsulinaemic conditions. Biochem. J. 432 (2), 333–341.

Gao, D., Bailey, C.J., Griffiths, H.R., 2009. Metabolic memory effect of the saturated fatty acid, palmitate, in monocytes. Biochem. Biophys. Res. Commun. 388 (2), 278–282. https://doi.org/10.1016/j.bbrc.2009.07.160.

Gao, C., Chen, G., Liu, L., Li, X., He, J., Jiang, L., Zhu, J., Xu, Y., 2013. Impact of high glucose and proteasome inhibitor MG132 on histone H2A and H2B ubiquitination in rat glomerular mesangial cells. J. Diabetes Res. 2013, 1–10. https://doi.org/10.1155/2013/589474.

Garay-Sevilla, M.E., Rojas, A., Portero-Otin, M., Uribarri, J., 2021. Dietary AGEs as exogenous boosters of inflammation. Nutrients 13 (8), 2802. https://doi.org/10.3390/nu13082802.

Genuth, S., Sun, W., Cleary, P., Gao, X., Sell, D.R., Lachin, J., Monnier, V.M., 2015. Skin advanced glycation end products glucosepane and methylglyoxal hydroimidazolone are independently associated with long-term microvascular complication progression of type 1 diabetes. Diabetes 64 (1), 266–278. https://doi.org/10.2337/db14-0215.

Geraldes, P., King, G.L., 2010. Activation of protein kinase C isoforms and its impact on diabetic complications. Circ. Res. 106 (8), 1319–1331. https://doi.org/10.1161/CIRCRESAHA.110.217117.

Giacco, F., Brownlee, M., Schmidt, A.M., 2010. Oxidative stress and diabetic complications. Circ. Res. 107 (9), 1058–1070. https://doi.org/10.1161/circresaha.110.223545.

Gomez-Arango, L.F., Barrett, H.L., McIntyre, H.D., Callaway, L.K., Morrison, M., Dekker Nitert, M., 2016. Increased systolic and diastolic blood pressure is associated with altered gut microbiota composition and butyrate production in early pregnancy. Hypertension 68 (4), 974–981. https://doi.org/10.1161/HYPERTENSIONAHA.116.07910.

Gowher, H., Jeltsch, A., 2018. Mammalian DNA methyltransferases: new discoveries and open questions. Biochem. Soc. Trans. 46 (5), 1191–1202. https://doi.org/10.1042/bst20170574.

Goyal, N., Kesharwani, D., Datta, M., 2018. Lnc-ing non-coding RNAs with metabolism and diabetes: roles of lncRNAs. Cell. Mol. Life Sci. 75 (10), 1827–1837. https://doi.org/10.1007/s00018-018-2760-9.

Guarner, V., Rubio-Ruiz, M.E., 2014. Low-grade systemic inflammation connects aging, metabolic syndrome and cardiovascular disease. Interdiscipl. Top. Gerontol. 40, 99–106. https://doi.org/10.1159/000364934.

Guttman, M., Rinn, J.L., 2012. Modular regulatory principles of large non-coding RNAs. Nature 482 (7385), 339–346. https://doi.org/10.1038/nature10887.

Harlan, S.M., Heinz-Taheny, K.M., Overstreet, J.M., Breyer, M.D., Harris, R.C., Heuer, J.G., 2018. Pathological and transcriptome changes in the ReninAAV db/db uNx model of advanced diabetic kidney disease exhibit features of human disease. Toxicol. Pathol. 46 (8), 991–998.

Hartig, S.M., Hamilton, M.P., Bader, D.A., McGuire, S.E., 2015. The miRNA interactome in metabolic homeostasis. Trends Endocrinol. Metabol. 26 (12), 733–745. https://doi.org/10.1016/j.tem.2015.09.006.

Hashimoto, H., Vertino, P.M., Cheng, X., 2010. Molecular coupling of DNA methylation and histone methylation. Epigenomics 2 (5), 657–669. https://doi.org/10.2217/epi.10.44.

He, Y., Dan, Y., Gao, X., Huang, L., Lv, H., Chen, J., 2021. DNMT1-mediated lncRNA MEG3 methylation accelerates endothelial-mesenchymal transition in diabetic retinopathy through the PI3K/Akt/mTOR signaling pathway. Am. J. Physiol. Endocrinol. Metabol. 320 (3), E598. https://doi.org/10.1152/ajpendo.00089.2020.

Henning, C., Glomb, M.A., 2016. Pathways of the Maillard reaction under physiological conditions. Glycoconjug. J. 33 (4), 499–512. https://doi.org/10.1007/s10719-016-9694-y.

Holman, R.R., 2013. Type 2 diabetes mellitus in 2012: optimal management of T2DM remains elusive. Nat. Rev. Endocrinol. 9 (2), 67–68. https://doi.org/10.1038/nrendo.2012.243.

Hu, X., Chen, W., Yang, M., Li, M., Li, X., Ouyang, S., 2025. IGFBP5 promotes EndoMT and renal fibrosis through H3K18 lactylation in diabetic nephropathy. Cell. Mol. Life Sci. 82 (1), 215.

Hudson, B.I., Lippman, M.E., 2018. Targeting RAGE signaling in inflammatory disease. Ann. Rev. Med. 69, 349–364. https://doi.org/10.1146/annurev-med-041316-085215.

Inoue, Y., Suzuki, Y., Kunishima, Y., Washio, T., Morishita, S., Takeda, H., 2023. High-fat diet in early life triggers both reversible and persistent epigenetic changes in the medaka fish (*Oryzias latipes*). BMC Genom. 24 (1). https://doi.org/10.1186/s12864-023-09557-1.

Intensive blood-glucose control with sulphonylureas or insulin compared with conventional treatment and risk of complications in patients with type 2 diabetes (UKPDS 33). UK Prospective Diabetes Study (UKPDS) Group. Lancet 352, 1998, 837–853.

Jia, Y., Reddy, M.A., Das, S., Oh, H.J., Abdollahi, M., Yuan, H., Zhang, E., Lanting, L., Wang, M., Natarajan, R., 2019. Dysregulation of histone H3 lysine 27 trimethylation in transforming growth factor-β1–induced gene expression in mesangial cells and diabetic kidney. J. Biol. Chem. 294 (34), 12695–12707. https://doi.org/10.1074/jbc.ra119.007575.

Jirtle, R.L., Skinner, M.K., 2007. Environmental epigenomics and disease susceptibility. Nat. Rev. Genet. 8 (4), 253–262. https://doi.org/10.1038/nrg2045.

Kato, M., Natarajan, R., 2014. Diabetic nephropathy—emerging epigenetic mechanisms. Nat. Rev. Nephrol. 10 (9), 517–530. https://doi.org/10.1038/nrneph.2014.116.

Kato, M., Natarajan, R., 2019. Epigenetics and epigenomics in diabetic kidney disease and metabolic memory. Nat. Rev. Nephrol. 15 (6), 327–345. https://doi.org/10.1038/s41581-019-0135-6.

Klose, R.J., Zhang, Y., 2007. Regulation of histone methylation by demethylimination and demethylation. Nat. Rev. Mol. Cell Biol. 8 (4), 307–318. https://doi.org/10.1038/nrm2143.

Koenen, M., Hill, M.A., Cohen, P., Sowers, J.R., 2021. Obesity, adipose tissue and vascular dysfunction. Circ. Res. 128 (7), 951–968. https://doi.org/10.1161/CIRCRESAHA.121.318093.

Kok, H.M., Falke, L.L., Goldschmeding, R., Nguyen, T.Q., 2014. Targeting CTGF, EGF and PDGF pathways to prevent progression of kidney disease. Nat. Rev. Nephrol. 10 (12), 700–711.

Komers, R., Mar, D., Denisenko, O., Xu, B., Oyama, T.T., Bomsztyk, K., 2013. Epigenetic changes in renal genes dysregulated in mouse and rat models of type 1 diabetes. Lab. Invest. 93 (5), 543–552. https://doi.org/10.1038/labinvest.2013.47.

Kowluru, R.A., Chakrabarti, S., Chen, S., 2004. Re-institution of good metabolic control in diabetic rats and activation of caspase-3 and nuclear transcriptional factor (NF-kB) in the retina. Acta Diabetol. 41 (4), 194–199. https://doi.org/10.1007/s00592-004-0165-8.

Lachin, J.M., Nathan, D.M., 2021. Understanding metabolic memory: the prolonged influence of glycemia during the diabetes control and complications trial (dcct) on future risks of complications during the study of the epidemiology of diabetes interventions and complications (edic). Diabetes Care 44 (10), 2216–2224.

Kushwaha, K., Garg, S.S., Mandal, D., Khurana, N., Gupta, J., 2024. Screening of natural epigenetic modifiers for managing glycemic memory and diabetic nephropathy. J. Drug Target. 32 (7), 807–819.

Lachin, J.M., Genuth, S., Cleary, P., Davis, M.D., Nathan, D.M., 2000. Retinopathy and nephropathy in patients with type I diabetes four years after a trial of intensive therapy. N. Engl. J. Med. 342 (6), 381–389. https://doi.org/10.1056/NEJM200002103420603.

Leung, A., Trac, C., Du, J., Natarajan, R., Schones, D.E., 2016. Persistent chromatin modifications induced by high fat diet. J. Biol. Chem. 291 (20), 10446–10455. https://doi.org/10.1074/jbc.m115.711028.

Li, M., Riddle, S., Zhang, H., D'Alessandro, A., Flockton, A., Serkova, N.J., Hansen, K.C., Moldovan, R., Alexandre McKeon, B., Frid, M., Kumar, S., Li, H., Liu, H., Caánovas, A., Medrano, J.F., Thomas, M.G., Iloska, D., Plecitá-Hlavatá, L., Ježek, P., Pullamsetti, S., Fini, M.A., El Kasmi, K.C., Zhang, Q.H., Stenmark, K.R., 2016a. Metabolic reprogramming regulates the proliferative and inflammatory phenotype of adventitial fibroblasts in pulmonary hypertension through the transcriptional corepressor C-terminal binding protein-1. Circulation 134 (15), 1105–1121. https://doi.org/10.1161/circulationaha.116.023171.

Li, X., Li, C., Sun, G., 2016b. Histone acetylation and its modifiers in the pathogenesis of diabetic nephropathy. J. Diabetes Res. 2016, 1–11. https://doi.org/10.1155/2016/4065382.

Li, K.Y., Tam, C.H.T., Liu, H., Day, S., Lim, C.K.P., So, W.Y., Huang, C., Jiang, G., Shi, M., Lee, H.M., Lan, H.y., Szeto, C.C., Hanson, R.L., Nelson, R.G., Susztak, K., Chan, J.C.N., Yip, K.Y., Ma, R.C.W., 2023. DNA methylation

markers for kidney function and progression of diabetic kidney disease. Nat. Commun. 14 (1). https://doi.org/10.1038/s41467-023-37837-7.
Liao, Y., et al., 2018. NADPH oxidase 4 and endothelial nitric oxide synthase contribute to endothelial dysfunction mediated by histone methylations in metabolic memory. Free Radic. Biol. Med. 115, 383–394.
Liu, J.J., Yeoh, L.Y., Sum, C.F., Tavintharan, S., Ng, X.W., Liu, S., Lee, S.B.M., Tang, W.E., Lim, S.C., 2015. Vascular cell adhesion molecule-1, but not intercellular adhesion molecule-1, is associated with diabetic kidney disease in Asians with type 2 diabetes. J. Diabetes Complicat. 29 (5), 707–712. https://doi.org/10.1016/j.jdiacomp.2015.02.011.
Lu, Q., Guo, P., Liu, A., Ares, I., María-Rosa Martínez-Larrañaga, Wang, X., Anadón, A., Aránzazu Martínez, M.-, 2021. The role of long noncoding RNA in lipid, cholesterol, and glucose metabolism and treatment of obesity syndrome. Med. Res. Rev. 41 (3), 1751–1774. https://doi.org/10.1002/med.21775.
Macvanin, M., Obradovic, M., Zafirovic, S., Stanimirovic, J., Isenovic, E.R., 2023. The role of miRNAs in metabolic diseases. Curr. Med. Chem. 30 (17), 1922–1944. https://doi.org/10.2174/0929867329666220801161536.
Maghbooli, Z., Larijani, B., Emamgholipour, S., Amini, M., Keshtkar, A., Pasalar, P., 2014. Aberrant DNA methylation patterns in diabetic nephropathy. J. Diabetes Metab. Disord. 13 (1). https://doi.org/10.1186/2251-6581-13-69.
Mishra, M., Duraisamy, A.J., Kowluru, R.A., 2018. Sirt1: a guardian of the development of diabetic retinopathy. Diabetes 67 (4), 745–754. https://doi.org/10.2337/db17-0996.
Mobbs, C.V., 2018. Glucose-induced transcriptional hysteresis: role in obesity, metabolic memory, diabetes, and aging. Front. Endocrinol. 9, 232.
Moore, L.D., Le, T., Fan, G., 2013. DNA methylation and its basic function. Neuropsychopharmacology 38 (1), 23–38. https://doi.org/10.1038/npp.2012.112.
Mossel, D.M., Moganti, K., Riabov, V., Weiss, C., Kopf, S., Cordero, J., Dobreva, G., Rots, M.G., Klüter, H., Harmsen, M.C., Kzhyshkowska, J., 2020. Epigenetic regulation of S100A9 and S100A12 expression in monocyte-macrophage system in hyperglycemic conditions. Front. Immunol. 11. https://doi.org/10.3389/fimmu.2020.01071.
Nathan, D.M., 1996. The Pathophysiology of Diabetic Complications: How Much Does the Glucose Hypothesis Explain? Ann. Intern. Med. 1, 86–89. https://doi.org/10.7326/0003-4819-124-1_part_2-199601011-00002, 124. http://annals.org/issues.aspx.
Nathan, D.M., 2014. The diabetes control and complications trial/epidemiology of diabetes interventions and complications study at 30 years: overview. Diabetes Care 37 (1), 9–16. https://doi.org/10.2337/dc13-2112.
Nojima, T., Proudfoot, N.J., 2022. Mechanisms of lncRNA biogenesis as revealed by nascent transcriptomics. Nat. Rev. Mol. Cell Biol. 23 (6), 389–406. https://doi.org/10.1038/s41580-021-00447-6.
Olsen, A.S., Sarras, M.P., Leontovich, A., Intine, R.V., 2012. Heritable transmission of diabetic metabolic memory in zebrafish correlates with DNA hypomethylation and aberrant gene expression. Diabetes 61 (2), 485–491. https://doi.org/10.2337/db11-0588.
Palazzo, A.F., Lee, E.S., 2015. Non-coding RNA: what is functional and what is junk? Front. Genet. 5. https://doi.org/10.3389/fgene.2015.00002. Available from: http://journal.frontiersin.org/article/10.3389/fgene.2015.00002/pdf.

Peng, K., Dong, W., Luo, T., Tang, H., Zhu, W., Huang, Y., Yang, X., 2023. Butyrate and obesity: current research status and future prospect. Front. Endocrinol. 14. https://doi.org/10.3389/fendo.2023.1098881.

Phillips, M.C., 2022. Metabolic strategies in healthcare: a new era. Aging and Dis. 13 (3), 655.

Pillai, P.U., Ray, A., Maan, M., Dutta, M., 2023. Repurposing drugs targeting metabolic diseases for cancer therapeutics. Drug Discov. Today 28 (9), 103684. https://doi.org/10.1016/j.drudis.2023.103684.

Portela, A., Esteller, M., 2010. Epigenetic modifications and human disease. Nat. Biotechnol. 28 (10), 1057–1068. https://doi.org/10.1038/nbt.1685.

Qian, Y., Feldman, E., Pennathur, S., Kretzler, M., Brosius, 2008. From fibrosis to sclerosis: mechanisms of glomerulosclerosis in diabetic nephropathy. Diabetes 57 (6), 1439–1445.

Qiu, G.Z., Tian, W., Fu, H.T., Li, C.P., Liu, B., 2016. Long noncoding RNA-MEG3 is involved in diabetes mellitus-related microvascular dysfunction. Biochem. Biophys. Res. Commun. 471 (1), 135–141. https://doi.org/10.1016/j.bbrc.2016.01.164.

Ramasamy, R., Vannucci, S.J., Shi Du Yan, S., Herold, K., Yan, S.F., Schmidt, A. M., 2005. Advanced glycation end products and RAGE: a common thread in aging, diabetes, neurodegeneration, and inflammation. Glycobiology 15 (7), 16R. https://doi.org/10.1093/glycob/cwi053.

Rana, G., Donizetti, A., Virelli, G., Piscopo, M., Viggiano, E., De Luca, B., Fucci, L., 2012. Cortical spreading depression differentially affects lysine methylation of H3 histone at neuroprotective genes and retrotransposon sequences. Brain Res. 1467, 113–119. https://doi.org/10.1016/j.brainres.2012.05.043.

Reddy, M.A., Natarajan, R., 2011. Epigenetic mechanisms in diabetic vascular complications. Cardiovasc. Res. 90 (3), 421–429. https://doi.org/10.1093/cvr/cvr024.

Savitha, S., Tamilselvan, J., Anusuyadevi, M., Panneerselvam, C., 2005. Oxidative stress on mitochondrial antioxidant defense system in the aging process: role of dl-α-lipoic acid and l-carnitine. Clin. Chim. Acta 355 (1–2), 173–180. https://doi.org/10.1016/j.cccn.2004.12.005.

Schmitz, S.U., Grote, P., Herrmann, B.G., 2016. Mechanisms of long noncoding RNA function in development and disease. Cell. Mol. Life Sci. 73 (13), 2491–2509. https://doi.org/10.1007/s00018-016-2174-5.

Schroen, B., Heymans, S., 2012. Small but smart—microRNAs in the centre of inflammatory processes during cardiovascular diseases, the metabolic syndrome, and ageing. Cardiovasc. Res. 93 (4), 605–613. https://doi.org/10.1093/cvr/cvr268.

Shantikumar, S., Caporali, A., Emanueli, C., 2012. Role of microRNAs in diabetes and its cardiovascular complications. Cardiovasc. Res. 93 (4), 583–593. https://doi.org/10.1093/cvr/cvr300.

Singh, R., Chandel, S., Dey, D., Ghosh, A., Roy, S., Ravichandiran, V., Ghosh, D., 2020. Epigenetic modification and therapeutic targets of diabetes mellitus. Biosci. Rep. 40 (9). https://doi.org/10.1042/bsr20202160.

Smith, B.W., Adams, L.A., 2011. Nonalcoholic fatty liver disease and diabetes mellitus: pathogenesis and treatment. Nat. Rev. Endocrinol. 7 (8), 456–465. https://doi.org/10.1038/nrendo.2011.72.

Stitt, A.W., Jenkins, A.J., Cooper, M.E., 2002. Advanced glycation end products and diabetic complications. Expert Opin. Invest. Drugs 11 (9), 1205–1223. https://doi.org/10.1517/13543784.11.9.1205.

Stokes, M.B., Holler, S., Cui, Y., Hudkins, K.L., Eitner, F., Fogo, A., Alpers, C.E., 2000. Expression of decorin, biglycan, and collagen type I in human renal fibrosing disease. Kidney Int. 57 (2), 487–498.

Sun, H., Saeedi, P., Karuranga, S., Pinkepank, M., Ogurtsova, K., Duncan, B.B., Stein, C., Basit, A., Chan, J.C.N., Mbanya, J.C., Pavkov, M.E., Ramachandaran, A., Wild, S.H., James, S., Herman, W.H., Zhang, P., Bommer, C., Kuo, S., Boyko, E.J., Magliano, D.J., 2022. IDF Diabetes Atlas: global, regional and country-level diabetes prevalence estimates for 2021 and projections for 2045. Diabetes Res. Clin. Pract. 183, 109119. https://doi.org/10.1016/j.diabres.2021.109119.

Sun, Y., Wang, H., Li, Y., Liu, S., Chen, J., Ying, H., 2018. miR-24 and miR-122 negatively regulate the transforming growth factor-β/Smad signaling pathway in skeletal muscle fibrosis. Mol. Ther. Nucleic Acids 11, 528–537.

Svikle, Z., Peterfelde, B., Sjakste, N., Baumane, K., Verkauskiene, R., Jeng, C.-J., Sokolovska, J., 2022. Ubiquitin-proteasome system in diabetic retinopathy. PeerJ (10), e13715. https://doi.org/10.7717/peerj.13715.

Taft, R.J., Pang, K.C., Mercer, T.R., Dinger, M., Mattick, J.S., 2010. Non-coding RNAs: regulators of disease. J. Pathol. 220 (2), 126–139. https://doi.org/10.1002/path.2638Australia.

Tao, H., Song, Z.Y., Ding, X.S., Yang, J.J., Shi, K.H., Li, J., 2018. Epigenetic signatures in cardiac fibrosis, special emphasis on DNA methylation and histone modification. Heart Fail. Rev. 23 (5), 789–799.

Tessarz, P., Kouzarides, T., 2014. Histone core modifications regulating nucleosome structure and dynamics. Nat. Rev. Mol. Cell Biol. 15 (11), 703–708. https://doi.org/10.1038/nrm3890.

The absence of a glycemic Threshold for the development of long-term complications: the perspective of the diabetes control and complications trial. Diabetes 45 (10), 1996, 1289–1298. https://doi.org/10.2337/diab.45.10.1289.

The Diabetes Control and Complications Trial (DCCT), 1986. Design and methodologic considerations for the feasibility phase. The DCCT Research Group. Diabetes 35, 530–545.

The relationship of glycemic exposure (HbA1c) to the risk of development and progression of retinopathy in the diabetes control and complications trial. Diabetes 44 (8), 1995, 968–983. https://doi.org/10.2337/diab.44.8.968.

Thomas, A.A., Feng, B., Chakrabarti, S., 2017. ANRIL: a regulator of VEGF in diabetic retinopathy. Investig. Ophthalmol. Visu. Sci. 58 (1), 470–480. https://doi.org/10.1167/iovs.16-20569.

Thompson, J.A., Webb, R.C., 2013. Potential role of toll-like receptors in programming of vascular dysfunction. Clin. Sci. 125 (1), 19–25. https://doi.org/10.1042/CS20120673.

Tian, L., Wu, D., Dasgupta, A., Chen, K.H., Mewburn, J., Potus, F., Lima, P.D.A., Hong, Z., Zhao, Y.Y., Hindmarch, C.C.T., Kutty, S., Provencher, S., Bonnet, S., Sutendra, G., Archer, S.L., 2020. Epigenetic metabolic reprogramming of right ventricular fibroblasts in pulmonary arterial hypertension: a pyruvate dehydrogenase kinase-dependent shift in mitochondrial metabolism promotes right ventricular fibrosis. Circ. Res. 126 (12), 1723–1745. https://doi.org/10.1161/CIRCRESAHA.120.316443.

Trumpower, B.L., 1990. The protonmotive Q cycle. Energy transduction by coupling of proton translocation to electron transfer by the cytochrome bc1 complex. J. Biol. Chem. 265 (20), 11409–11412. https://doi.org/10.1016/s0021-9258(19)38410-8.

Tu, Y., Song, E., Wang, Z., Ji, N., Zhu, L., Wang, K., Sun, H., Zhang, Y., Zhu, Q., Liu, X., Zhu, M., 2021. Melatonin attenuates oxidative stress and inflammation of Müller cells in diabetic retinopathy via activating the Sirt1 pathway. Biomed. Pharmacother. 137, 111274. https://doi.org/10.1016/j.biopha.2021.111274.

van Diepen, J.A., Thiem, K., Stienstra, R., Riksen, N.P., Tack, C.J., Netea, M.G., 2016. Diabetes propels the risk for cardiovascular disease: sweet monocytes becoming aggressive? Cell. Mol. Life Sci. 73 (24), 4675–4684. https://doi.org/10.1007/s00018-016-2316-9.

Vasishta, S., Umakanth, S., Adiga, P., Joshi, M.B., 2022. Extrinsic and intrinsic factors influencing metabolic memory in type 2 diabetes. Vasc. Pharmacol. 142, 106933. https://doi.org/10.1016/j.vph.2021.106933.

Villeneuve, L.M., Reddy, M.A., Lanting, L.L., Wang, M., Meng, L., Natarajan, R., 2008. Epigenetic histone H3 lysine 9 methylation in metabolic memory and inflammatory phenotype of vascular smooth muscle cells in diabetes. Proc. Natl. Acad. Sci. U. S. A 105 (26), 9047–9052. https://doi.org/10.1073/pnas.0803623105.

Wang, J., Wu, Z., Li, D., Li, N., Dindot, S.V., Carey Satterfield, M., Bazer, F.W., Wu, G., 2012. Nutrition, epigenetics, and metabolic syndrome. Antioxid. Redox Signaling 17 (2), 282–301. https://doi.org/10.1089/ars.2011.4381.

Wang, X., Liu, J., Zhen, J., Zhang, C., Wan, Q., Liu, G., Wei, X., Zhang, Y., Wang, Z., Han, H., Xu, H., Bao, C., Song, Z., Zhang, X., Li, N., Yi, F., 2014. Histone deacetylase 4 selectively contributes to podocyte injury in diabetic nephropathy. Kidney Int. 86 (4), 712–725. https://doi.org/10.1038/ki.2014.111.

Wang, J., Song, Y.-X., Ma, B., Wang, J.-J., Sun, J.-X., Chen, X.-W., Zhao, J.-H., Yang, Y.-C., Wang, Z.-N., 2015. Regulatory roles of non-coding RNAs in colorectal cancer. Int. J. Mol. Sci. 16 (8), 19886–19919. https://doi.org/10.3390/ijms160819886.

Wang, Y., Tar, M.T., Davies, K.P., 2020a. Hyperglycemic memory in the rat bladder detrusor is associated with a persistent hypomethylated state. Physiol. Rep. 8 (22). https://doi.org/10.14814/phy2.14614. Available from: http://physoc.onlinelibrary.wiley.com/hub/journal/10.1002/(ISSN)2051-817X/.

Wang, Z., Zhao, Y., Phipps-Green, A., Bryan, R.L.-, Ceponis, A., Boyle, D.L., Wang, J., Merriman, T.R., Wang, W., Terkeltaub, R., 2020b. Differential DNA methylation of networked signaling, transcriptional, innate and adaptive immunity, and osteoclastogenesis genes and pathways in gout. Arthritis Rheumatol. 72 (5), 802–814. https://doi.org/10.1002/art.41173.

Wankhade, U.D., Zhong, Y., Kang, P., Alfaro, M., Chintapalli, S.V., Thakali, K.M., Shankar, K., Ashton, N., 2017. Enhanced offspring predisposition to steatohepatitis with maternal high-fat diet is associated with epigenetic and microbiome alterations. PLoS One 12 (4), e0175675. https://doi.org/10.1371/journal.pone.0175675.

Watanabe, Y., Tsuchiya, A., Seino, S., Kawata, Y., Kojima, Y., Ikarashi, S., Terai, S., 2019. Mesenchymal stem cells and induced bone marrow-derived macrophages synergistically improve liver fibrosis in mice. Stem Cells Transl. Med. 8 (3), 271–284.

Watson, C.J., Collier, P., Tea, I., Neary, R., Watson, J.A., Robinson, C., Phelan, D., Ledwidge, M.T., Mcdonald, K.M., Mccann, A., Sharaf, O., Baugh, J.A., 2014. Hypoxia-induced epigenetic modifications are associated with cardiac tissue fibrosis and the development of a myofibroblast-like phenotype. Hum. Mol. Genet. 23 (8), 2176–2188. https://doi.org/10.1093/hmg/ddt614.

Whitelaw, N.C., Whitelaw, E., 2008. Transgenerational epigenetic inheritance in health and disease. Curr. Opin. Genet. Dev. 18 (3), 273–279. https://doi.org/10.1016/j.gde.2008.07.001.

Writing Team for the diabetes control and complications trial/epidemiology of diabetes interventions and complications research group. Sustained effect of intensive treatment of type 1 diabetes mellitus on development and progression of diabetic nephropathy: the epidemiology of diabetes interventions and complications (EDIC) study. J. Am. Med. Assoc. 290, 2003, 2159–2167.

Wu, Q., Han, L., Yan, W., Ji, X., Han, R., Yang, J., Ni, C., 2016. miR-489 inhibits silica-induced pulmonary fibrosis by targeting MyD88 and Smad3 and is negatively regulated by lncRNA CHRF. Sci. Rep. 6 (1), 30921.

Wu, Y.L., Lin, Z.J., Li, C.C., Lin, X., Shan, S.K., Guo, B., Zheng, M.H., Li, F., Yuan, L.Q., Li, Z.h., 2023. Epigenetic regulation in metabolic diseases: mechanisms and advances in clinical study. Signal Trans. Target. Therapy 8 (1). https://doi.org/10.1038/s41392-023-01333-7. Available from: https://www.nature.com/sigtrans.

Wu, D., Lu, P., Mi, X., Miao, J., 2018. Exosomal miR-214 from endometrial stromal cells inhibits endometriosis fibrosis. MHR: Basic Sci. Reprod. Med. 24 (7), 357–365.

Xu, H., Wu, X., Qin, H., Tian, W., Chen, J., Sun, L., Xu, Y., 2015. Myocardin-related transcription factor A epigenetically regulates renal fibrosis in diabetic nephropathy. J. Am. Soc. Nephrol. 26 (7), 1648–1660.

Yamagishi, S.-ichi, 2011. Role of advanced glycation end products (AGEs) and receptor for AGEs (RAGE) in vascular damage in diabetes. Exp. Gerontol. 46 (4), 217–224. https://doi.org/10.1016/j.exger.2010.11.007.

Yang, J., Liu, F., Wang, Y., Qu, L., Lin, A., 2022. LncRNAs in tumor metabolic reprogramming and immune microenvironment remodeling. Cancer Lett. 543, 215798. https://doi.org/10.1016/j.canlet.2022.215798.

Yao, Y., Song, Q., Hu, C., Da, X., Yu, Y., He, Z., Xu, C., Chen, Q., Wang, Q.K., 2022. Endothelial cell metabolic memory causes cardiovascular dysfunction in diabetes. Cardiovasc. Res. 118 (1), 196–211. https://doi.org/10.1093/cvr/cvab013.

Yun, J.M., Jialal, I., Devaraj, S., 2011. Epigenetic regulation of high glucose-induced proinflammatory cytokine production in monocytes by curcumin. JNB (J. Nutr. Biochem.) 22 (5), 450–458. https://doi.org/10.1016/j.jnutbio.2010.03.014.

Zhang, Di, Tang, Z., Huang, H., Zhou, G., Cui, C., Weng, Y., Liu, W., Kim, S., Lee, S., Perez-Neut, M., Ding, J., Czyz, D., Hu, R., Ye, Z., He, M., Zheng, Y.G., Shuman, H.A., Dai, L., Ren, B., Roeder, R.G., Becker, L., Zhao, Y., 2019. Metabolic regulation of gene expression by histone lactylation. Nature 574 (7779), 575–580. https://doi.org/10.1038/s41586-019-1678-1.

Zhao, X.Y., Lin, J.D., 2015. Long noncoding RNAs: a new regulatory code in metabolic control. Trends Biochem. Sci. 40 (10), 586–596. https://doi.org/10.1016/j.tibs.2015.08.002.

Zhang, Y., Wang, Y., Qiao, Y., Liu, L., Zhao, H., Jin, Q., Li, P., 2026. Targeting the NAD+-SIRT3 axis to mitigate metabolic memory in diabetic kidney disease. Renal Failure 48 (1), 2648912.

Zhao, S., Li, T., Li, J., Lu, Q., Han, C., Wang, N., Qiu, Q., Cao, H., Xu, X., Chen, H., Zheng, Z., 2016. miR-23b-3p induces the cellular metabolic memory of high glucose in diabetic retinopathy through a SIRT1-dependent signalling pathway. Diabetologia 59 (3), 644–654. https://doi.org/10.1007/s00125-015-3832-0.

Zheng, Z., Chen, H., Li, J., Li, T., Zheng, B., Zheng, Y., Jin, H., He, Y., Gu, Q., Xu, X., 2012. Sirtuin 1–mediated cellular metabolic memory of high glucose via the LKB1/AMPK/ROS pathway and therapeutic effects of metformin. Diabetes 61 (1), 217–228. https://doi.org/10.2337/db11-0416.

Zhong, X., Chung, A.C.K., Chen, H.Y., Dong, Y., Meng, X.M., Li, R., Yang, W., Hou, F.F., Lan, H.Y., 2013. miR-21 is a key therapeutic target for renal injury in a mouse model of type 2 diabetes. Diabetologia 56 (3), 663–674. https://doi.org/10.1007/s00125-012-2804-x.

Zhuo, C., Feng, M., Andrew, D.P., John, M.L., Lingxiao, Z., Dustin, E.S., Xiwei, W., Jinhui, W., Joshua, D.T., Saul, G., Barbara, H.B., Arthur, D.R., Rama, N., 2016. Epigenomic profiling reveals an association between persistence of DNA methylation and metabolic memory in the DCCT/EDIC type 1 diabetes cohort. Proc. Natl. Acad. Sci. U. S. A. 113 (21), E3002. https://doi.org/10.1073/pnas.1603712113.

2

Biochemical pathways and regulation of metabolic memory

1. Introduction

Metabolic memory refers to the persistent cellular and molecular alterations caused by prior hyperglycemia, even after glycemic control is achieved. This phenomenon is driven by interconnected biochemical pathways, including the accumulation of advanced glycation end-products (AGEs), oxidative stress, mitochondrial dysfunction, and epigenetic modifications, all of which contribute to sustained inflammation and vascular damage (Dong et al., 2024) Additionally, the polyol pathway exacerbates oxidative stress, further accelerating diabetic complications such as nephropathy, retinopathy, neuropathy, and cardiovascular disease (Garg and Gupta, 2022).

A critical driver of metabolic memory is the formation of advanced glycation end-products (AGEs), which result from the non-enzymatic modification of proteins, lipids, and nucleic acids by sugars (Aragno and Mastrocola, 2017). AGEs interact with their receptor (RAGE), initiating a cascade of oxidative stress, inflammation, and endothelial dysfunction. This AGE-RAGE axis plays a pivotal role in sustaining metabolic dysfunction and chronic disease states (Cannizzaro et al., 2017). Another key pathway involved in metabolic memory is oxidative stress and mitochondrial dysfunction. Hyperglycemia-induced overproduction of reactive oxygen species (ROS) damages cellular components, disrupts mitochondrial function, and activates inflammatory pathways such as NF-κB and MAPK (Pal et al., 2020). This oxidative environment further amplifies AGE accumulation and sustains metabolic memory, even in the absence of continued hyperglycemia (Nowotny et al., 2015). Epigenetic modifications also contribute significantly to metabolic memory by regulating gene expression through DNA methylation, histone modifications, and non-coding RNAs. These alterations reinforce pro-inflammatory and pro-oxidative gene expression, promoting

Metabolic Memory. https://doi.org/10.1016/B978-0-443-44591-0.00002-3

long-term metabolic dysfunction and vascular complications (Klimczak and Śliwińska, 2024).

Additionally, the polyol pathway exacerbates metabolic memory by converting excess glucose into sorbitol, leading to osmotic stress, NADPH depletion, and oxidative damage (Tigchelaar et al., 2022). This pathway is particularly relevant in diabetic complications affecting the retina, kidneys, and peripheral nerves (Asnaghi et al., 2003).

Understanding these interconnected pathways provides crucial insights into the mechanisms sustaining metabolic memory and highlights the need for targeted therapeutic strategies. This chapter explores key regulatory pathways involved in metabolic memory, focusing on antioxidant defense mechanisms, epigenetic interventions, pharmacological strategies, and lifestyle modifications. Enzymatic and non-enzymatic antioxidants help counteract oxidative stress, while epigenetic therapies offer promising avenues to reverse pathological gene expression. Pharmacological agents, including metformin and SGLT2 inhibitors, modulate oxidative stress and inflammation, whereas dietary and lifestyle modifications, such as caloric restriction and exercise, enhance metabolic resilience (Troise et al., 2024). By integrating these approaches, more effective strategies can be developed to counteract metabolic memory and improve long-term metabolic health.

2. Biochemical pathways involved in metabolic memory

2.1 Advanced glycation end-products (AGEs) pathway

Advanced glycation end-products (AGEs) are harmful compounds formed when sugars non-enzymatically modify proteins, lipids, and nucleic acids. Elevated AGEs are linked to aging, diabetes mellitus (DM) (Kim et al., 2017), and autoimmune diseases such as lupus, rheumatoid arthritis, systemic sclerosis, and psoriasis (Vlassara and Striker, 2013; Nowak et al., 2020). Over 20 advanced glycation end-products (AGEs) are found in food, blood, and tissues, formed by sugar-protein/lipid interactions. They are categorized into fluorescent AGEs (e.g., pentosidine, methylglyoxal-derived lysine dimer [MOLD]) and nonfluorescent AGEs (e.g., Nε-(carboxymethyl)lysine [CML], Nε-(carboxyethyl) lysine [CEL]). (e.g., pyrraline, CML, CEL) (Sharma et al., 2015; Suzuki et al., 1997; Luevano-Contreras and Chapman-

Novakofski, 2010). AGEs are metabolized in renal tubular cells and excreted via the kidneys (Vlassara et al., 2008).

AGEs bind to the receptor Receptor for Advanced Glycation End-products (RAGE)., triggering oxidative stress, inflammation, hyperglycemia, and endothelial dysfunction (Del Turco and Basta, 2012). Their formation is accelerated by sedentary lifestyles, high-calorie diets, processed foods, and smoking (Perrone et al., 2020). Infant formulas, particularly soy-based and hydrolyzed protein formulas, have higher AGE levels than cow- or goat-based formulas, with lactose-containing formulas being more prone to glycation (Xie et al., 2023). Bakery products also generate AGEs during baking, but phenolic additives like ferulic acid and dihydromyricetin can reduce their formation (Boz, 2023). Optimizing food processing may help minimize AGEs and their health risks (Gill et al., 2019).

RAGE, a key immunoglobulin superfamily receptor, is expressed on various cells, including macrophages and endothelial cells (Boyer et al., 2015). The AGE-RAGE interaction activates signaling pathways leading to oxidative stress, inflammation, and chronic diseases such as diabetes, Alzheimer's, and cancer (Barlovic et al., 2011). RAGE also binds endogenous ligands like S100/calgranulins and HMGB1, further amplifying inflammation and tissue damage (Zhang et al., 2017). Additionally, RAGE activation stimulates NF-κB, upregulating its own expression under hyperglycemic conditions, perpetuating chronic inflammation (Xie et al., 2013).

2.1.1 Maillard reaction and AGE formation

The Maillard reaction (MR) is a key process in AGE formation, influenced by protein glycation, turnover rates, hyperglycemia, and oxidative stress (Peppa and Vlassara, 2005). It occurs in three stages (Fig. 2.1). In the initial phase, reducing sugars like glucose and fructose react with protein amino groups (lysine, arginine) to form a Schiff base, which later converts into stable but reversible Amadori products (APs) capable of generating free radicals and protein crosslinks (Bonnefont-Rousselot, 2016). During the proliferation phase, APs undergo further modifications, forming reactive dicarbonyl intermediates such as glyoxal, methylglyoxal, and 3-deoxyglucosone. These intermediates accumulate as "carbonyl stress", reacting with proteins and causing browning and crosslinking (Thorpe and Baynes, 2003). In the advanced phase, dicarbonyls undergo oxidation, glycation, dehydration, and other modifications, leading to the formation of stable,

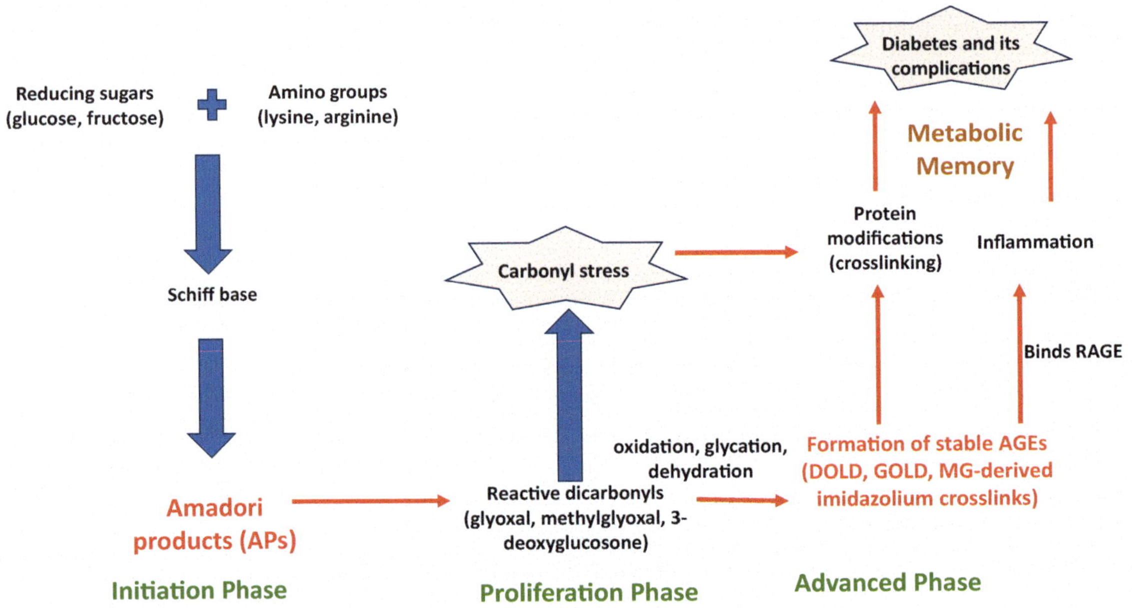

Figure 2.1 Pathophysiology of AGE formation in metabolic memory.

irreversible AGEs like DOLD, GOLD, and MG-derived imidazolium crosslinks, which contribute to various pathological conditions.

These modifications accumulate over time and contribute to metabolic memory by altering protein function and stability, leading to structural and functional impairments in key enzymes and receptors. They also activate the receptor for AGEs (RAGE), triggering intracellular signaling cascades involving NF-κB, which increases the transcription of pro-inflammatory cytokines such as TNF-α, IL-6, and IL-1β. Additionally, these modifications induce epigenetic changes that sustain pro-inflammatory states by modifying histones and DNA methylation patterns, further exacerbating metabolic dysfunction.

The interaction of AGEs with RAGE leads to sustained cellular dysfunction, metabolic memory, where accumulated AGEs maintain RAGE overexpression, NF-κB activation, oxidative stress, and inflammation, even after hyperglycemia is reversed (Yamagishi et al., 2015). This AGEs/RAGE axis is central to diabetes complications, including macrovascular and microvascular diseases, which contribute to increased morbidity, mortality, and healthcare costs (Dal Canto et al., 2019). Type 2 diabetes patients have a higher cardiovascular mortality risk due to hyperglycemia-induced vascular damage mediated by AGEs/RAGE activation of

NF-κB, MAPK, and oxidative stress pathways. This promotes inflammatory markers like VCAM-1, ICAM-1, MCP-1, and PAI-1, contributing to arterial stiffness, vascular calcification, and atherosclerosis (Glovaci et al., 2019). Additionally, oxidized LDL, acting as a RAGE ligand, amplifies inflammatory signaling, leading to vascular dysfunction and CVD progression (Kay et al., 2016). AGEs also modify collagen and lipoproteins in blood vessels, increasing arterial stiffness and endothelial dysfunction, key factors in arteriosclerosis and organ damage, including nephropathy and retinopathy (Yamagishi and Matsui, 2018; Sanajou et al., 2018). In diabetes, AGEs accumulate in the kidneys, activating RAGE and oxidative stress pathways, reducing antioxidant defences, and triggering inflammation, leading to renal fibrosis and kidney dysfunction, a major cause of end-stage renal disease (ESRD) (Jitraknatee et al., 2020; London, 2018). AGEs also degrade the glomerular filtration barrier, worsening diabetic nephropathy (Suryavanshi and Kulkarni, 2017; An et al., 2018).

The AGEs/RAGE axis, along with environmental and metabolic factors, contributes to metabolic memory, which perpetuates diabetic complications through epigenetic modifications like DNA methylation and histone alterations, further driving NF-κB activation and chronic inflammation (Berezin, 2016; Al-Haddad et al., 2016). AGEs influence epigenetic modifications by inducing DNA methylation, histone modifications, and non-coding RNA regulation, all of which alter gene expression patterns linked to inflammation and metabolic disorders (Prandi et al., 2022). Increased DNA methylation of key antioxidant and anti-inflammatory genes, such as Nrf2 and SOD2, results in their suppression, reducing cellular defense mechanisms against oxidative stress (Zhao et al., 2018; Wang et al., 2018a). Meanwhile, histone modifications, such as H3K9 and H3K27 methylation, lead to chromatin condensation, repressing genes involved in insulin signaling and vascular repair, while histone acetylation at H3K9 enhances the expression of pro-inflammatory genes like TNF-α and IL-6, amplifying chronic inflammation (Bahman et al., 2024) Additionally, AGEs modulate non-coding RNAs, such as miR-21, miR-146a, and miR-155, which regulate key pathways involved in endothelial dysfunction, fibrosis, and diabetic complications (Desantis et al., 2023). Through these epigenetic alterations, AGEs reinforce metabolic memory, sustaining pathological gene expression and exacerbating conditions like diabetic nephropathy, neuropathy, retinopathy, and cardiovascular disease, even after hyperglycemia is controlled. This highlights the need for targeted therapeutic strategies, such as epigenetic inhibitors, sirtuin activators, and AGE inhibitors like aminoguanidine, to mitigate AGE-induced epigenetic dysregulation and its long-term consequences.

2.2 Oxidative stress and mitochondrial dysfunction

When blood sugar levels are elevated (hyperglycemia), excessive glucose metabolism generates reactive oxygen species (ROS) within mitochondria, leading to oxidative stress. This oxidative burden damages cellular components such as proteins, lipids, and DNA, resulting in structural and functional impairments (Mukai et al., 2022). Additionally, hyperglycemia-induced AGE formation further exacerbates oxidative stress and inflammation by engaging the receptor for AGEs (RAGE), perpetuating cellular dysfunction (Shen et al., 2020). Oxidative stress also acts as a mediator of epigenetic modifications, altering DNA methylation, histone modifications, and non-coding RNA expression. It induces hypermethylation of genes that regulate antioxidant defences while promoting histone acetylation at pro-inflammatory genes, sustaining their overexpression (Gu et al., 2013). Non-coding RNAs, such as microRNAs, contribute to this process by suppressing antioxidant pathways and enhancing inflammatory gene expression, thereby reinforcing the metabolic memory effect even after glucose levels normalize (Jakubik et al., 2021). Organs with high metabolic activity, such as the heart, kidneys, and blood vessels, are particularly vulnerable to metabolic memory due to their sensitivity to oxidative stress (Popolo et al., 2013). In the heart, oxidative damage leads to myocardial fibrosis, endothelial dysfunction, and left ventricular hypertrophy, increasing cardiovascular risk. The kidneys suffer glomerular and tubular damage, contributing to diabetic nephropathy, while in blood vessels, oxidative stress accelerates endothelial dysfunction, arterial stiffness, and plaque formation, heightening the risk of atherosclerosis and microvascular complications.

2.2.1 How oxidative stress contributes to metabolic memory

2.2.1.1 Mitochondrial dysfunction

Excessive reactive oxygen species (ROS) disrupt mitochondrial function by impairing oxidative phosphorylation and ATP production through direct damage to key electron transport chain (ETC) complexes, such as Complex I and Complex III (Ralph et al., 2011). This leads to electron leakage, further amplifying ROS production in a vicious cycle. Mitochondrial DNA (mtDNA), which lacks protective histones and has limited repair mechanisms, is particularly vulnerable to oxidative damage

(Mikhed et al., 2015). Oxidized mtDNA can result in mutations that impair mitochondrial gene expression, disrupt protein synthesis, and lead to defective ETC function. These alterations further compromise mitochondrial efficiency, reduce ATP availability, and increase cellular stress, contributing to apoptosis, inflammation, and metabolic disorders.

2.2.1.2 Activation of inflammatory pathways

Oxidative stress activates key inflammatory signaling cascades, including NF-κB, JNK, and p38 MAPK, by stimulating upstream kinases such as IKK and ASK1 (Kojima et al., 2021). This activation leads to increased transcription of pro-inflammatory mediators, including cytokines (TNF-α, IL-6, IL-1β), adhesion molecules (ICAM-1, VCAM-1), and chemokines (MCP-1) (Kim et al., 2008; Suzuki et al., 2012). These factors promote leukocyte recruitment, endothelial activation, and vascular inflammation, contributing to endothelial dysfunction. Chronic activation of these pathways leads to increased vascular permeability, impaired nitric oxide (NO) production, and heightened oxidative stress, which collectively drive the progression of diabetic complications such as atherosclerosis, nephropathy, and retinopathy (Teodoro et al., 2019). Additionally, persistent NF-κB activation sustains metabolic memory, perpetuating inflammation even after glucose levels normalize (Cai et al., 2011).

2.2.1.3 Protein glycation

Elevated glucose levels promote the non-enzymatic glycation of proteins, leading to the formation of AGEs through a series of oxidative and non-oxidative reactions. AGEs interact with their receptor (RAGE), triggering intracellular signaling cascades such as NF-κB, MAPK, and JNK, which amplify oxidative stress by increasing reactive oxygen species (ROS) production. This oxidative environment further accelerates AGE accumulation, perpetuating a cycle of cellular damage (Boyer et al., 2015). Additionally, AGEs induce cross-linking of extracellular matrix (ECM) proteins like collagen and elastin, reducing tissue elasticity and increasing stiffness. This cross-linking disrupts normal cellular interactions, impairs endothelial function, and contributes to vascular calcification and fibrosis, particularly in diabetic organs such as the heart, kidneys, and blood vessels (Kesava Reddy, 2004). The structural and functional (alterations induced by AGEs are key drivers of complications like nephropathy, retinopathy, and atherosclerosis, leading to progressive organ dysfunction.

2.2.2 Important pathways involved in oxidative stress and metabolic memory

2.2.2.1 NADPH oxidase

NADPH oxidase is a major enzymatic source of ROS production, particularly under hyperglycemic conditions. Its overactivation in endothelial cells, macrophages, and kidney cells leads to excessive superoxide anion (O_2^-) generation, which disrupts redox homeostasis and exacerbates oxidative stress (Teshima et al., 2014). In diabetic nephropathy, NADPH oxidase-derived ROS contribute to glomerular injury by promoting mesangial cell proliferation, extracellular matrix expansion, and podocyte dysfunction, ultimately leading to proteinuria and renal fibrosis (Lee and Jose, 2021). In diabetic retinopathy, increased ROS production damages retinal capillary endothelial cells, induces pericyte apoptosis, and enhances vascular permeability, resulting in retinal edema, neovascularization, and vision loss (Mrugacz et al., 2021). Furthermore, NADPH oxidase activation stimulates pro-inflammatory pathways such as NF-κB and AP-1, increasing the expression of cytokines (TNF-α, IL-6), adhesion molecules (ICAM-1, VCAM-1), and pro-fibrotic factors (TGF-β, CTGF), which further drive chronic inflammation and microvascular complications in diabetes (Fakhri et al., 2024).

2.2.2.2 Mitochondrial electron transport chain (ETC)

Under hyperglycemic conditions, excessive glucose metabolism drives an overload of electron donors (NADH and $FADH_2$) into the mitochondrial electron transport chain (ETC). This excessive flux increases electron leakage at complexes I and III, generating superoxide (O_2^-), a highly reactive ROS. The accumulation of superoxide disrupts mitochondrial function by impairing oxidative phosphorylation, reducing ATP synthesis, and triggering mitochondrial permeability transition pore (mPTP) opening, which can lead to cytochrome *c* release and apoptosis (Cortés-Rojo et al., 2020).

Moreover, superoxide reacts with nitric oxide (NO) to form peroxynitrite ($ONOO^-$), a potent oxidant that damages mitochondrial DNA (mtDNA), proteins, and lipids, further impairing mitochondrial efficiency (Piacenza et al., 2022). This oxidative stress perpetuates metabolic memory by sustaining inflammation, activating redox-sensitive transcription factors such as NF-κB and AP-1, and enhancing the formation of AGEs, which in turn maintain RAGE activation (An et al., 2018). This chronic mitochondrial dysfunction fosters sustained ROS production even after glycemic control is restored, contributing to long-term diabetic complications such as nephropathy, retinopathy, and cardiovascular disease.

2.2.2.3 Protein kinase C (PKC)

Protein kinase C (PKC) activation in diabetes plays a pivotal role in oxidative stress and vascular dysfunction. Chronic hyperglycemia leads to excessive diacylglycerol (DAG) accumulation, which persistently activates PKC isoforms, particularly PKC-β and PKC-δ (Gupta et al., 2010). Activated PKC enhances ROS production by stimulating NADPH oxidase, increasing superoxide (O_2^-) generation in endothelial cells, macrophages, and renal mesangial cells (Rathore et al., 2008). This oxidative burst not only exacerbates mitochondrial dysfunction but also reduces nitric oxide (NO) bioavailability by promoting NO degradation through peroxynitrite ($ONOO^-$) formation, leading to endothelial dysfunction and impaired vasodilation (Roy et al., 2023).

Beyond oxidative stress, PKC signaling modulates the expression of several pro-inflammatory and pro-fibrotic mediators. It upregulates vascular endothelial growth factor (VEGF), monocyte chemoattractant protein-1 (MCP-1), and transforming growth factor-beta (TGF-β), fostering chronic inflammation, vascular permeability, and extracellular matrix deposition (Fui et al., 2019). These changes contribute to diabetic complications such as nephropathy (glomerular fibrosis and albuminuria), retinopathy (increased angiogenesis and vascular leakage), and atherosclerosis (vascular calcification and plaque instability). Additionally, PKC activation exacerbates metabolic memory by sustaining NF-κB-driven inflammation and AGEs-RAGE signaling, prolonging tissue damage even after glycemic control is restored (Sivandzade et al., 2019).

These mechanisms collectively reinforce the persistent impact of metabolic memory, prolonging oxidative damage and inflammation even after glycemic control is restored, thereby increasing the risk of long-term diabetic complications.

2.3 Epigenetic modifications

Epigenetic mechanisms, including DNA methylation, histone modifications, and non-coding RNAs, play a crucial role in sustaining metabolic memory, perpetuating diabetic complications even after glucose levels normalize (Fig. 2.2).

Histone modifications contribute significantly to metabolic memory, with persistent histone acetylation at inflammatory gene promoters, such as *NF-κB, TNF-α,* and *IL-6,* maintaining

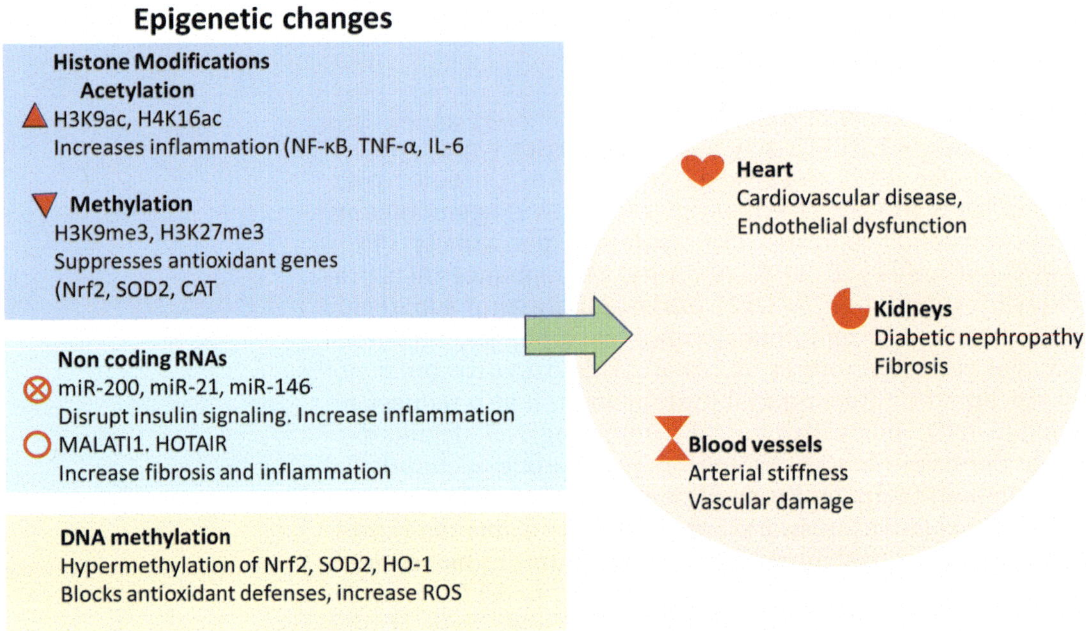

Figure 2.2 Epigenetic mechanisms in metabolic memory.

their active transcription (Xu et al., 2015). This is largely mediated by histone acetyltransferases (HATs), such as p300/CBP and PCAF, which deposit acetyl groups on histone tails (e.g., H3K9ac and H4K16ac), enhancing chromatin accessibility and recruiting transcription factors that sustain chronic inflammation and endothelial dysfunction in diabetic tissues (Wang et al., 2021). This prolonged inflammatory signaling leads to increased expression of adhesion molecules such as VCAM-1 and ICAM-1, promoting leukocyte adhesion and vascular damage (Olivares-Silva et al., 2018). Conversely, histone methylation acts in an opposing manner, with repressive marks like H3K9me2/3 and H3K27me3 deposited by histone methyltransferases (HMTs) such as SUV39H1 and EZH2, leading to the silencing of key antioxidant defense genes, including *Nrf2, SOD2,* and *Catalase (CAT)* (Yi et al., 2022). The repression of *Nrf2*, a master regulator of antioxidant responses, reduces the transcription of downstream detoxifying enzymes like *HO-1 and GPx,* impairing the cell's ability to neutralize reactive oxygen species (ROS) and exacerbating oxidative stress (Zhang et al., 2018). This imbalance between pro-inflammatory histone acetylation and repressive histone methylation fosters a pro-oxidant, pro-inflammatory environment, perpetuating vascular complications and metabolic dysfunction in diabetes.

DNA methylation further reinforces metabolic memory by increasing methylation of key antioxidant and detoxifying genes like *Nrf2* and *SOD2*, leading to their transcriptional repression. This process is mediated by DNA methyltransferases (DNMTs), such as DNMT1 and DNMT3A, which add methyl groups to CpG islands in the promoter regions of these genes, preventing transcription factor binding and reducing gene expression (Silva-Llanes et al., 2023). Hypermethylation of *Nrf2*, a master regulator of the cellular antioxidant response, decreases the transcription of its downstream targets, including *HO-1*, *GPx*, and *NQO1*, weakening the cell's ability to detoxify reactive oxygen species (ROS) (Taheri et al., 2020). Similarly, silencing of *SOD2*, which encodes mitochondrial superoxide dismutase, disrupts the conversion of superoxide radicals into less harmful molecules, further amplifying oxidative stress. These DNA methylation-driven changes persist even after glycemic normalization, sustaining ROS accumulation and inflammation, thereby contributing to long-term endothelial dysfunction, vascular stiffness, and progression of diabetic complications such as nephropathy and retinopathy (Balasubramanian et al., 2021).

Non-coding RNAs, particularly dysregulated microRNAs (miRNAs) and long non-coding RNAs (lncRNAs), play a crucial role in amplifying metabolic dysfunction by modulating gene expression at the post-transcriptional level. MiRNAs such as *miR-200*, *miR-21*, and *miR-146* disrupt key metabolic and inflammatory pathways by binding to target mRNAs, leading to their degradation or translational repression. MiR-200 negatively regulates *ZEB1* and *ZEB2*, impairing insulin signaling and promoting β-cell dysfunction (Chen et al., 2022). MiR-21 suppresses *PTEN* and *FOXO1*, which enhances pro-inflammatory cytokine production and contributes to insulin resistance (Liu et al., 2020). MiR-146a, involved in immune regulation, inhibits *TRAF6* and *IRAK1*, disrupting NF-κB signaling but paradoxically sustaining chronic low-grade inflammation in diabetic tissues (He et al., 2021).

Similarly, lncRNAs like *MALAT1* and *HOTAIR* exacerbate inflammation and fibrosis in diabetic tissues. MALAT1, highly expressed in endothelial and renal cells, acts as a competing endogenous RNA (ceRNA) by sponging miR-146a, thereby sustaining NF-κB activation and inflammatory cytokine production (e.g., IL-6, TNF-α, IL-1β), leading to endothelial dysfunction and diabetic nephropathy (Dai et al., 2018). HOTAIR, a chromatin-modifying lncRNA, interacts with Polycomb Repressive Complex

2 (PRC2) to promote H3K27me3-mediated silencing of antifibrotic genes, thereby driving fibrosis in diabetic kidneys and contributing to renal dysfunction (Majumder et al., 2019). These persistent alterations in non-coding RNA expression perpetuate metabolic memory, exacerbating inflammation, oxidative stress, and fibrosis even after glucose normalization, ultimately accelerating diabetic complications such as nephropathy, retinopathy, and cardiovascular disease.

Collectively, these epigenetic alterations create a self-perpetuating cycle of oxidative stress, inflammation, and metabolic dysfunction, driving the progression of diabetic complications despite glycemic control.

2.4 Polyol pathway and sorbitol accumulation

Under hyperglycemic conditions, the enzyme aldose reductase plays a pivotal role in the activation of the polyol pathway by catalyzing the conversion of excess intracellular glucose into sorbitol. This metabolic diversion contributes significantly to the development of diabetic complications through multiple interconnected mechanisms. Firstly, sorbitol accumulation induces osmotic stress by increasing intracellular osmotic pressure, leading to cellular swelling and dysfunction. This effect is especially detrimental in tissues with low levels of sorbitol dehydrogenase, such as the retina, kidneys, and peripheral nerves, thereby contributing to diabetic retinopathy, diabetic nephropathy, and diabetic neuropathy, respectively (Obrosova, 2005). Secondly, the polyol pathway consumes NADPH, a critical cofactor required for the regeneration of glutathione (GSH), one of the cell's primary antioxidants. The resultant depletion of GSH weakens the cell's defense against reactive oxygen species (ROS), intensifying oxidative stress and leading to endothelial dysfunction, a key feature in the progression of microvascular damage (Thorne et al., 2024). Additionally, the diversion of glucose into this alternative pathway causes metabolic imbalance by reducing the flux through glycolysis and impairing ATP production, which in turn aggravates mitochondrial dysfunction (Yan, 2018). This metabolic disturbance perpetuates a cycle of oxidative stress, inflammation, and metabolic memory, all of which are central to the chronic progression of diabetic complications. The persistent activation of the polyol pathway under hyperglycemic conditions underscores its critical role in the pathogenesis of diabetic microvascular diseases and positions aldose reductase as a promising therapeutic target for intervention in diabetes-related tissue damage.

2.5 Protein kinase C (PKC) activation

Under hyperglycemic conditions, protein kinase C (PKC) isoforms become activated and play a significant role in driving various diabetes-related pathophysiological processes. One major consequence of PKC activation is vascular inflammation, wherein the expression of adhesion molecules such as intercellular adhesion molecule-1 (ICAM-1) and vascular cell adhesion molecule-1 (VCAM-1) is upregulated (Jubaidi et al., 2022). This promotes the adhesion and infiltration of leukocytes into the vascular endothelium, initiating chronic inflammation, impairing endothelial function, and contributing to atherosclerotic plaque formation, all of which are key features of diabetic vascular complications (Jubaidi et al., 2022).

Additionally, PKC activation leads to endothelial dysfunction by disrupting nitric oxide (NO) signaling. This occurs through enhanced production of endothelin-1 (ET-1) and increased degradation of NO due to elevated levels of reactive oxygen species (ROS). The resultant vasoconstriction, reduced blood flow, and increased vascular resistance contribute to hypertension and elevate the risk of cardiovascular disease in individuals with diabetes (Chen et al., 2014).

PKC also impairs metabolic regulation by promoting insulin resistance. It does so by phosphorylating insulin receptor substrate proteins (IRS-1 and IRS-2), thereby disrupting downstream insulin signaling. This inhibits the translocation of glucose transporter type 4 (GLUT4) in skeletal muscle and adipose tissue, reducing glucose uptake and exacerbating hyperglycemia, a hallmark of type 2 diabetes (Rabiee et al., 2018).

Collectively, the activation of PKC isoforms amplifies oxidative stress, inflammation, and metabolic dysfunction, positioning PKC as a critical contributor to diabetic complications and a potential therapeutic target for mitigating the progression of diabetes and its associated vascular and metabolic disorders. Top of Form.

3. Regulation of metabolic memory

Several regulatory mechanisms modulate metabolic memory, offering potential therapeutic targets (Table 2.1).

3.1 Antioxidant défense mechanisms

Cells utilize both enzymatic and non-enzymatic antioxidant systems to mitigate oxidative stress and maintain cellular

Table 2.1 Regulatory mechanisms targeting metabolic memory: Antioxidant, epigenetic, pharmacological, and lifestyle interventions.

Mechanism	Specific components/ Interventions	Mode of action	Target outcomes	References
Antioxidant defense mechanisms (enzymatic)	Superoxide dismutase (SOD)	Converts superoxide radicals (O_2^-) into hydrogen peroxide (H_2O_2), reducing oxidative stress.	Prevents ROS-induced cellular damage.	Ighodaro and Akinloye (2018)
	Catalase (CAT)	Breaks down H_2O_2 into water and oxygen.	Reduces oxidative stress and protects cells.	Ighodaro and Akinloye (2018)
	Glutathione peroxidase (GPx)	Converts H_2O_2 and lipid peroxides to non-toxic products using glutathione.	Maintains redox homeostasis.	Ighodaro and Akinloye (2018)
Antioxidant defense mechanisms (non-enzymatic)	Vitamin C, vitamin E	Act as free radical scavengers, protect lipid membranes from peroxidation.	Prevent lipid peroxidation and oxidative damage.	Ahamad et al. (2019)
	Polyphenols, carotenoids	Plant-based antioxidants providing additional ROS neutralization.	Lower chronic oxidative stress.	Ahamad et al. (2019)
Nrf2-mediated antioxidant response	Nrf2 activation, HO-1, NQO1, GCLM induction	Nrf2 dissociates from Keap1, binds AREs, and induces antioxidant genes.	Enhances natural defense, reduces oxidative damage.	Liu et al. (2025)
Epigenetic interventions (histone modifications)	HDAC inhibitors (valproic acid, trichostatin A)	Maintain histone acetylation at anti-inflammatory promoters, suppress cytokines (TNF-α, IL-6).	Restore chromatin structure, reduce inflammation.	Zhang et al. (2024)
Epigenetic interventions (DNA methylation)	DNMT inhibitors (5-azacytidine, decitabine)	Reverse hypermethylation-induced silencing of antioxidant genes like Nrf2.	Improve antioxidant response, reduce oxidative stress.	Hsieh et al. (2022)
Epigenetic interventions (miRNA therapy)	Antagomirs (anti–miR-21)	Inhibit fibrosis and inflammation.	Improve tissue healing and vascular function.	An et al. (2018)
	miR-126 enhancement	Improves endothelial function and vascular repair.	Restore vascular homeostasis.	An et al. (2018)

Table 2.1 Regulatory mechanisms targeting metabolic memory: Antioxidant, epigenetic, pharmacological, and lifestyle interventions.—*continued*

Mechanism	Specific components/ Interventions	Mode of action	Target outcomes	References
Pharmacological interventions	Metformin	Inhibits mitochondrial complex I → ↓ ROS, suppresses AGE formation.	Improves metabolic control, reduces oxidative stress.	Zuliani et al. (2020)
	SGLT2 inhibitors	Lower glucose, modulate epigenetic pathways, reduce inflammation.	Improve glycemic control and vascular health.	Pignatelli et al. (2022)
	Anti-RAGE therapies (sRAGE, small molecules)	Block AGE-RAGE interaction, attenuate inflammation and vascular damage.	Prevent vascular complications.	Egaña-Gorroño et al. (2020)
	Antioxidants (alpha-lipoic acid, resveratrol)	Neutralize ROS, enhance Nrf2-mediated defense, improve endothelial function.	Counteract oxidative stress-driven complications.	Attia et al. (2020)
Lifestyle & dietary modifications (diet)	Caloric restriction/ intermittent fasting	Improve insulin sensitivity, promote autophagy.	Reduce oxidative stress, improve metabolic efficiency.	Yuan et al. (2021)
	Omega-3 fatty acids (fish oil, flaxseeds)	Anti-inflammatory, enhance mitochondrial function.	Mitigate oxidative damage induced by metabolic memory.	Borja-Magno et al. (2023)
Lifestyle & dietary modifications (exercise)	Regular physical activity	Stimulates mitochondrial biogenesis, increases antioxidant enzymes (via PGC-1α).	Improve metabolic efficiency and reduce long-term hyperglycemia effects.	Jia et al. (2019)

homeostasis. Enzymatic antioxidants such as superoxide dismutase (SOD), catalase (CAT), and glutathione peroxidase (GPx) play crucial roles in neutralizing reactive oxygen species (ROS). SOD converts superoxide radicals (O_2^-) into hydrogen peroxide (H_2O_2), which is then broken down by CAT and GPx to prevent cellular damage (Ighodaro and Akinloye, 2018). Non-enzymatic antioxidants, including vitamins C and E, act as free radical scavengers, protecting lipid membranes from peroxidation. Additionally, polyphenols and carotenoids from plant-based foods provide further antioxidant protection (Ahamad et al., 2019). A key regulatory pathway in oxidative stress defense is the Nrf2-mediated antioxidant response. Under oxidative stress, nuclear factor erythroid 2-related factor 2 (Nrf2) dissociates from its cytoplasmic inhibitor Keap1, translocates to the nucleus, and binds to antioxidant response elements (AREs), inducing genes such as HO-1, NQO1, and GCLM (Liu et al., 2022). This activation enhances the cell's natural defense mechanisms against oxidative damage and inflammation. By integrating these antioxidant strategies, cells effectively counteract ROS accumulation, reduce oxidative damage, and mitigate the progression of oxidative stress-related diseases such as diabetes and neurodegenerative disorders.

3.2 Epigenetic interventions

Therapeutic modulation of epigenetic marks offers promising strategies to reverse metabolic memory and mitigate diabetes-related complications. Histone deacetylase (HDAC) inhibitors, such as valproic acid and trichostatin A, work by maintaining histone acetylation at critical anti-inflammatory gene promoters, thereby suppressing pro-inflammatory cytokine expression (e.g., TNF-α, IL-6) and restoring normal chromatin structure (Zhang et al., 2024). DNA methyltransferase (DNMT) inhibitors, like 5-azacytidine and decitabine, can reverse hypermethylation-induced silencing of genes involved in antioxidant defense (e.g., Nrf2), improving the cellular response to oxidative stress (Hsieh et al., 2022). Additionally, miRNA-based therapies, such as antagomirs or miRNA mimics, target key metabolic regulators. For instance, inhibiting miR-21 can reduce fibrosis and inflammation, while enhancing miR-126 can improve endothelial function and vascular repair (Wang et al., 2018b). These approaches collectively aim to reprogram pathological gene expression, reduce chronic inflammation, and restore metabolic homeostasis, offering potential therapeutic benefits for diabetic complications.

3.3 Pharmacological interventions

Several drugs have been investigated for their potential to mitigate metabolic memory and its associated complications. Metformin, a first-line antidiabetic drug, reduces oxidative stress by inhibiting mitochondrial complex I, thereby decreasing ROS production (Zuliani et al., 2020). It also suppresses AGE formation and enhances mitochondrial function, contributing to improved metabolic control. Sodium-glucose cotransporter 2 (SGLT2) inhibitors not only lower blood glucose levels by promoting renal glucose excretion but also modulate epigenetic pathways, reducing inflammation and oxidative stress (Pignatelli et al., 2022). Anti-RAGE therapies, such as soluble RAGE (sRAGE) and small-molecule inhibitors, block the interaction between AGEs and their receptor (RAGE), thereby attenuating inflammatory and vascular damage (Egaña-Gorroño et al., 2020). Additionally, antioxidants like alpha-lipoic acid (ALA) and resveratrol neutralize ROS, enhance Nrf2-mediated antioxidant defense, and improve endothelial function, collectively helping to counteract metabolic imbalances and oxidative stress-driven diabetic complications (Attia et al., 2020).

3.4 Lifestyle and dietary modifications

Long-term glycemic control and dietary interventions are essential in preventing metabolic memory and its long-lasting effects on cellular function. Caloric restriction and intermittent fasting improve insulin sensitivity by reducing systemic glucose levels and enhancing cellular energy efficiency. These dietary approaches also promote autophagy, a critical process that clears damaged organelles, including dysfunctional mitochondria, thereby mitigating oxidative stress (Yuan et al., 2021). Omega-3 fatty acids, found in fish oil and flaxseeds, have anti-inflammatory properties that help regulate immune responses, enhance mitochondrial function, and counteract oxidative damage induced by metabolic memory (Borja-Magno et al., 2023). Additionally, regular physical activity plays a pivotal role by stimulating mitochondrial biogenesis, increasing antioxidant enzyme expression, and improving metabolic efficiency. Exercise-induced activation of pathways such as PGC-1α enhances cellular resilience against oxidative stress, reducing the long-term impact of hyperglycemia on metabolic and vascular health (Jia et al., 2019).

4. Conclusion

Metabolic memory is a critical factor in the progression of chronic metabolic diseases, with long-term consequences even after metabolic normalization. The biochemical pathways underlying this phenomenon involve oxidative stress, epigenetic regulation, and chronic inflammation. Understanding the regulatory mechanisms provides opportunities for targeted therapeutic strategies to mitigate the effects of metabolic memory and improve long-term metabolic health.

5. Future directions

Further research is essential to develop more effective strategies for mitigating metabolic memory and its role in chronic metabolic diseases. Targeted epigenetic therapies, such as histone modification modulators and miRNA-based interventions, hold promise for reversing metabolic memory and restoring normal gene function. Additionally, exploring novel antioxidant compounds with sustained efficacy could provide long-term protection against oxidative stress and inflammation, key drivers of metabolic dysfunction. The gut microbiota also plays a crucial role in metabolic regulation, and understanding its influence on metabolic memory could lead to microbiome-based therapeutic interventions. Furthermore, integrating personalized medicine approaches—leveraging genomic and epigenetic profiling—will allow for tailored interventions that optimize treatment outcomes. By addressing these research areas, we can enhance our ability to prevent and manage the long-term consequences of metabolic disorders effectively.

References

Ahamad, T., Ansari, W.A., Singh Negi, D., Khan, M.F., 2019. Non-enzymatic natural reactive oxygen scavengers (ROS): a review on structures and mode of action. Era's Journal of Medical Research 6 (2), 103–112. https://doi.org/10.24041/ejmr2019.139.

Al-Haddad, R., Karnib, N., Assaad, R.A., Bilen, Y., Emmanuel, N., Ghanem, A., Younes, J., Zibara, V., Stephan, J.S., Sleiman, S.F., 2016. Epigenetic changes in diabetes. Neurosci. Lett. 625, 64–69. https://doi.org/10.1016/j.neulet.2016.04.046.

An, X., Zhang, L., Yao, Q., Li, L., Wang, B., Zhang, J., He, M., Zhang, J., 2018. The receptor for advanced glycation endproducts mediates podocyte heparanase expression through NF-κB signaling pathway. Mol. Cell. Endocrinol. 470, 14–25. https://doi.org/10.1016/j.mce.2017.05.004.

Aragno, M., Mastrocola, R., 2017. Dietary sugars and endogenous formation of advanced glycation endproducts: emerging mechanisms of disease. Nutrients 9 (4), 385. https://doi.org/10.3390/nu9040385.

Asnaghi, V., Gerhardinger, C., Todd, H., Adeboje, A., Lorenzi, M., 2003. A role for the polyol pathway in the early neuroretinal apoptosis and glial changes induced by diabetes in the rat. Diabetes 52 (2), 506–511. https://doi.org/10.2337/diabetes.52.2.506.

Attia, M., Essa, E.A., Zaki, R.M., Elkordy, A.A., 2020. An overview of the antioxidant effects of ascorbic acid and alpha lipoic acid (In liposomal forms) as adjuvant in cancer treatment. Antioxidants 9 (5). https://doi.org/10.3390/antiox9050359.

Bahman, F., Al-Roub, A., Akhter, N., Al Madhoun, A., Wilson, A., Almansour, N., Al-Rashed, F., Sindhu, S., Al-Mulla, F., Ahmad, R., 2024. TNF-α/Stearate induced H3K9/18 histone acetylation amplifies IL-6 expression in 3T3-L1 mouse adipocytes. Int. J. Mol. Sci. 25 (12). https://doi.org/10.3390/ijms25126776.

Balasubramanian, N., Sagarkar, S., Choudhary, A.G., Kokare, D.M., Sakharkar, A. J., 2021. Epigenetic blockade of hippocampal SOD2 via DNMT3b-mediated DNA methylation: implications in mild traumatic brain injury-induced persistent oxidative damage. Mol. Neurobiol. 58 (3), 1162–1184. https://doi.org/10.1007/s12035-020-02166-z.

Barlovic, D.P., Soro-Paavonen, A., Jandeleit-Dahm, K.A.M., 2011. RAGE biology, atherosclerosis and diabetes. Clin. Sci. 121 (2), 43–55. https://doi.org/10.1042/CS20100501Slovenia.

Berezin, A., 2016. Metabolic memory phenomenon in diabetes mellitus: achieving and perspectives. Diabetes Metabol. Syndr.: Clin. Res. Rev. 10 (2), S176. https://doi.org/10.1016/j.dsx.2016.03.016.

Bonnefont-Rousselot, D., 2016. Resveratrol and cardiovascular diseases. Nutrients 8. https://doi.org/10.3390/nu8050250 ([DOI] [PMC free article] [PubMed] [Google Scholar]).

Borja-Magno, A.I., Furuzawa-Carballeda, J., Guevara-Cruz, M., Arias, C., Granados, J., Bourges, H., Tovar, A.R., Sears, B., Noriega, L.G., Gómez, F.E., 2023. Supplementation with EPA and DHA omega-3 fatty acids improves peripheral immune cell mitochondrial dysfunction and inflammation in subjects with obesity. JNB (J. Nutr. Biochem.) 120. https://doi.org/10.1016/j.jnutbio.2023.109415.

Boyer, F., Vidot, J.B., Dubourg, A.G., Rondeau, P., Essop, M.F., Bourdon, E., 2015. Oxidative stress and adipocyte biology: focus on the role of AGEs. Oxid. Med. Cell. Longev. 2015. https://doi.org/10.1155/2015/534873.

Boz, H., 2023. N ϵ -(carboxymethyl)lysine in bakery products: a review. J. Food Sci. 88 (3), 901–908. https://doi.org/10.1111/1750-3841.16475.

Cai, Z., Zhao, Y., Yao, S., Zhao, B., 2011. Increases in β-amyloid protein in the hippocampus caused by diabetic metabolic disorder are blocked by minocycline through inhibition of NF-κB pathway activation. Pharmacol. Rep. 63 (2), 381–391. https://doi.org/10.1016/s1734-1140(11)70504-7.

Cannizzaro, L., Rossoni, G., Savi, F., Altomare, A., Marinello, C., Saethang, T., Carini, M., Payne, D.M., Pisitkun, T., Aldini, G., Leelahavanichkul, A., 2017. Regulatory landscape of AGE-RAGE-oxidative stress axis and its modulation by PPARγ activation in high fructose diet-induced metabolic syndrome. Nutr. Metabol. 14 (1). https://doi.org/10.1186/s12986-016-0149-z.

Chen, F., Kumar, S., Yu, Y., Aggarwal, S., Gross, C., Wang, Y., Chakraborty, T., Verin, A.D., Catravas, J.D., Rudolf, L., Black, S.M., Fulton, D.J.R., Dang, Y.-hui, 2014. PKC-dependent phosphorylation of eNOS at T495 regulates eNOS coupling and endothelial barrier function in response to G+ -toxins. PLoS One 9 (7), e99823. https://doi.org/10.1371/journal.pone.0099823.

Chen, W., Jiang, W., Dong, J., Wang, J., Wang, B., 2022. miR-200b-3p induces the formation of insulin-producing cells from umbilical cord mesenchymal stem cells by targeting ZEB2. Crit. Rev. Eukaryot. Gene Expr. 32 (6), 33–46. https://doi.org/10.1615/critreveukaryotgeneexpr.2022041822.

Cortés-Rojo, C., Vargas-Vargas, M.A., Olmos-Orizaba, B.E., Rodríguez-Orozco, A. R., Calderón-Cortés, E., 2020. Interplay between NADH oxidation by complex I, glutathione redox state and sirtuin-3, and its role in the development of insulin resistance. Biochim. Biophys. Acta (BBA) - Mol. Basis Dis. 1866 (8). https://doi.org/10.1016/j.bbadis.2020.165801.

Dai, L., Zhang, G., Cheng, Z., Wang, X., Jia, L., Jing, X., Wang, H., Zhang, R., Liu, M., Jiang, T., Yang, Y., Yang, M., 2018. Knockdown of LncRNA MALAT1 contributes to the suppression of inflammatory responses by up-regulating miR-146a in LPS-induced acute lung injury. Connect. Tissue Res. 59 (6), 581–592. https://doi.org/10.1080/03008207.2018.1439480.

Dal Canto, E., Ceriello, A., Rydén, L., Ferrini, M., Hansen, T.B., Schnell, O., Standl, E., Beulens, J.W.J., 2019. Diabetes as a cardiovascular risk factor: an overview of global trends of macro and micro vascular complications. Eur. J. Prev. Cardiol. 26 (2), 25–32. https://doi.org/10.1177/2047487319878371.

Del Turco, S., Basta, G., 2012. An update on advanced glycation endproducts and atherosclerosis. Biofactors 38 (4), 266–274. https://doi.org/10.1002/biof.1018.

Desantis, V., Potenza, M.A., Sgarra, L., Nacci, C., Scaringella, A., Cicco, S., Solimando, A.G., Vacca, A., Montagnani, M., 2023. microRNAs as biomarkers of endothelial dysfunction and therapeutic target in the pathogenesis of atrial fibrillation. Int. J. Mol. Sci. 24 (6), 5307. https://doi.org/10.3390/ijms24065307.

Dong, H., Sun, Y., Nie, L., Cui, A., Zhao, P., Leung, W.K., Wang, Q., 2024. Metabolic memory: mechanisms and diseases. Signal Transduct. Targeted Ther. 9 (1). https://doi.org/10.1038/s41392-024-01755-x.

Egaña-Gorroño, L., López-Díez, R., Yepuri, G., Ramirez, L.S., Reverdatto, S., Gugger, P.F., Shekhtman, A., Ramasamy, R., Schmidt, A.M., 2020. Receptor for advanced glycation end products (Rage) and mechanisms and therapeutic opportunities in diabetes and cardiovascular disease: insights from human subjects and animal models. Front. Cardiovasc. Med. 7. https://doi.org/10.3389/fcvm.2020.00037.

Fakhri, S., Moradi, S.Z., Nouri, Z., Cao, H., Wang, H., Khan, H., Xiao, J., 2024. Modulation of integrin receptor by polyphenols: downstream Nrf2-Keap1/ARE and associated cross-talk mediators in cardiovascular diseases. Crit. Rev. Food Sci. Nutr. 64 (6), 1592–1616. https://doi.org/10.1080/10408398.2022.2118226.

Fui, L.W., Lok, M.P.W., Govindasamy, V., Yong, T.K., Lek, T.K., Das, A.K., 2019. Understanding the multifaceted mechanisms of diabetic wound healing and therapeutic application of stem cells conditioned medium in the healing process. J. Tissue Eng. Regen. Med. 13 (12), 2218–2233. https://doi.org/10.1002/term.2966.

Garg, S.S., Gupta, J., 2022. Polyol pathway and redox balance in diabetes. Pharmacol. Res. 182. https://doi.org/10.1016/j.phrs.2022.106326.

Gill, V., Kumar, V., Singh, K., Kumar, A., Kim, J.J., 2019. Advanced glycation end products (AGEs) may be a striking link between modern diet and health. Biomolecules 9 (12). https://doi.org/10.3390/biom9120888.

Glovaci, D., Fan, W., Wong, N.D., 2019. Epidemiology of diabetes mellitus and cardiovascular disease. Curr. Cardiol. Rep. 21 (4). https://doi.org/10.1007/s11886-019-1107-y.

Gu, X., Sun, J., Li, S., Wu, X., Li, L., 2013. Oxidative stress induces DNA demethylation and histone acetylation in SH-SY5Y cells: potential epigenetic mechanisms in gene transcription in Aβ production. Neurobiol. Aging 34 (4), 1069–1079. https://doi.org/10.1016/j.neurobiolaging.2012.10.013.

Gupta, J., Gaikwad, A.B., Tikoo, K., 2010. Hepatic expression profiling shows involvement of PKC epsilon, DGK eta, Tnfaip, and Rho kinase in type 2 diabetic nephropathy rats. J. Cell. Biochem. 111 (4), 944–954. https://doi.org/10.1002/jcb.22783.

He, L., Wang, Z., Zhou, R., Xiong, W., Yang, Y., Song, N., Qian, J., 2021. Dexmedetomidine exerts cardioprotective effect through miR-146a-3p targeting IRAK1 and TRAF6 via inhibition of the NF-κB pathway. Biomed. Pharmacother. 133, 110993. https://doi.org/10.1016/j.biopha.2020.110993.

Hsieh, C.H., Kuan, W.H., Chang, W.L., Kuo, I.Y., Liu, H., Shieh, D.B., Liu, H., Tan, B., Wang, Y.C., 2022. Dysregulation of SOX17/NRF2 axis confers chemoradiotherapy resistance and emerges as a novel therapeutic target in esophageal squamous cell carcinoma. J. Biomed. Sci. 29 (1).

Ighodaro, O.M., Akinloye, O.A., 2018. First line defence antioxidants-superoxide dismutase (SOD), catalase (CAT) and glutathione peroxidase (GPX): their fundamental role in the entire antioxidant defence grid. Alexandria Journal of Medicine 54 (4), 287–293. https://doi.org/10.1016/j.ajme.2017.09.001.

Jakubik, D., Fitas, A., Eyileten, C., Jarosz-Popek, J., Nowak, A., Czajka, P., Wicik, Z., Sourij, H., Siller-Matula, J.M., Rosa, S.De, Postula, M., 2021. MicroRNAs and long non-coding RNAs in the pathophysiological processes of diabetic cardiomyopathy: emerging biomarkers and potential therapeutics. Cardiovasc. Diabetol. 20 (1). https://doi.org/10.1186/s12933-021-01245-2.

Jia, D., Lu, H., Lv, Y., Xi, L., Tian, Z., 2019. Postinfarction exercise training alleviates cardiac dysfunction and adverse remodeling via mitochondrial biogenesis and SIRT1/PGC-1α/PI3K/Akt signaling. J. Cell. Physiol. 234 (12), 23705–23718. https://doi.org/10.1002/jcp.28939.

Jitraknatee, J., Ruengorn, C., Nochaiwong, S., 2020. Prevalence and risk factors of chronic kidney disease among type 2 diabetes patients: a cross-sectional study in primary care practice. Sci. Rep. 10 (1). https://doi.org/10.1038/s41598-020-63443-4.

Jubaidi, F.F., Zainalabidin, S., Taib, I.S., Abdul Hamid, Z., Mohamad Anuar, N. N., Jalil, J., Mohd Nor, N.A., Budin, S.B., 2022. The role of PKC-MAPK signalling pathways in the development of hyperglycemia-induced cardiovascular complications. Int. J. Mol. Sci. 23 (15). https://doi.org/10.3390/ijms23158582.

Kesava Reddy, G., 2004. AGE-related cross-linking of collagen is associated with aortic wall matrix stiffness in the pathogenesis of drug-induced diabetes in rats. Microvasc. Res. 68 (2), 132–142. https://doi.org/10.1016/j.mvr.2004.04.002.

Kim, S.R., Bae, Y.H., Bae, S.K., Choi, K.S., Yoon, K.H., Koo, T.H., Jang, H.O., Yun, I., Kim, K.W., Kwon, Y.G., Yoo, M.A., Bae, M.K., 2008. Visfatin enhances ICAM-1 and VCAM-1 expression through ROS-dependent NF-κB activation in endothelial cells. Biochim. Biophys. Acta Mol. Cell Res. 1783 (5), 886–895. https://doi.org/10.1016/j.bbamcr.2008.01.004.

Kim, C.S., Park, S., Kim, J., 2017. The role of glycation in the pathogenesis of aging and its prevention through herbal products and physical exercise. J Exerc Nutrition Biochem. 21, 55–61. https://doi.org/10.20463/jenb.2017.0027 ([DOI] [PMC free article] [PubMed] [Google Scholar]).

Klimczak, S., Śliwińska, A., 2024. Epigenetic regulation of inflammation in insulin resistance. Semin. Cell Dev. Biol. 154, 185–192. https://doi.org/10.1016/j.semcdb.2022.09.004.

Kojima, K., Ichijo, H., Naguro, I., 2021. Molecular functions of ASK family in diseases caused by stress-induced inflammation and apoptosis. J. Biochem. 169 (4), 395–407. https://doi.org/10.1093/jb/mvaa145.

Lee, H., Jose, P.A., 2021. Coordinated contribution of NADPH oxidase- and mitochondria-derived reactive oxygen species in metabolic syndrome and its implication in renal dysfunction. Front. Pharmacol. 12. https://doi.org/10.3389/fphar.2021.670076.

Liu, J.H., Li, C., Zhang, C.H., Zhang, Z.H., 2020. LncRNA-CASC7 enhances corticosteroid sensitivity via inhibiting the PI3K/AKT signaling pathway by targeting miR-21 in severe asthma. Pulmonology 26 (1), 18–26. https://doi.org/10.1016/j.pulmoe.2019.07.001.

Liu, L., Xiao, D., Yuan, M., Zhi, L., Qin, Q., Huang, X., Huang, Y., 2025. Nrf2 exerted potential antioxidant and anti-inflammatory activities to inhibit SGIV replication in vitro. Aquaculture 607, 742686.

London, G.M., 2018. Arterial stiffness in chronic kidney disease and end-stage renal disease. Blood Purif. 45 (1–3), 154–158. https://doi.org/10.1159/000485146.

Luevano-Contreras, C., Chapman-Novakofski, K., 2010. Dietary advanced glycation end products and aging. Nutrients 2 (12), 1247–1265. https://doi.org/10.3390/nu2121247.

Majumder, S., Hadden, M.J., Thieme, K., Batchu, S.N., Niveditha, D., Chowdhury, S., Yerra, V.G., Advani, S.L., Bowskill, B.B., Liu, Y., Vakili, H., Alghamdi, T.A., White, K.E., Geldenhuys, L., Siddiqi, F.S., Advani, A., 2019. Dysregulated expression but redundant function of the long non-coding RNA HOTAIR in diabetic kidney disease. Diabetologia 62 (11), 2129–2142. https://doi.org/10.1007/s00125-019-4967-1.

Mikhed, Y., Daiber, A., Steven, S., 2015. Mitochondrial oxidative stress, mitochondrial DNA damage and their role in age-related vascular dysfunction. Int. J. Mol. Sci. 16 (7), 15918–15953. https://doi.org/10.3390/ijms160715918.

Mrugacz, M., Bryl, A., Zorena, K., 2021. Retinal vascular endothelial cell dysfunction and neuroretinal degeneration in diabetic patients. J. Clin. Med. 10 (3), 458. https://doi.org/10.3390/jcm10030458.

Mukai, E., Fujimoto, S., Inagaki, N., 2022. Role of reactive oxygen species in glucose metabolism disorder in diabetic pancreatic β-cells. Biomolecules 12 (9), 1228. https://doi.org/10.3390/biom12091228.

Nowak, A., Przywara-Chowaniec, B., Tyrpień-Golder, K., Nowalany-Kozielska, E., 2020. Systemic lupus erythematosus and glycation process. Cent. Eur. J. Immunol. 45 (1), 93–98. https://doi.org/10.5114/CEJI.2018.77875.

Nowotny, K., Jung, T., Höhn, A., Weber, D., Grune, T., 2015. Advanced glycation end products and oxidative stress in type 2 diabetes mellitus. Biomolecules 5 (1), 194–222. https://doi.org/10.3390/biom5010194.

Obrosova, I.G., 2005. Increased sorbitol pathway activity generates oxidative stress in tissue sites for diabetic complications. Antioxidants Redox Signal. 7 (11–12), 1543–1552. https://doi.org/10.1089/ars.2005.7.1543.

Olivares-Silva, F., Landaeta, R., Aránguiz, P., Bolivar, S., Humeres, C., Anfossi, R., Vivar, R., Boza, P., Muñoz, C., Pardo-Jiménez, V., Peiró, C., Sánchez-Ferrer, C.F., Díaz-Araya, G., 2018. Heparan sulfate potentiates leukocyte adhesion on cardiac fibroblast by enhancing Vcam-1 and Icam-1 expression. Biochim. Biophys. Acta Mol. Basis Dis. 1864 (3), 831–842. https://doi.org/10.1016/j.bbadis.2017.12.002.

Pal, S., Rao, G.N., Pal, A., 2020. High glucose-induced ROS accumulation is a critical regulator of ERK1/2-Akt-tuberin-mTOR signalling in RGC-5 cells. Life Sci. 256. https://doi.org/10.1016/j.lfs.2020.117914.

Peppa, M., Vlassara, H., 2005. Advanced glycation end products and diabetic complications: a General overview. Hormones (Basel) 4 (1), 28–37. https://doi.org/10.14310/horm.2002.11140.

Perrone, A., Giovino, A., Benny, J., Martinelli, F., 2020. Advanced glycation end products (AGEs): biochemistry, signaling, analytical methods, and epigenetic effects. Oxid. Med. Cell. Longev. 2020, 1–18. https://doi.org/10.1155/2020/3818196.

Piacenza, L., Zeida, A., Trujillo, M., Radi, R., 2022. The superoxide radical switch in the biology of nitric oxide and peroxynitrite. Physiol. Rev. 102 (4), 1881–1906. https://doi.org/10.1152/physrev.00005.2022.

Pignatelli, P., Baratta, F., Buzzetti, R., D'Amico, A., Castellani, V., Bartimoccia, S., Siena, A., D'Onofrio, L., Maddaloni, E., Pingitore, A., Chiariello, G.A., Santilli, F., Pastori, D., Cocomello, N., Violi, F., Del Ben, M., Cammisotto, V., Carnevale, R., 2022. The sodium–glucose Co-Transporter-2 (SGLT2) inhibitors reduce platelet activation and thrombus formation by lowering NOX2-related oxidative stress: a pilot study. Antioxidants 11 (10), 1878. https://doi.org/10.3390/antiox11101878.

Popolo, A., Autore, G., Pinto, A., Marzocco, S., 2013. Oxidative stress in patients with cardiovascular disease and chronic renal failure. Free Radic. Res. 47 (5), 346–356. https://doi.org/10.3109/10715762.2013.779373.

Prandi, F.R., Lecis, D., Illuminato, F., Milite, M., Celotto, R., Lerakis, S., Romeo, F., Barillà, F., 2022. Epigenetic modifications and non-coding RNA in diabetes-mellitus-induced coronary artery disease: pathophysiological link and new therapeutic frontiers. Int. J. Mol. Sci. 23 (9), 4589. https://doi.org/10.3390/ijms23094589.

Rabiee, A., Krüger, M., Ardenkjær-Larsen, J., Kahn, C.R., Emanuelli, B., 2018. Distinct signalling properties of insulin receptor substrate (IRS)-1 and IRS-2 in mediating insulin/IGF-1 action. Cell. Signal. 47, 1–15. https://doi.org/10.1016/j.cellsig.2018.03.003.

Ralph, S.J., Moreno-Sánchez, R., Neuzil, J., Rodríguez-Enríquez, S., 2011. Inhibitors of succinate: quinone reductase/Complex II regulate production of mitochondrial reactive oxygen species and protect normal cells from ischemic damage but induce specific cancer cell death. Pharm. Res. 28 (11), 2695–2730. https://doi.org/10.1007/s11095-011-0566-7.

Rathore, R., Zheng, Y.M., Niu, C.F., Liu, Q.H., Korde, A., Ho, Y.S., Wang, Y.X., 2008. Hypoxia activates NADPH oxidase to increase [ROS]i and [Ca2+]i through the mitochondrial ROS-PKCe{open} signaling axis in pulmonary artery smooth muscle cells. Free Radic. Biol. Med. 45 (9), 1223–1231. https://doi.org/10.1016/j.freeradbiomed.2008.06.012.

Roy, R., Wilcox, J., Webb, A.J., O'Gallagher, K., 2023. Dysfunctional and dysregulated nitric oxide synthases in cardiovascular disease: mechanisms and therapeutic potential. Int. J. Mol. Sci. 24 (20), 15200. https://doi.org/10.3390/ijms242015200.

Sanajou, D., Haghjo, A.G., Argani, H., Aslani, S., 2018. AGE-RAGE Axis blockade in diabetic nephropathy: current status and future directions. Eur. J. Pharmacol. 833, 158–164 ([Google Scholar] [CrossRef] [PubMed]).

Sharma, C., Kaur, A., Thind, S.S., Singh, B., Raina, S., 2015. Advanced glycation End-products (AGEs): an emerging concern for processed food industries. J. Food Sci. Technol. 52 (12), 7561–7576. https://doi.org/10.1007/s13197-015-1851-y.

Shen, C.Y., Lu, C.H., Wu, C.H., Li, K.J., Kuo, Y.M., Hsieh, S.C., Yu, C.L., 2020. The development of maillard reaction, and advanced glycation end product (Age)-receptor for age (rage) signaling inhibitors as novel therapeutic strategies for patients with age-related diseases. Molecules 25 (23). https://doi.org/10.3390/molecules25235591.

Silva-Llanes, I., Shin, C.H., Jiménez-Villegas, J., Gorospe, M., Lastres-Becker, I., 2023. The transcription factor NRF2 has epigenetic regulatory functions modulating HDACs, DNMTs, and miRNA biogenesis. Antioxidants 12 (3), 641. https://doi.org/10.3390/antiox12030641.

Sivandzade, F., Prasad, S., Bhalerao, A., Cucullo, L., 2019. NRF2 and NF-κB interplay in cerebrovascular and neurodegenerative disorders: molecular mechanisms and possible therapeutic approaches. Redox Biol. 21, 101059. https://doi.org/10.1016/j.redox.2018.11.017.

Suryavanshi, S.V., Kulkarni, Y.A., 2017. NF-κβ: a potential target in the management of vascular complications of diabetes. Front. Pharmacol. 8. https://doi.org/10.3389/fphar.2017.00798.

Suzuki, H., Kurihara, Y., Takeya, M., Kamada, N., Kataoka, M., Jishage, K., Ueda, O., Sakaguchi, H., Higashi, T., Suzuki, T., Takashima, Y., Kawabe, Y., Cynshi, O., Wada, Y., Honda, M., Kurihara, H., Aburatani, H., Doi, T., Matsumoto, A., Azuma, S., Noda, T., Toyoda, Y., Itakura, H., Yazaki, Y., Horiuchi, S., Takahashi, K., Kruijt, J.K., Van Berkel, T.J.C., Steinbrecher, U.P., Ishibashi, S., Maeda, N., Gordon, S., Kodama, T., 1997. A role for macrophage scavenger receptors in atherosclerosis and susceptibility to infection. Nature 386 (6622), 292–296. https://doi.org/10.1038/386292a0.

Suzuki, M., Tsujikawa, M., Itabe, H., Du, Z.J., Xie, P., Matsumura, N., Fu, X., Zhang, R., Sonoda, K.H., Egashira, K., Hazen, S.L., Kamei, M., 2012. Chronic photo-oxidative stress and subsequent MCP-1 activation as causative factors for age-related macular degeneration. J. Cell Sci. 125 (10), 2407–2415. https://doi.org/10.1242/jcs.097683Japan.

Taheri, Z., Aghdaei, H.A., Irani, S., Modarressi, M.H., Noormohammadi, Z., 2020. Evaluation of the epigenetic demethylation of NRF2, a master transcription factor for antioxidant enzymes, in colorectal cancer. Reports of Biochemistry and Molecular Biology 9 (1), 33–39. https://doi.org/10.29252/rbmb.9.1.33.

Teodoro, J.S., Nunes, S., Rolo, A.P., Reis, F., Palmeira, C.M., 2019. Therapeutic options targeting oxidative stress, mitochondrial dysfunction and inflammation to hinder the progression of vascular complications of diabetes. Front. Physiol. 10. https://doi.org/10.3389/fphys.2018.01857.

Teshima, Y., Takahashi, N., Nishio, S., Saito, S., Kondo, H., Fukui, A., Aoki, K., Yufu, K., Nakagawa, M., Saikawa, T., 2014. Production of reactive oxygen species in the diabetic heart: roles of mitochondria and NADPH oxidase. Circ. J. 78 (2), 300–306. https://doi.org/10.1253/circj.CJ-13-1187Japan.

Thorne, C.A., Grey, A.C., Lim, J.C., Donaldson, P.J., 2024. The synergistic effects of polyol pathway-induced oxidative and osmotic stress in the aetiology of diabetic cataracts. Int. J. Mol. Sci. 25 (16). https://doi.org/10.3390/ijms25169042.

Thorpe, S.R., Baynes, J.W., 2003. Maillard reaction products in tissue proteins: new products and new perspectives. Amino Acids 25 (3–4), 275–281. https://doi.org/10.1007/s00726-003-0017-9.

Tigchelaar, C., van Zuylen, M.L., Hulst, A.H., Preckel, B., van Beek, A.P., Kema, I. P., Hermanides, J., Absalom, A.R., 2022. Elevated cerebrospinal fluid glucose levels and diabetes mellitus are associated with activation of the neurotoxic polyol pathway. Diabetologia 65 (7), 1098–1107. https://doi.org/10.1007/s00125-022-05693-7.

Troise, D., Mercuri, S., Infante, B., Losappio, V., Cirolla, L., Netti, G.S., Ranieri, E., Stallone, G., 2024. mTOR and SGLT-2 inhibitors: their synergistic effect on age-related processes. Int. J. Mol. Sci. 25 (16). https://doi.org/10.3390/ijms25168676.

Vlassara, H., Uribarri, J., Cai, W., Striker, G., 2008. Advanced glycation end product homeostasis: exogenous oxidants and innate defenses. Ann. N. Y. Acad. Sci. 1126, 46–52. https://doi.org/10.1196/annals.1433.055.

Vlassara, H., Striker, G.E., 2013. Advanced glycation endproducts in diabetes and diabetic complications. Endocrinol Metab. Clin. N. Am. 42, 697–719. https://doi.org/10.1016/j.ecl.2013.07.005 ([DOI] [PubMed] [Google Scholar]).

Wang, S., Liao, J., Huang, J., Yin, H., Yang, W., Hu, M., 2018a. miR-214 and miR-126 were associated with restoration of endothelial function in obesity after exercise and dietary intervention. J. Appl. Biomed. 16 (1), 34–39. https://doi.org/10.1016/j.jab.2017.10.003.

Wang, X., Li, H., Chen, S., He, J., Chen, W., Ding, Y., Huang, J., 2021. P300/CBP-associated factor (PCAF) attenuated M1 macrophage inflammatory responses possibly through KLF2 and KLF4. Immunol. Cell Biol. 99 (7), 724–736. https://doi.org/10.1111/imcb.12455.

Wang, Z., Zhao, H., Guan, W., Kang, X., Tai, X., Shen, Y., 2018b. Metabolic memory in mitochondrial oxidative damage triggers diabetic retinopathy. BMC Ophthalmol. 18, 1–7.

Xie, J., Méndez, J.D., Méndez-Valenzuela, V., Aguilar-Hernández, M.M., 2013. Cellular signalling of the receptor for advanced glycation end products (RAGE). Cell. Signal. 25 (11), 2185–2197. https://doi.org/10.1016/j.cellsig.2013.06.013.

Xie, Y., van der Fels-Klerx, H.J., van Leeuwen, S.P.J., 2023. Vincenzo Fogliano, Occurrence of dietary advanced glycation end-products in commercial cow, goat and soy protein based infant formulas. Food Chem. 411, 135424. https://doi.org/10.1016/j.foodchem.2023.135424.

Xu, G., Liu, G., Xiong, S., Liu, H., Chen, X., Zheng, B., 2015. The histone methyltransferase Smyd2 is a negative regulator of macrophage activation by suppressing interleukin 6 (IL-6) and tumor necrosis factor α (TNF-α) production. J. Biol. Chem. 290 (9), 5414–5423. https://doi.org/10.1074/jbc.m114.610345.

Yamagishi, S.-ichi, Fukami, K., Matsui, T., 2015. Crosstalk between advanced glycation end products (AGEs)-receptor RAGE axis and dipeptidyl peptidase-4-incretin system in diabetic vascular complications. Cardiovasc. Diabetol. 14 (1), 2. https://doi.org/10.1186/s12933-015-0176-5.

Yamagishi, S.-ichi, Matsui, T., 2018. Role of ligands of receptor for advanced glycation end products (RAGE) in peripheral artery disease. Rejuvenation Res. 21 (5), 456–463. https://doi.org/10.1089/rej.2017.2025.

Yan, L.j., 2018. Redox imbalance stress in diabetes mellitus: role of the polyol pathway. Animal Model. Exp. Med. 1 (1), 7–13. https://doi.org/10.1002/ame2.12001.

Yi, X., Zhu, Q.X., Wu, X.L., Tan, T.T., Jiang, X.J., 2022. Histone methylation and oxidative stress in cardiovascular diseases. Oxid. Med. Cell. Longev. 2022. https://doi.org/10.1155/2022/6023710.

Yuan, W., He, X., Morin, D., Barrière, G., Liu, X., Li, J., Zhu, Y., 2021. Autophagy induction contributes to the neuroprotective impact of intermittent fasting on the acutely injured spinal cord. J. Neurotrauma 38 (3), 373–384. https://doi.org/10.1089/neu.2020.7166.

Zhang, J., Zhang, L., Zhang, S., Yu, Q., Xiong, F., Huang, K., Wang, C.Y., Yang, P., 2017. HMGB1, an innate alarmin, plays a critical role in chronic inflammation of adipose tissue in obesity. Mol. Cell. Endocrinol. 454, 103–111. https://doi.org/10.1016/j.mce.2017.06.012.

Zhang, J.F., Bai, K.W., Su, W.P., Wang, A.A., Zhang, L.L., Huang, K.H., Wang, T., 2018. Curcumin attenuates heat-stress-induced oxidant damage by simultaneous activation of GSH-related antioxidant enzymes and Nrf2-mediated phase II detoxifying enzyme systems in broiler chickens. Poult. Sci. 97 (4), 1209–1219. https://doi.org/10.3382/ps/pex408.

Zhang, S.Y., Zhang, L.Y., Wen, R., Yang, N., Zhang, T.N., 2024. Histone deacetylases and their inhibitors in inflammatory diseases. Biomed. Pharmacother. 179. https://doi.org/10.1016/j.biopha.2024.117295.

Zhao, F., Zhang, J., Chang, N., 2018. Epigenetic modification of Nrf2 by sulforaphane increases the antioxidative and anti-inflammatory capacity in a cellular model of Alzheimer's disease. Eur. J. Pharmacol. 824, 1–10. https://doi.org/10.1016/j.ejphar.2018.01.046.

Zuliani, I., Urbinati, C., Valenti, D., Quattrini, M.C., Medici, V., Cosentino, L., Pietraforte, D., Di Domenico, F., Perluigi, M., Vacca, R.A., De Filippis, B., 2020. The anti-diabetic drug metformin rescues aberrant mitochondrial activity and restrains oxidative stress in a female mouse model of rett syndrome. J. Clin. Med. 9 (6), 1669. https://doi.org/10.3390/jcm9061669.

3

DNA methylation mechanisms and their contribution to metabolic pathophysiology

1. Introduction

Epigenetics has emerged as one of the most transformative concepts in modern biology, reshaping our understanding of how cells establish, maintain, and modify patterns of gene expression without altering the underlying DNA sequence. Among all epigenetic mechanisms, DNA methylation stands out as one of the most extensively studied and biologically influential. It fundamentally affects chromatin architecture, gene regulation, cellular identity, and long term physiological adaptation. DNA methylation provides a means for cells to interpret and respond to environmental cues, translating nutritional, hormonal, and metabolic signals into persistent molecular memory (Moore et al., 2013). This capacity makes DNA methylation a critical factor not only in development and differentiation but also in metabolic diseases such as type 2 diabetes, obesity, non alcoholic fatty liver disease (NAFLD), and gestational diabetes mellitus (GDM) (Barres and Zierath, 2011). Understanding the principles, patterns, and consequences of DNA methylation is therefore essential for unraveling the complex interactions between genetics, environment, and disease.

At the core of DNA methylation lies a simple yet powerful chemical modification: the addition of a methyl group (-CH_3) to the fifth carbon of the cytosine ring, forming 5-methylcytosine (5mC). This reaction occurs primarily at cytosine guanine (CpG) dinucleotides and is catalyzed by a highly conserved family of DNA methyltransferases (DNMTs). Despite its chemical simplicity, this modification profoundly influences

Metabolic Memory. https://doi.org/10.1016/B978-0-443-44591-0.00011-4

the epigenetic landscape by shaping chromatin accessibility, transcription factor binding, and higherorder genome organization (Klemm et al., 2019). CpG sites are relatively rare in the genome; however, clusters of CpGs, known as CpG islands, are enriched in gene promoters and are typically unmethylated in transcriptionally active regions. The strategic positioning of methylation within promoters, enhancers, gene bodies, and repetitive elements underscores its versatility as a regulatory mechanism (Vavouri and Lehner, 2012). Moreover, the availability of the methyl donor S adenosylmethionine (SAM) directly links DNA methylation to one carbon metabolism, diet, and cellular metabolic state, illustrating the intimate interplay between epigenetics and physiology (Yu et al., 2019).

Although DNA methylation is frequently characterized as a stable and heritable mark, advances in molecular biology have revealed that methylation patterns are far more dynamic than once believed. During early embryogenesis, the mammalian genome undergoes waves of demethylation and de novo methylation, establishing lineage-specific patterns that guide organ development and long-term metabolic programming. Specialized enzymes such as DNMT3A and DNMT3B create new methylation signatures, while DNMT1 faithfully maintains these patterns during cell division (Tajima et al., 2022). The discovery of ten-eleven translocation (TET) enzymes in the late 2000s revolutionized the field by demonstrating that methylation marks can also be actively removed through oxidation processes that generate 5-hydroxymethylcytosine (5hmC) and other intermediates (Ismail et al., 2020). These insights have reframed DNA methylation as part of a dynamic, reversible system capable of responding to internal physiological changes and external environmental exposures.

The history of DNA methylation research spans more than a century, evolving from obscure biochemical observations into a central pillar of modern epigenetics. The discovery of 5mC in 1925 initially held little biological meaning, but gradual technological progress, including restriction enzyme mapping, bisulphite conversion, and high-throughput sequencing, transformed the landscape of epigenetic research. By the early 1990s, the identification and cloning of DNMTs, unravelling of imprinting mechanisms, and insights into X-chromosome inactivation established DNA methylation as a heritable regulatory system integral to developmental biology (Mattei et al., 2022). The 2000s brought about genome-wide methylation maps, revealing the complexity of methylation patterns across tissues, developmental stages, and disease states. These milestones shifted the perception of DNA methylation from a gene-silencing mark to a multifaceted regulatory mechanism intricately linked with chromatin remodelling, transcription factor networks, and metabolic signaling pathways (Mattei et al., 2022).

Over the past 2 decades, the relevance of DNA methylation to metabolic health and disease has emerged with unprecedented clarity. Environmental and lifestyle factors like nutrition, physical activity, stress, pollutants, and early-life exposures, exert profound epigenetic effects on metabolic tissues such as liver, skeletal muscle, adipose tissue, and pancreatic β-cells (Kadayifci et al., 2019). These epigenetic changes can activate or silence genes involved in insulin secretion, glucose uptake, lipid metabolism, oxidative stress responses, and inflammation. Aberrant methylation of key metabolic regulators, including PPARγ, PDX1, GLUT4, IRS1, and PGC-1α, has been identified as a hallmark of metabolic dysfunction (Wu et al., 2023). Notably, persistent methylation signatures contribute to the phenomenon of metabolic memory, wherein prior episodes of hyperglycemia or unhealthy diet leave enduring epigenetic "scars" that sustain disease processes even after biochemical normalization (Chen et al., 2016). This phenomenon highlights the long-lasting impact of epigenetic perturbations and underscores the importance of early interventions in metabolic disease prevention.

The developmental origins of health and disease (DOHaD) hypothesis further emphasize the role of DNA methylation in shaping lifelong metabolic trajectories. During critical windows of fetal development, epigenetic plasticity is at its peak. Maternal diet, body weight, stress levels, and glucose control can alter methylation marks in the fetus, influencing organ development, hormone sensitivity, appetite regulation, and metabolic set points (Hagemann et al., 2021). Differential methylation of genes such as IGF2, HNF4A, LEP, and ADIPOQ can predispose offspring to obesity, insulin resistance, and diabetes, revealing a transgenerational epigenetic dimension to metabolic disease risk (Houshmand-Oeregaard et al., 2017; Ghosh et al., 2023).

Technological advancements have also propelled DNA methylation into the realm of diagnostics and precision medicine. Blood-based methylation markers measured in circulating cell-free DNA offer minimally invasive tools for early detection of metabolic disorders, assessment of disease progression, and prediction of therapeutic outcomes (de Vos et al., 2017). Tissue-specific methylation signatures, in β-cells, adipocytes, and hepatic cells, provide high-resolution insights into metabolic dysfunction and potential therapeutic targets (Sala et al., 2017). The emergence of multi-omics approaches integrating methylomics with transcriptomics, proteomics, and metabolomics has deepened our understanding of the complex interplay between epigenetic modifications and metabolic pathways (Sanches et al., 2024). These integrative frameworks set the stage for personalized epigenetic therapies capable of reversing maladaptive methylation signatures.

As research continues to expand, DNA methylation stands at the forefront of epigenetic investigation, offering critical insights into how the environment shapes metabolic health across the lifespan. This chapter explores the fundamental principles, enzymatic machinery, genomic distribution, regulatory mechanisms, and functional implications of DNA methylation, with particular emphasis on its role in metabolism and metabolic disease. By bridging molecular detail with physiological relevance, it aims to provide a comprehensive understanding of how DNA methylation governs metabolic homeostasis and how its dysregulation contributes to disease, a foundation essential for the development of targeted epigenetic diagnostics and therapeutics.

2. Fundamentals of DNA methylation

2.1 Definition

DNA methylation is a covalent epigenetic modification in which a methyl group (-CH_3) is enzymatically transferred from S-adenosylmethionine (SAM) to the carbon-5 position of cytosine residues, leading to the formation of 5-methylcytosine (5mC). This reaction occurs predominantly in CpG dinucleotides, where a cytosine is immediately followed by a guanine. Although CpG sites are under-represented in the mammalian genome, they cluster into CpG-rich regions known as CpG islands (CGIs), which are frequently found in gene promoter regions and are typically unmethylated in actively transcribed genes (Long et al., 2016). The methyl donor SAM is produced from the interconnected folate and methionine cycles, making DNA methylation highly sensitive to nutritional status, one-carbon metabolism, and cellular metabolic state (Abbasi et al., 2018). Importantly, 5mC is a stable and heritable epigenetic mark that persists during cell division due to faithful copying of methylation patterns, thus forming a molecular basis for cellular memory (Zheng et al., 2024). In addition to classical CpG methylation, non-CpG methylation (CpH, where H = A, T, or C) is observed in embryonic stem cells, neurons, and metabolically stressed tissues, indicating functional specialization beyond canonical methylation patterns (Lee et al., 2017). Functionally, DNA methylation contributes to long-term gene silencing, preservation of genomic stability, suppression of transposable elements, establishment of tissue-specific gene expression programs, and the integration of environmental, nutritional, and metabolic cues into the genome.

2.1.1 Historical perspective

The understanding of DNA methylation and its implications in human disease has evolved over more than a century, beginning with early biochemical investigations that unintentionally laid the groundwork for modern epigenetics. Although 5-methylcytosine (5mC) was first detected in *Mycobacterium tuberculosis* DNA in 1925, its biological significance remained unknown for decades due to limited analytical tools (Johnson and Coghill, 1925). After DNA was firmly established as the genetic material in the 1940s and its double-helical structure was elucidated in 1953, attention gradually turned toward exploring chemical modifications embedded within the genome (Watson and Crick, 1953). In the 1960s, pivotal studies in bacteria revealed that methylation played a protective role by distinguishing self-DNA from invading phage DNA, thereby guiding restriction enzymes. This discovery not only demonstrated that methylation was enzymatically regulated but also suggested its involvement in essential cellular processes such as DNA replication and repair (Billen, 1968; Sager and Kitchin, 1975). Through the 1970s, advancements in chromatography and sequencing enabled widespread mapping of methylation patterns across tissues and species. Researchers noticed that methylation did not occur randomly but was enriched in CpG dinucleotides and varied predictably with gene activity, development, and tissue specificity (Riggs, 2004). The development of methylation-sensitive restriction enzymes, particularly the HpaII/MspI system, allowed targeted analysis of CpG-rich regions, later termed CpG islands, which became central to understanding transcriptional regulation (Singer et al., 1979).

The 1970s also introduced 5-azacytidine, a nucleoside analog that inhibits DNA methyltransferases (DNMTs), leading to passive demethylation. Its ability to reactivate silenced genes, including developmental regulators and tumor suppressors, provided the first experimental evidence that methylation could directly silence transcription (Friedman, 1979). During the 1980s, locus-specific studies established that hypermethylation of promoter CpG islands often suppressed gene expression, confirming DNA methylation as a stable epigenetic mark controlling transcription (Kruczek and Doerfler, 1983). Yet exceptions, such as methylation in gene bodies and repetitive regions, highlighted its context-dependent effects, including roles in splicing, genome stability, and prevention of transposable element activation (Niwa et al., 1983). The decade also saw major conceptual breakthroughs, including understanding dynamic methylation changes during embryogenesis, imprinting, and X-chromosome inactivation (Galupa and Heard, 2018; Andergassen et al., 2021). The cloning of the first mammalian DNA methyltransferase, Dnmt1, further clarified that maintenance and de novo methylation were carried out by specialized enzymes, each essential for epigenetic fidelity (Lauster et al., 1989).

The decade from 1990 to 1999 marked a transformative period in understanding eukaryotic DNA methylation, defined by the discovery, cloning, and functional characterization of mammalian and plant DNA methyltransferases (Dnmts), alongside major advances in imprinting, X-chromosome inactivation, and the molecular mechanisms safeguarding or altering cytosine methylation. During this period, foundational work on genomic imprinting revealed that parent-of-origin–specific methylation patterns are established by DNMT3A and DNMT3L in oocytes and sperm, with key imprinted loci such as Igf2, H19, Snrpn, and Peg1 mapped in mouse and human (Okano et al., 1999). Although early speculation suggested methylation could drive X-inactivation, subsequent studies clarified that DNA methylation contributes to the maintenance, but not initiation, of X-chromosome silencing (Jones et al., 1982; Lee and Bartolomei, 2013). Parallel observations by the Bird lab showed that CpG islands (CGIs) remained unmethylated in vivo but were prone to aberrant methylation in cell culture, suggesting the existence of active protection mechanisms (Bird, 1986). In 1992, groundbreaking knockout studies of Dnmt1 demonstrated that global DNA methylation is essential for embryonic development, as Dnmt1-deficient embryonic stem cells survived only in the undifferentiated state, while knockout embryos exhibited severe developmental failure (Li et al., 1992). Attempts to rescue Dnmt1-null cells revealed that imprinting methylation could not be restored without germline passage, establishing the unique inheritance logic of imprinted marks. Structural biology also progressed substantially, with the 1993 determination of the first crystal structure of a DNA methyltransferase (M.HhaI), revealing base flipping and confirming a covalent catalytic intermediate in cytosine methylation (Cheng et al., 1993).

These findings prompted searches for additional eukaryotic methyltransferases, leading to the independent identification of Dnmt2, Dnmt3a, and Dnmt3b, with the latter two shown to perform true de novo methylation and to be essential, partially redundant enzymes during embryogenesis. The discovery of methyl-CpG binding proteins (MBDs) such as MeCP1 and MeCP2 established that transcriptional repression by DNA methylation is largely indirect and mediated through methyl-binding proteins that recruit histone deacetylase complexes, highlighting one of the earliest mechanistic links between DNA methylation and chromatin modifications (Ng et al., 1999). In plants, *Arabidopsis thaliana* emerged as a powerful genetic model for epigenetic research, leading to the cloning of MET1 (the plant DNMT1 homolog) and the discovery of DDM1, a SWI2/SNF2 chromatin remodeler essential for repeat methylation (Vongs et al., 1993). Plant studies showed that both CpG and non-CpG (CpXpG) methylation persist across generations without complete resetting, unlike in mammals (Jackson et al., 2002). By the late 1990s, Arabidopsis researchers uncovered three major classes of plant methyltransferases, MET1, CMTs, and DRMs, with the latter possessing rearranged catalytic motifs, representing a unique plant-specific innovation (Genger et al., 1999; Cao et al., 2000). Despite tremendous progress, the decade ended with ongoing debates about the primary biological function of methylation, particularly whether it mainly represses retrotransposons or broadly regulates gene expression, alongside the unresolved question of how active DNA demethylation occurs (Bird, 1997).

The 2000–09 era brought a revolution in epigenomics, driven by genome sequencing, bisulfite sequencing, and the first generation of genome-wide DNA methylation maps (Frommer et al., 1992). With the release of Arabidopsis, mouse, and human genome assemblies, researchers could extend insights from single genes to genome-scale patterns (Pennacchio, 2003). The first methylomes, produced via antibody- and enzyme-enriched microarrays, revealed that plant gene bodies were methylated while promoter regions remained largely unmethylated, and that transposons displayed dense cytosine methylation (Tran et al., 2005). Human methylation maps confirmed that promoter CpG islands are mostly unmethylated in normal cells yet aberrantly hypermethylated in certain cancers, while large genomic domains, including the inactive X, were hypomethylated (Antequera et al., 1990). The development of reduced representation bisulfite sequencing (RRBS) and whole-genome bisulfite sequencing (WGBS) enabled single-base resolution methylation landscapes in mammals, showing dynamic methylation at enhancers, focal changes during differentiation, and extensive hypomethylation in immortalized cells forming partially methylated domains (PMDs) (Meissner et al., 2008; Ziller et al., 2013).

Mechanistic advances paralleled these mapping efforts. Work in Neurospora and Arabidopsis demonstrated that histone H3K9 methylation guides DNA methylation, providing evidence that Dnmts interface directly with chromatin states (Tamaru and

Selker, 2001). Structural studies revealed that DNMT3L, although catalytically inactive, regulates imprint establishment through interactions inhibited by H3K4 methylation, thereby explaining how H3K4me protects CpG islands from de novo methylation. The discovery of the DNMT1 cofactor UHRF1, which binds hemimethylated DNA and is required for DNMT1 recruitment, clarified how maintenance methylation is executed during replication (Bostick et al., 2007). Studies of the H19/Igf2 imprinting control region (ICR) demonstrated that methylation-sensitive CTCF binding controls long-range enhancer–promoter interactions, underscoring that methylation outside promoters can regulate higher-order chromatin looping (Hark et al., 2000). Computational studies categorized human promoters into high-CpG and low-CpG classes, revealing that most high-CpG promoters remain unmethylated regardless of transcriptional state and are protected by H3K4 methylation, further shifting focus away from promoter methylation as a universal regulatory mechanism (Saxonov et al., 2006).

The decade concluded with the landmark discovery of TET enzymes (TET1/2/3), which convert 5-methylcytosine to 5-hydroxymethylcytosine (5hmC), finally providing a biochemical basis for active DNA demethylation after decades of controversy (Tahiliani et al., 2009). This discovery, along with the recognition that 5hmC is abundant in neurons, opened a new dimension in epigenetics involving iterative oxidation and base excision repair (Kriaucionis and Heintz, 2009). Together, the combined structural, genetic, and genome-wide studies of the 1990 and 2000s transformed DNA methylation from a promoter-centric, static mark into a dynamic, context-dependent, chromatin-integrated epigenetic system central to development, genome defense, and long-range gene regulation.

As research advanced into the late 20th and early 21st centuries, DNA methylation emerged as a critical factor linking environmental exposures with long-term metabolic health (Li et al., 2003). Studies revealed that nutrient availability, hormonal signals, early-life stress, and toxic environmental factors could alter methylation patterns in key metabolic tissues such as liver, muscle, adipose tissue, and pancreatic β-cells (Yang et al., 2012). Such changes influence genes controlling insulin secretion, glucose uptake, mitochondrial function, lipid metabolism, inflammation, and oxidative stress (Kuroda et al., 2009; Hall et al., 2018). Persistent methylation "scars" in metabolic pathways provide a molecular basis for metabolic memory (Chen et al., 2016). Aberrant methylation of key genes such as *PPARγ*, *IRS1*, *GLUT4*, *FTO*, and *IGF2* has been implicated in obesity, insulin resistance, type 2 diabetes, dyslipidemia, and non-alcoholic fatty liver disease (Gao et al., 2022). Moreover, high-throughput technologies like bisulfite sequencing and epigenome-wide association studies (EWAS) have revealed distinct methylation signatures predictive of metabolic disease risk, progression, and therapeutic response (Chen et al., 2020).

2.2 Key enzymes involved in DNA methylation and demethylation

2.2.1 DNMT1-maintenance methyltransferase

DNMT1 is principally responsible for maintaining DNA methylation patterns during DNA replication. It recognizes hemi-methylated DNA, where the parental strand is methylated but the newly synthesized daughter strand is not, and restores symmetrical methylation to preserve epigenetic fidelity throughout cell division (He et al., 2019). This makes DNMT1 essential for sustaining stable, lineage-specific gene expression programs, including metabolic pathways in hepatocytes, adipocytes, β-cells, and muscle cells (Liu et al., 2016). Alterations in DNMT1 expression or activity can disrupt the stability of gene networks involved in glucose metabolism and inflammation. In metabolic disorders, DNMT1 often becomes hyperactive, contributing to the "metabolic memory" phenomenon seen in chronic hyperglycemia, where cells retain pathological transcriptional patterns even after glycemic control is restored (Kameswaran et al., 2018). Overexpression of DNMT1 also promotes the methylation-mediated silencing of anti inflammatory and antioxidant genes, exacerbating oxidative stress and chronic inflammation in diabetes (Cai et al., 2020).

2.2.2 DNMT3A and DNMT3B—De novo methyltransferases

DNMT3A and DNMT3B are responsible for establishing new methylation patterns during early development and in response to environmental changes. DNMT3A, in particular, plays central roles in adipocyte differentiation, hepatic metabolic regulation, and pancreatic β-cell development (Guo et al., 2016; Kim et al., 2020). Proper activity of DNMT3A and DNMT3B ensures the correct methylation of enhancers, promoters, and CpG islands that regulate metabolic genes involved in lipid storage, insulin secretion, mitochondrial biogenesis, and oxidative phosphorylation (Barrès et al., 2009). Mutations or dysregulation of these enzymes lead to aberrant de novo methylation, which disrupts lipid metabolism, impairs mitochondrial function, and contributes to insulin resistance (Li et al., 2022). DNMT3B mutations are also associated with genome-wide methylation imbalances, resulting in impaired metabolic tissue remodeling and greater susceptibility to metabolic syndrome (Park et al., 2021).

2.2.3 DNMT3L—Regulatory cofactor

DNMT3L is a catalytically inactive protein that interacts with DNMT3A and DNMT3B to enhance their enzymatic activity and stabilize their association with DNA (Pacaud et al., 2014). Although it lacks intrinsic methyltransferase activity, DNMT3L plays a critical role in controlling DNA methylation in the germline, particularly in the establishment of imprinting marks that influence embryonic development and metabolic programming (Heo et al., 2017). By shaping the epigenetic landscape of gametes, DNMT3L indirectly contributes to intergenerational metabolic risk transmission (Stenz et al., 2018). Impairments in DNMT3L function can lead to incomplete imprinting, abnormal methylation patterns, and transgenerational inheritance of metabolic phenotypes, such as altered glucose tolerance and increased susceptibility to obesity (Bozdemir et al., 2025).

2.2.4 TET enzymes (TET1, TET2, TET3)—Active demethylation

The TET family of dioxygenase enzymes catalyzes active DNA demethylation through a series of oxidative reactions that convert 5mC into 5-hydroxymethylcytosine (5hmC), 5-formylcytosine (5fC), and 5-carboxylcytosine (5caC) (Wu and Zhang, 2017). These oxidized intermediates are subsequently replaced with unmethylated cytosines by the base excision repair machinery. Beyond merely erasing methylation, TET enzymes also modulate chromatin structure by generating 5hmC, which acts as a stable epigenetic mark associated with active transcription (Salmeron-Barcenas et al., 2023). TET2 plays a vital role in regulating adipogenesis, mitochondrial function, and systemic insulin sensitivity, whereas TET3 is crucial for maintaining β-cell identity and appropriate insulin secretion in response to glucose (Liu et al., 2023; Cai et al., 2025). Loss or dysfunction of TET enzymes disrupts methylation–demethylation balance, leading to chronic inflammation, impaired oxidative metabolism, and the development of insulin resistance and dyslipidemia (Fig. 3.1).

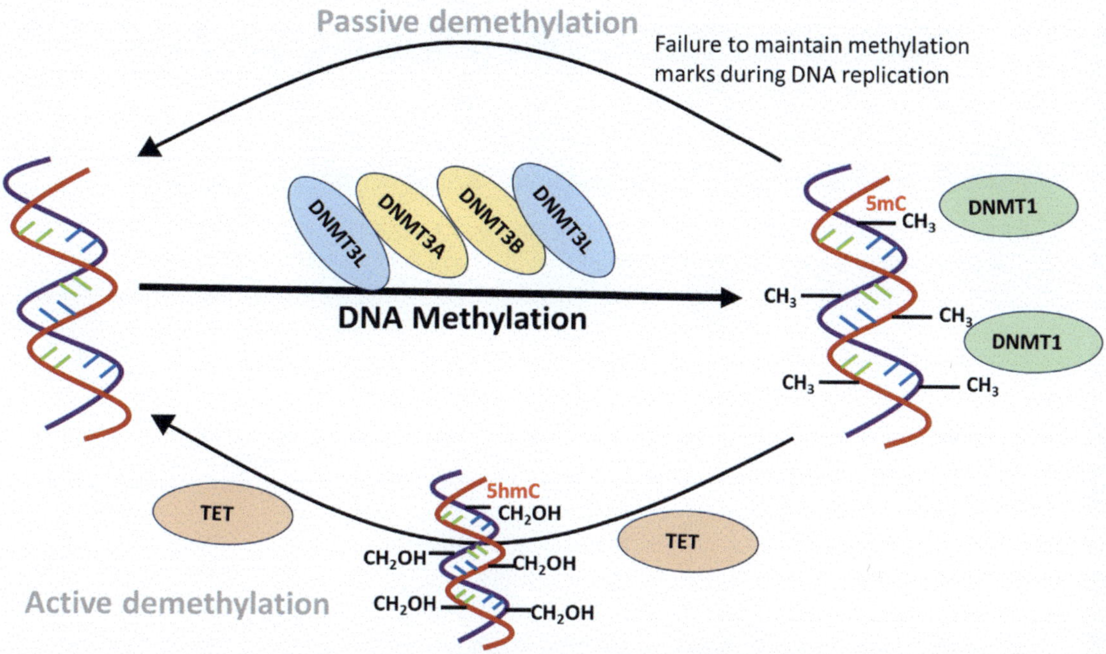

Figure 3.1 Mechanisms of DNA methylation, maintenance, and active versus Passive demethylation the figure shows how DNA methylation is added, maintained, or removed in cells. DNMT3A/3B (with DNMT3L) establish new methylation, while DNMT1 maintains these marks during replication; if DNMT1 fails, methylation is gradually lost through passive demethylation. In contrast, TET enzymes actively remove methylation by converting 5-methylcytosine into oxidized forms that are replaced with unmethylated cytosine.

2.3 Genomic distribution of DNA methylation

2.3.1 Promoters and CpG islands

Promoter regions and CpG islands are typically unmethylated in actively transcribed genes, allowing transcription factors and the transcriptional machinery to bind effectively. However, methylation of CpG islands leads to robust and often irreversible gene silencing. In metabolic diseases, aberrant promoter methylation alters the expression of genes essential for glucose homeostasis, lipid metabolism, and inflammation. For example, hypermethylation of the PDX1 promoter reduces β-cell insulin production in diabetes (Li et al., 2021), while methylation of PPARγ disrupts adipocyte differentiation and contributes to obesity (Table 3.1). In an ex vivo model, mesenchymal stem cells from subcutaneous and visceral adipose tissues were exposed to palmitic acid to induce Insulin resistance. Analysis revealed increased global DNA methylation in IR adipocytes after 72 h, along with hypermethylation of key insulin-regulating genes

Table 3.1 Genomic distribution of DNA methylation in metabolic disorders.

Genomic region	Key role	Impact in metabolic disorders	References
Promoters & CpG islands	Control gene initiation; usually unmethylated in active genes.	Hypermethylation silences metabolic genes (PDX1, PPARG, GLUT4), contributing to insulin resistance and inflammation.	Li et al. (2021), Małodobra-Mazur et al. (2021), Karin and Shalapour (2022)
Enhancers	Regulate tissue-specific gene expression and promoter–enhancer interactions.	Methylation changes alter lipid metabolism, adipogenesis (TET3–C/EBPδ), and hepatic glycolysis in obesity.	Howard et al. (2014), Park et al. (2022), Kirchner et al. (2016)
Gene bodies	Support active transcription and regulate alternative splicing.	Altered methylation affects OXPHOS, insulin signaling; T2D shows TSS hypomethylation and gene-body hypermethylation.	Shayevitch et al. (2018), Dayeh et al. (2014), Ejarque et al. (2019)
Repetitive elements	Maintain genomic stability by silencing transposons.	Hypomethylation activates LINE/SINE elements, causing inflammation, DNA damage, and metabolic complications.	Kanholm et al. (2023), Sae-Lee et al. (2020)

CpG, cytosine–phosphate–guanine dinucleotide; *PDX1*, pancreatic and duodenal homeobox 1; *PPARG/PPARγ*, peroxisome proliferator-activated receptor gamma; *SLC2A4/GLUT4*, solute carrier family 2 member 4/glucose transporter type 4; *ADIPOQ*, adiponectin gene; *TET3*, ten-eleven translocation methylcytosine dioxygenase 3; *C/EBPδ*, CCAAT/enhancer-binding protein delta; *PUFA*, polyunsaturated fatty acids; *T2D*, type 2 diabetes; *TSS*, transcription start site; *LINEs*, long interspersed nuclear elements; *SINEs*, short interspersed nuclear elements; *LTRs*, long terminal repeats.

such as PPARG, SLC2A4 (GLUT4), and ADIPOQ. PPARG showed the earliest and most prominent site-specific methylation changes. These epigenetic modifications appear to be driven mainly by DNMT1 activity. DNA methylation is thus a critical contributor to IR pathogenesis, with early PPARG methylation emerging as a central event in newly developing insulin resistance (Małodobra-Mazur et al., 2021). Similarly, tumor suppressors and anti inflammatory genes are frequently silenced via promoter methylation, promoting metabolic dysfunction and chronic inflammation (Karin and Shalapour, 2022).

2.3.2 Enhancers

Enhancers are distal regulatory elements that shape tissue-specific transcriptional programs by facilitating long-range interactions with promoters. DNA methylation at enhancer regions modulates transcription factor accessibility, chromatin loop formation, and allele-specific expression, such as in imprinted genes. Enhancers relevant to metabolic tissues, such as those regulating lipid storage, mitochondrial activity, or inflammatory responses, undergo dynamic methylation changes in response to diet, hormones, and metabolic stress. For example, a genome-wide DNA methylation study in 144 human liver samples showed that the fatty acid desaturase (FADS) gene variant rs174537 correlates with altered methylation of CpG sites within an enhancer region of the FADS cluster, and these methylation differences are linked to changes in polyunsaturated fatty acid levels (Howard et al., 2014). Altered enhancer methylation disrupts adipocyte remodeling, impairs hepatic glucose production control, and exacerbates inflammation in obesity and metabolic syndrome. Whole-genome bisulfite sequencing shows that during adipogenesis, DNA methylation decreases specifically at adipocyte-related loci containing **C/EBP binding motifs**, aligning with increased activity of adipogenic promoters and enhancers. Mechanistically, C/EBPδ recruits **TET3** to these motifs, driving targeted DNA demethylation and activating key adipogenic genes. Overexpression of TET3 enhances adipocyte differentiation both in vitro and in vivo and restores reduced adipogenic capacity in aging mice and humans. Overall, the findings reveal that precise reprogramming of DNA methylation through C/EBPδ–TET3 cooperation is a central mechanism controlling adipocyte differentiation (Park et al., 2022). Severely obese and diabetic individuals show hypomethylation of hepatic glycolytic and insulin-regulating genes enhancers, leading to their overexpression. Obesity-driven epigenetic shifts at ATF-motif CpGs reprogram the liver toward enhanced glycolysis and lipogenesis, promoting insulin resistance (Kirchner et al., 2016).

2.3.3 Gene bodies

Gene-body methylation, in contrast to promoter methylation, is often associated with active transcription. It helps maintain transcriptional fidelity by preventing inappropriate initiation within gene bodies and by influencing alternative splicing. Site-specific editing of DNA methylation using dCas9-methylation enzymes showed that altering methylation on alternatively spliced exons, but not constitutive exons or introns, directly changes exon inclusion (Shayevitch et al., 2018). In metabolic tissues like skeletal muscle and liver, gene-body methylation regulates genes involved in oxidative phosphorylation, fatty acid β-oxidation, mitochondrial dynamics, and insulin signaling. In pancreatic islet cells genomic regions near the transcription start site of TSS1500, TSS200 were found hypomethylated, while distal regions (gene body, 3′UTR, intergenic areas) showed higher methylation in type 2 diabetic individuals (Dayeh et al., 2014). Changes in gene-body methylation contribute to mitochondrial dysfunction, reduced energy expenditure, and impaired glucose utilization, key pathological features of metabolic disord (Kanholm et al., 2023; Ejarque et al., 2019).

2.3.4 Repetitive elements and transposable elements

Repetitive genomic elements, including LINEs, SINEs, LTRs, and satellite DNA, are normally heavily methylated to prevent their transcription and mobility. This methylation preserves genomic stability by suppressing transposon activation. However, metabolic stress conditions such as chronic hyperglycemia, oxidative stress, and inflammation frequently lead to global hypomethylation (Kanholm et al., 2023). Hypomethylated transposable elements can become transcriptionally active, generating DNA damage, inflammatory signals, and chromatin instability. A study found 714 locus-specific methylation changes in LINE-1 and Alu elements in T2D patients who developed presymptomatic dementia, many linked to genes involved in Alzheimer's risk, and some of these changes were modifiable through folate and vitamin B12 supplementation (Sae-Lee et al., 2020). Such events exacerbate metabolic dysfunction and promote complications such as diabetic cardiovascular disease and tissue fibrosis.

3. Regulation of gene expression via DNA methylation

DNA methylation is a dynamic and multilayered regulatory system that modulates gene expression in response to nutritional, hormonal, and metabolic cues. It shapes gene activity through direct effects on transcription factor binding, recruitment of methyl-binding proteins, chromatin remodeling, and reorganization of three-dimensional genome architecture (Fig. 3.2). These mechanisms collectively influence metabolic pathways involved in glucose uptake, insulin signaling, lipid homeostasis, oxidative stress management, and inflammatory responses.

3.1 Blocking transcription factor binding

Methylation of cytosines within or near promoter regions can directly hinder the binding of key transcription factors such as CREB, NF-κB, and C/EBP (Nerlich et al., 2021). When

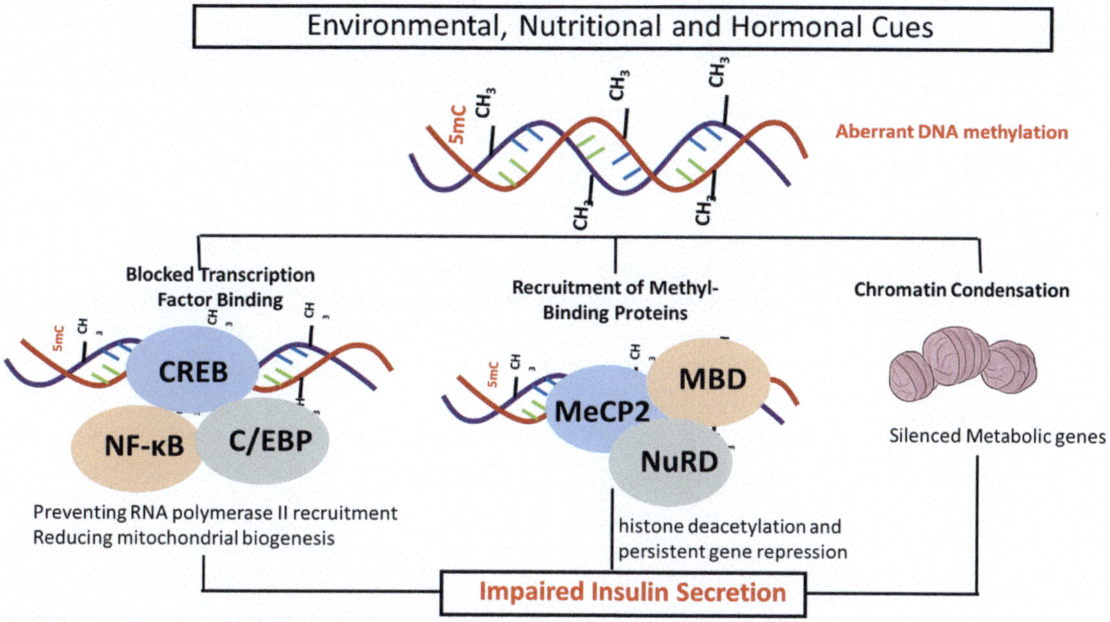

Figure 3.2 Multi-level regulation of gene expression by DNA methylation and its impact on metabolic pathways this figure illustrates how DNA methylation regulates gene expression through transcription factor blocking, recruitment of methyl-binding proteins, chromatin condensation, and alterations in 3D genome architecture. These epigenetic mechanisms collectively disrupt insulin signaling, lipid metabolism, inflammatory pathways, and antioxidant defense, contributing to metabolic dysfunction. *CREB*, cAMP response element–binding protein; *NF-κB*, nuclear factor kappa-light-chain-enhancer of activated B cells; *C/EBP*, CCAAT/enhancer-binding protein; *MeCP2*, methyl-CpG binding protein 2; *MBD*, methyl-CpG binding domain protein; *NuRD*, nucleosome remodeling and deacetylase complex.

transcription factors cannot bind to their recognition motifs, RNA polymerase II recruitment is impaired, resulting in reduced gene transcription. This mechanism plays a central role in metabolic diseases: for instance, methylation of the PPARGC1A (PGC-1α) promoter in skeletal muscle diminishes transcription factor binding and reduces mitochondrial biogenesis, ultimately contributing to insulin resistance and energy imbalance (Popov et al., 2017).

3.2 Recruitment of methyl-binding proteins

Methylated DNA serves as a docking platform for methyl-binding proteins such as MeCP2 and members of the MBD family (MBD1, MBD2, MBD4). These proteins recruit corepressor complexes containing histone deacetylases (HDACs), histone methyltransferases (HMTs), and ATP-dependent chromatin remodelers. A study identifies a previously uncharacterized intrinsically disordered region (MBD2IDR) in MBD2 that enhances its binding to methylated DNA and recruits the NuRD histone deacetylase core through two key residues, Arg286 and Leu287. Mutating these residues disrupts NuRD interaction and impairs repression of the methylated tumor suppressor PRSS8, revealing structural and functional insights into MBD2-NuRD regulation (Desai et al., 2015). The resulting chromatin condensation leads to long-term gene repression. In metabolic disorders, this mechanism silences antioxidant and anti inflammatory genes, thereby amplifying oxidative stress and creating a self-sustaining cycle of metabolic dysfunction (Paluvai et al., 2023).

3.3 Chromatin condensation

DNA methylation promotes the formation of tightly packed heterochromatin, reducing nucleosome mobility and limiting accessibility of transcriptional regulators. Persistent chromatin compaction contributes to sustained silencing of metabolic genes involved in insulin signaling, mitochondrial function, and lipid oxidation (Morrison, 2020). Additionally, heterochromatin accumulation enhances activation of inflammatory gene clusters, creating a chronic pro-inflammatory state characteristic of obesity and type 2 diabetes (Xu et al., 2017).

3.4 Modulation of 3D genome architecture

DNA methylation influences higher-order chromatin organization by modifying topologically associated domain (TAD) boundaries, enhancer–promoter looping, and genomic compartmentalization (Clemens et al., 2020). These structural changes impact coordinated transcription of metabolic gene networks. For example, altered 3D chromatin structure in pancreatic β-cells affects insulin secretion pathways, while similar disruptions in adipocytes impair lipid storage regulation (Miguel-Escalada et al., 2019; Jin et al., 2023). In hepatocytes, methylation-driven architectural changes modify the expression of genes governing gluconeogenesis, contributing to hyperglycemia (Honma et al., 2017).

3.5 Impact on metabolic pathways

Altered DNA methylation profiles regulate key metabolic pathways. In insulin signaling, methylation of genes such as

IRS1, AKT2, and GLUT4 reduces glucose uptake and contributes to insulin resistance (Zimmerman, 2022). In lipid metabolism, methylation of PPARγ, SREBP-1c, and FASN alters adipogenesis, lipogenesis, and lipid storage (Wu and Liu, 2021). Methylation of inflammatory genes such as TNF-α and IL-6 promotes chronic low-grade inflammation, a hallmark of metabolic syndrome (Indumathi et al., 2022). Meanwhile, methylation-induced suppression of antioxidant genes like SOD2, GPx1, and NRF2 diminishes cellular defenses against oxidative stress, exacerbating mitochondrial dysfunction (Balasubramanian et al., 2021). Together, these methylation-driven changes in gene expression act as a molecular bridge between environmental exposures and metabolic phenotypes, shaping the development and progression of metabolic disorders.

4. Environmental and lifestyle influences on DNA methylation

4.1 Nutrition

Nutrition plays a central role in shaping DNA methylation patterns because it directly influences the biochemical availability of methyl donors required for epigenetic reactions. Key nutrients such as folate, vitamin B12, choline, betaine, and methionine participate in the one-carbon metabolism cycle, which generates S-adenosylmethionine (SAM), the universal methyl donor for DNA and histone methyltransferases (Łoboś and Regulska-Ilow, 2021). Deficiencies or imbalances in these nutrients can reduce SAM levels or alter the S-adenosylhomocysteine (SAH)/SAM ratio, thereby inhibiting DNA methyltransferase (DNMT) activity and leading to aberrant methylation. Beyond micronutrients, macronutrient composition significantly affects epigenetic regulation. High-fat and high-sugar diets induce hypermethylation of key metabolic genes such as GLUT4 in muscle, impairing glucose uptake, while hypomethylation of lipogenic regulators like SREBP-1c and FASN promotes hepatic lipid accumulation (Hor et al., 2025). Diet-induced methylation changes in PGC-1α, a master regulator of mitochondrial biogenesis, reduce oxidative metabolism and contribute to insulin resistance (Laker et al., 2014). Chronic overnutrition also modifies methylation of inflammatory genes, amplifying systemic inflammation and accelerating metabolic syndrome progression (Bollati et al., 2014). Thus, nutritional exposures act as powerful environmental epigenetic modulators capable of reprogramming metabolic health across the lifespan.

4.2 Early-life programming

Early developmental stages represent a critical window of epigenetic plasticity during which environmental and nutritional stimuli can leave long-lasting methylation marks. Maternal undernutrition, obesity, stress, gestational diabetes, or hyperglycemia can trigger persistent epigenetic reprogramming of metabolic genes in the fetus (Li et al., 2021). These methylation changes can alter organ development, hormone sensitivity, and metabolic set points, predisposing offspring to chronic diseases such as obesity, dyslipidemia, and type 2 diabetes. Landmark examples include differential methylation of IGF2, a gene essential for fetal growth; LEP (leptin), which regulates appetite and adiposity; PPARγ, a key adipogenic transcription factor; and HNF4A, critical for pancreatic β-cell function and glucose homeostasis (Montoya-Williams et al., 2018; Kadakia et al., 2017; Du et al., 2020). Epigenetic alterations established during gestation can persist into adulthood and even across multiple generations through germline methylation changes, contributing to the intergenerational transmission of metabolic disease risk. These findings highlight the concept of developmental origins of health and disease (DOHaD), emphasizing that metabolic disorders often begin with epigenetic events set early in life (Lacagnina, 2020).

4.3 Physical activity

Physical activity is one of the most potent lifestyle interventions capable of modulating DNA methylation in metabolic tissues such as skeletal muscle, liver, and adipose tissue. Exercise induces rapid and dynamic demethylation of regulatory regions within genes controlling oxidative metabolism, mitochondrial biogenesis, and glucose transport (Świątowy et al., 2021). Notably, endurance exercise has been shown to decrease methylation of promoters such as PGC-1α, enhancing mitochondrial function and oxidative phosphorylation (Lochmann et al., 2015). Reduced methylation of genes such as GLUT4 and AMPK subunits improves insulin sensitivity and enhances cellular glucose uptake (King-Himmelreich et al., 2016). Both acute and chronic exercise also modulate methylation of inflammatory genes, shifting the metabolic environment toward a less inflammatory state (Hunter et al., 2023). Moreover, exercise-induced epigenetic remodeling is partly mediated by increased levels of TET enzymes, improved NAD^+ metabolism, and enhanced chromatin accessibility (Bittel and Chen, 2024). Over time, these epigenetic modifications contribute to long-term improvements in metabolic flexibility, making physical activity a powerful regulator of epigenetic health.

4.4 Stress and endocrine disruptors

Chronic psychological stress and exposure to environmental toxins significantly influence DNA methylation patterns, often in ways that promote metabolic dysfunction. Elevated cortisol levels during stress activate glucocorticoid signaling pathways that can alter DNMT expression and lead to methylation changes in genes regulating appetite, glucose metabolism, and adipocyte differentiation (Wrigglesworth et al., 2019). Persistent stress is associated with methylation of FKBP5, a regulator of glucocorticoid sensitivity, thereby disrupting metabolic and inflammatory responses (Miller et al., 2020). Additionally, numerous environmental pollutants and endocrine-disrupting chemicals (EDCs) such as bisphenol A (BPA), phthalates, pesticides, and heavy metals interfere with methyl donor availability, DNMT/TET activity, or chromatin structure (El Henafy et al., 2020). BPA, for example, has been shown to modify methylation of genes involved in adipogenesis (e.g., PPARγ, C/EBPα) and pancreatic function, increasing susceptibility to obesity and insulin resistance (Dalamaga et al., 2024). Exposure to air pollutants and particulate matter can hypomethylate genes linked to oxidative stress and inflammation, contributing to metabolic syndrome development (Poursafa et al., 2022). Collectively, stress and environmental contaminants reprogram epigenetic regulation in metabolic tissues, amplifying disease risk across multiple biological systems.

5. DNA methylation in major metabolic disorders

5.1 Type 2 diabetes mellitus (T2DM)

DNA methylation plays a crucial role in the onset and progression of Type 2 Diabetes Mellitus by altering gene expression in key metabolic tissues including pancreatic β-cells, skeletal muscle, liver, and adipose tissue (Fig. 3.1). In pancreatic β-cells, aberrant methylation patterns disrupt insulin production and glucose sensing. Pancreatic β-cells include a small TH+ subset, a special subset of β-cells, those that express tyrosine hydroxylase (TH), affects insulin secretion. TH is an enzyme normally involved in producing catecholamines (like dopamine), which *suppress* insulin release. So, when more β-cells express TH, the pancreas secretes less insulin. Keeping TH+ cells numbers low is essential for normal islet function. DNA methylation, especially controlled by Dnmt3a, silences TH during β-cell development, preventing excess TH+ cells. When this methylation is lost, either genetically or due to overnutrition, TH+ β-cells increase and β-cell function becomes impaired (Parveen et al., 2023). Similarly, a subset of Pancreatic β-cells expressing the imprinted gene Nnat also shows specialized roles in insulin production. This NNAT+ subpopulation is developmentally established and controlled by DNMT3A-dependent DNA methylation, which defines their transcriptome and reduces their likelihood of becoming highly connected "hub" cells. Disruption of Nnat methylation alters β-cell hierarchy and may weaken insulin secretion, contributing to diabetes (Yu et al., 2024).

Hypermethylation of the Pdx1 promoter leads to diminished PDX1 expression, destabilizing β-cell identity and impairing insulin transcriptional regulation (Yang et al., 2012). Similarly, methylation of the Ins1/Ins2 loci decreases insulin gene expression, while hypermethylation of GLUT2, a glucose transporter essential for β-cell glucose sensing, reduces glucose uptake and insulin secretory responses (Carry et al., 2020; Rajagopal et al., 2019). In skeletal muscle, an important tissue for insulin-mediated glucose disposal, genome-wide studies reveal hypermethylation of PPARGC1A (PGC-1α), resulting in impaired mitochondrial biogenesis and reduced oxidative phosphorylation (Ribel-Madsen et al., 2012). Additional methylation alterations in IRS1 and AKT2, key components of the insulin signaling cascade, further contribute to insulin resistance (Krause et al., 2020). In the liver, hypermethylation of gluconeogenic genes such as FOXO1 and G6PC dysregulates glucose homeostasis, while hypomethylation of inflammatory genes exacerbates hepatic insulin resistance (Horiguchi et al., 2021). Adipose tissue demonstrates differential methylation of adipokine genes including LEP and ADIPOQ, promoting chronic inflammation and metabolic dysfunction (Weyman-Vela et al., 2025). Collectively, these methylation changes disrupt insulin dynamics across tissues, establishing DNA methylation as a central regulator in T2DM pathology.

5.2 Obesity

Obesity is accompanied by widespread epigenetic remodeling that affects genes governing energy balance, adipocyte biology, inflammation, and appetite regulation. Epigenome-wide association studies (EWAS) consistently identify obesity-related differential methylation in genes such as FTO, which is strongly associated with BMI and energy intake regulation (Osório, 2014). Altered methylation in LEP and LEPR affects leptin signaling, impairing satiety sensing and promoting overeating (Weyman-Vela et al., 2025). Hypermethylation or hypomethylation in PPARγ, a master regulator of adipogenesis, leads to dysfunctional adipocyte differentiation and lipid storage, contributing to the expansion of hypertrophic, pro-inflammatory fat cells (Volberg et al., 2017). Inflammatory mediators such as TNF-α also show methylation shifts, perpetuating chronic low-grade inflammation characteristic of obesity (Boonrong et al., 2024). These combined methylation changes reinforce adipocyte dysfunction, metabolic inflexibility, and the progressive nature of obesity as an epigenetically modulated disorder.

5.3 Non-alcoholic fatty liver disease (NAFLD)

In NAFLD, DNA methylation modulates key pathways involved in lipid synthesis, oxidative stress responses, and fibrogenesis within the liver. Hypermethylation of lipid metabolism regulators such as SREBP-2 and ACC disrupts lipid homeostasis and drives hepatic triglyceride accumulation (Li et al., 2019). Fibrosis-associated genes including TGF-β and COL1A also undergo methylation changes, promoting extracellular matrix deposition and the transition to non-alcoholic steatohepatitis (NASH) (Lyu et al., 2023). Additionally, methylation alterations in oxidative stress–related pathways, including Nrf2, compromise antioxidant defenses and enhance susceptibility to oxidative damage (Hosseini et al., 2020). Recent studies indicate that blood-based methylation signatures of these genes serve as potential non-invasive biomarkers for early NAFLD detection and staging, highlighting the translational significance of methylation research in liver disease (Zeng et al., 2024).

5.4 Gestational diabetes mellitus (GDM)

GDM exerts profound epigenetic effects on the placenta, cord blood, and fetal metabolic tissues, setting the stage for long-term metabolic consequences in offspring. Elevated maternal glucose

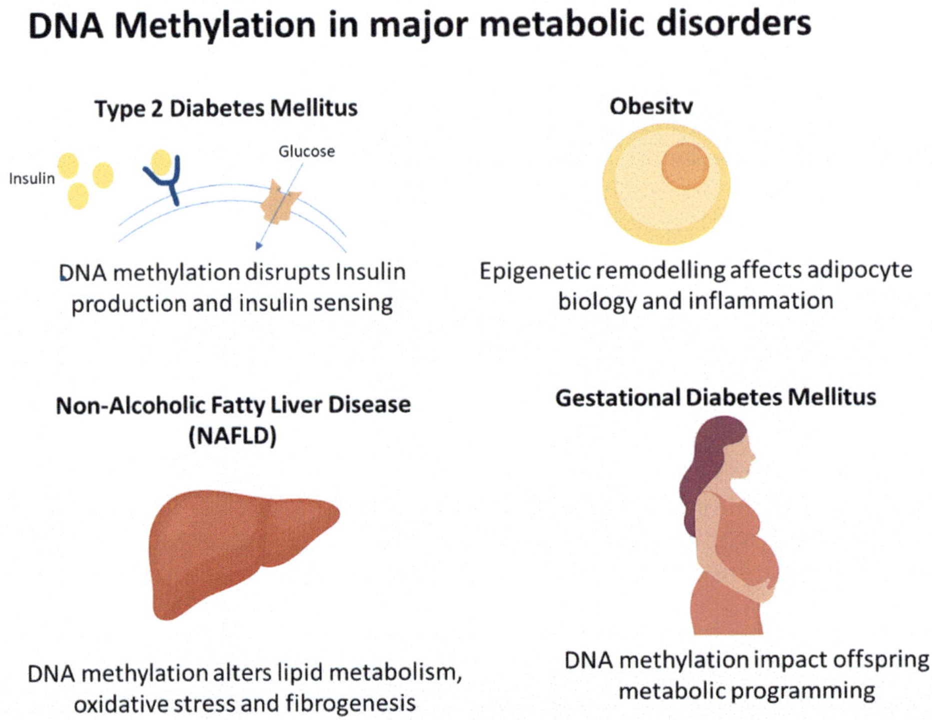

Figure 3.3 DNA methylation alterations across major metabolic disorder this figure illustrates how DNA methylation abnormalities contribute to four major metabolic conditions: Type 2 diabetes, obesity, non-alcoholic fatty liver disease (NAFLD), and gestational diabetes mellitus (GDM). Epigenetic modifications in key tissues—including pancreatic β-cells, adipose tissue, liver, and the placenta—drive impaired insulin signaling, altered lipid metabolism, inflammation, and intergenerational metabolic risk.

levels induce hyper- and hypo-methylation of genes involved in pancreatic development, glucose transport, and adiposity regulation (Howe et al., 2020). These alterations persist beyond birth, affecting childhood growth trajectories and increasing the risk of obesity and T2DM later in life, a phenomenon known as intergenerational metabolic memory (Ren et al., 2018). Methylation changes in genes governing insulin sensitivity, appetite regulation, and energy expenditure underscore the enduring impact of intrauterine glycemic exposure on offspring metabolic programming (Fig. 3.3).

6. Advances in methylation biomarkers for metabolic diseases

6.1 Blood-based methylation markers

Circulating methylation signatures in cell-free DNA offer a minimally invasive approach for early detection and monitoring of metabolic diseases. Methylation patterns associated with T2DM risk, obesity subtypes, and response to pharmacological or lifestyle interventions provide promising tools for personalized medicine (Willmer et al., 2018; Day et al., 2017). These blood-based markers reflect methylation changes in metabolic tissues and potentially enable real-time monitoring of disease progression.

6.2 Tissue-specific signatures

Beyond blood markers, tissue-specific methylation patterns offer deep insights into metabolic dysfunction. β-cell–specific methylation of INS, GCK, and PDX1 provides valuable indicators of β-cell stress and insulin secretory capacity (Yang et al., 2012; Carry et al., 2020; Rajagopal et al., 2019). In skeletal muscle, methylation signatures can predict individual responsiveness to exercise training (Sharples and Seaborne, 2019). These tissue-level insights support the development of precision diagnostics tailored to specific metabolic phenotypes.

6.3 Multi-omics approaches

Integrating DNA methylation data with transcriptomics, metabolomics, proteomics, and chromatin accessibility maps enhances the predictive power and biological understanding of metabolic diseases (Bizzarri et al., 2024; Agarwal et al., 2022). Such integrative approaches uncover complex regulatory networks and help distinguish causal methylation changes from secondary adaptations, enabling more accurate disease modeling and biomarker discovery.

7. Therapeutic targeting of DNA methylation

7.1 Epigenetic drugs

Epigenetic therapies targeting DNA methylation represent a promising frontier in metabolic disease treatment. DNMT inhibitors such as 5-azacytidine and decitabine, though primarily used in cancer therapy, are being explored for metabolic disorders (Du et al., 2023; Liu et al., 2025). However, their limited specificity and off-target effects pose challenges for clinical translation. In contrast, TET activators and nutraceutical compounds capable of promoting active demethylation are emerging as safer alternatives with metabolic benefits (Rui et al., 2021; Liang et al., 2021).

7.2 Nutritional interventions

Dietary modulation of the one-carbon metabolism pathway provides an accessible strategy to influence DNA methylation. Nutrients including folate, choline, betaine, and vitamin B12 support SAM production and sustain balanced methylation. Bioactive dietary components such as EGCG (green tea), resveratrol, and curcumin can modulate DNMT and TET enzyme activity, offering promising nutraceutical approaches to restore healthy epigenetic patterns (Remely et al., 2017; Li et al., 2018; Hosseini et al., 2020).

7.3 Lifestyle modifications

Lifestyle interventions, particularly physical activity, weight loss, caloric restriction, and intermittent fasting, exert powerful effects on DNA methylation (Waziry et al., 2023; Selvaraji et al., 2021). These interventions can reverse aberrant methylation patterns in metabolic tissues, improve insulin sensitivity, and enhance mitochondrial function. Exercise-induced demethylation of key metabolic genes underscores the therapeutic potential of lifestyle-driven epigenetic remodeling (Vasileva et al., 2024).

7.4 Microbiome-based approaches

The gut microbiome significantly influences host DNA methylation through microbial metabolites such as short-chain fatty acids (SCFAs), folate, betaine, and B vitamins (Martínez-Montoro et al., 2024). Butyrate, for example, functions as both an HDAC inhibitor and a methylation modulator, improving insulin sensitivity and reducing inflammation (Khan and Jena, 2015). These findings position the microbiome as an innovative target for epigenetic therapy in metabolic disease.

8. Future perspectives

Emerging technologies such as single-cell methylomics, long-read sequencing, and CRISPR-based epigenome editing are revolutionizing our ability to characterize and manipulate methylation landscapes (Fadul et al., 2023). These tools enable cell-type specific mapping of methylation changes, high-resolution tracking of epigenetic evolution during disease progression, and precise reprogramming of epigenetic states in metabolic tissues. While these innovations promise breakthroughs in personalized metabolic medicine, a major challenge remains, distinguishing whether methylation changes are causal drivers of metabolic dysfunction or merely reflective of disease states. Addressing this question will be key to developing safe and effective epigenetic therapies.

9. Conclusion

DNA methylation is a central regulator of metabolic health, influencing gene expression programs involved in insulin secretion, glucose regulation, lipid metabolism, inflammation, and mitochondrial function. Environmental exposures, diet, physical activity, stress, and developmental factors dynamically shape methylation landscapes, establishing both short-term metabolic responses and long-term metabolic memory. Understanding the epigenetic mechanisms underlying metabolic disorders provides new opportunities for diagnostics, prevention, and therapeutic innovation. As technologies advance, the integration of methylation profiling into precision medicine holds great promise for transforming the management of metabolic diseases.

References

Abbasi, I.H.R., Abbasi, F., Wang, L., Abd El Hack, M.E., Swelum, A.A., Hao, R., Yao, J., Cao, Y., 2018. Folate promotes S-adenosyl methionine reactions and the microbial methylation cycle and boosts ruminants production and reproduction. AMB Express 8 (1). https://doi.org/10.1186/s13568-018-0592-5. Available from: http://www.amb-express.com/.

Agarwal, P., Wicklow, B.A., Dart, A.B., Hizon, N.A., Sellers, E.A.C., McGavock, J. M., Talbot, C.P.J., Fonseca, M.A., Xu, W., Davie, J.R., Jones, M.J., Acharjee, A., Dolinsky, V.W., 2022. Integrative analysis reveals novel associations between DNA methylation and the serum metabolome of adolescents with type 2 diabetes: a cross-sectional study. Front. Endocrinol. 13. https://doi.org/10.3389/fendo.2022.934706. Available from: https://www.frontiersin.org/journals/endocrinology#.

Andergassen, D., Smith, Z.D., Kretzmer, H., Rinn, J.L., Meissner, A., 2021. Diverse epigenetic mechanisms maintain parental imprints within the embryonic and extraembryonic lineages. Dev. Cell 56 (21), 2995. https://doi.org/10.1016/j.devcel.2021.10.010.

Antequera, F., Boyes, J., Bird, A., 1990. High levels of de novo methylation and altered chromatin structure at CpG islands in cell lines. Cell 62 (3), 503–514. https://doi.org/10.1016/0092-8674(90)90015-7.

Balasubramanian, N., Sagarkar, S., Choudhary, A.G., Kokare, D.M., Sakharkar, A. J., 2021. Epigenetic blockade of hippocampal SOD2 via DNMT3b-mediated DNA methylation: implications in mild traumatic brain injury-induced persistent oxidative damage. Mol. Neurobiol. 58 (3), 1162–1184. https://doi.org/10.1007/s12035-020-02166-z.

Barres, R., Zierath, J.R., 2011. DNA methylation in metabolic disorders. Am. J. Clin. Nutr. 93 (4), 897S. https://doi.org/10.3945/ajcn.110.001933.

Barrès, R., Osler, M.E., Yan, J., Rune, A., Fritz, T., Caidahl, K., Krook, A., Zierath, J.R., 2009. Non-CpG methylation of the PGC-1α promoter through DNMT3B controls mitochondrial density. Cell Metab. 10 (3), 189–198. https://doi.org/10.1016/j.cmet.2009.07.011.

Billen, D., 1968. Methylation of the bacterial chromosome: an event at the "replication point"? J. Mol. Biol. 31 (3), 477–486. https://doi.org/10.1016/0022-2836(68)90422-1.

Bird, A.P., 1986. CpG-Rich islands and the function of DNA methylation. Nature 321 (6067), 209–213. https://doi.org/10.1038/321209a0.

Bird, A., 1997. Does DNA methylation control transposition of selfish elements in the germline? Trends Genet. 13 (12), 469–470. https://doi.org/10.1016/s0168-9525(97)01310-3.

Bittel, A.J., Chen, Y.W., 2024. DNA methylation in the adaptive response to exercise. Sports Med. 54 (6), 1419–1458. https://doi.org/10.1007/s40279-024-02011-6.

Bizzarri, D., Reinders, M.J.T., Kuiper, L., Beekman, M., Deelen, J., van Meurs, J. B.J., van Dongen, J., Pool, R., Boomsma, D.I., Ghanbari, M., Franke, L., Geleijnse, J.M., Boersma, E., van Spil, W.E., van Greevenbroek, M.M.J., Stehouwer, C.D.A., van der Kallen, C.J.H., Arts, I.C.W., Rutters, F., Beulens, J. W.J., Muilwijk, M., Elders, P.J.M., t Hart, L.M., Ghanbari, M., Ikram, M.A., Netea, M.G., Kloppenburg, M., Ramos, Y.F.M., Bomer, N., Meulenbelt, I., Stronks, K., Snijder, M.B., Zwinderman, A.H., Heijmans, B.T., Lumey, L.H., Wijmenga, C., Fu, J., Zhernakova, A., Deelen, J., Mooijaart, S.P., Beekman, M., Onderwater, G.L.J., van den Maagdenberg, A.M.J.M., Terwindt, G.M., Thesing, C., Bot, M., Penninx, B.W.J.H., Trompet, S., Jukema, J.W., Sattar, N., van der Horst, I.C.C., van der Harst, P., So-Osman, C., van Hilten, J.A., Nelissen, R.G.H.H., Höfer, I.E., Asselbergs, F.W., Scheltens, P., Teunissen, C.E., van der Flier, W.M., van Dongen, J., Pool, R., Willemsen, A.H.M., Boomsma, D.I., Suchiman, H.E.D., Barkey Wolf, J.J.H., Cats, D., Mei, H., Slofstra, M., Swertz, M., Reinders, M.J.T., van den Akker, E. B., Slagboom, P.E., van den Akker, E.B., 2024. NMR metabolomics-guided DNA methylation mortality predictors. EBioMedicine 107. https://doi.org/10.1016/j.ebiom.2024.105279. Available from: https://www.sciencedirect.com/science/journal/23523964.

Bollati, V., Favero, C., Albetti, B., Tarantini, L., Moroni, A., Byun, H.M., Motta, V., Conti, D.M., Tirelli, A.S., Vigna, L., Bertazzi, P.A., Pesatori, A.C., 2014. Nutrients intake is associated with DNA methylation of candidate inflammatory genes in a population of obese subjects. Nutrients 6 (10), 4625–4639. https://doi.org/10.3390/nu6104625.

Boonrong, C., Roytrakul, S., Shantavasinkul, P.C., Sritara, P., Sirivarasai, J., 2024. Role of dietary factors on DNA methylation levels of TNF-alpha gene and proteome profiles in obese men. Nutrients 16 (6), 877. https://doi.org/10.3390/nu16060877.

Bostick, M., Jong, K.K., Estève, P.O., Clark, A., Pradhan, S., Jacobsen, S.E., 2007. UHRF1 plays a role in maintaining DNA methylation in mammalian cells. Science 317 (5845), 1760–1764. https://doi.org/10.1126/science.1147939.

Bozdemir, N., Sukur, G., Kablan, T., Cinar, O., Uysal, F., Martin, G., 2025. Obesity induced by a high-fat diet is associated with changes in the expression levels of Dnmt3b and Dnmt3l proteins in mouse testes. Reproduction. Fertility and Development 37 (10). https://doi.org/10.1071/rd24194.

Cai, L., Zhan, M., Li, Q., Li, D., Xu, Q., 2020. DNA methyltransferase DNMT1 inhibits lipopolysaccharide-induced inflammatory response in human dental pulp cells involving the methylation changes of IL-6 and TRAF6. Mol. Med. Rep. 21 (2), 959–968. https://doi.org/10.3892/mmr.2019.10860.

Cai, W., Song, Q., Mo, X., Li, H., Song, Y., Yin, L., 2025. TET2-mediated epigenetic modification promotes stress senescence of pancreatic β cells in type 2 diabetes mellitus. eLife. https://doi.org/10.7554/eLife.104550.1. Available from: https://elifesciences.org/.

Cao, X., Springer, N.M., Muszynski, M.G., Phillips, R.L., Kaeppler, S., Jacobsen, S.E., 2000. Conserved plant genes with similarity to mammalian de novo DNA methyltransferases. Proc. Natl. Acad. Sci. 97 (9), 4979–4984. https://doi.org/10.1073/pnas.97.9.4979.

Carry, P.M., Vanderlinden, L.A., Johnson, R.K., Dong, F., Steck, A.K., Frohnert, B. I., Rewers, M., Yang, I.V., Kechris, K., Norris, J.M., 2020. DNA methylation near the INS gene is associated with INS genetic variation (rs689) and type 1 diabetes in the Diabetes Autoimmunity Study in the Young. Pediatr. Diabetes 21 (4), 597–605. https://doi.org/10.1111/pedi.12995. Available from: http://onlinelibrary.wiley.com/journal/10.1111/(ISSN)1399-5448.

Chen, Z., Miao, F., Paterson, A.D., Lachin, J.M., Zhang, L., Schones, D.E., Wu, X., Wang, J., Tompkins, J.D., Genuth, S., Braffett, B.H., Riggs, A.D., Natarajan, R., Nathan, D.M., Zinman, B., Crofford, O., Genuth, S., Brown-Friday, J., Crandall, J., Engel, H., Engel, S., Martinez, H., Phillips, M., Reid, M., Shamoon, H., Sheindlin, J., Gubitosi-Klug, R., Mayer, L., Pendegast, S., Zegarra, H., Miller, D., Singerman, L., Smith-Brewer, S., Novak, M., Quin, J., Genuth, S., Palmert, M., Brown, E., McConnell, J., Pugsley, P., Crawford, P., Dahms, W., Brillon, D., Lackaye, M.E., Kiss, S., Chan, R., Orlin, A., Rubin, M., Reppucci, V., Lee, T., Heinemann, M., Chang, S., Levy, B., Jovanovic, L., Richardson, M., Bosco, B., Dwoskin, A., Hanna, R., Barron, S., Campbell, R., Bhan, A., Kruger, D., Jones, J.K., Edwards, P.A., Bhan, A., Carey, J.D., Angus, E., Thomas, A., Galprin, A., McLellan, M., Whitehouse, F., Bergenstal, R., Johnson, M., Gunyou, K., Thomas, L., Laechelt, J., Hollander, P., Spencer, M., Kendall, D., Cuddihy, R., Callahan, P., List, S., Gott, J., Rude, N., Olson, B., Franz, M., Castle, G., Birk, R., Nelson, J., Freking, D., Gill, L., Mestrezat, W., Etzwiler, D., Morgan, K., Aiello, L.P., Golden, E., Arrigg, P., Asuquo, V., Beaser, R., Bestourous, L., Cavallerano, J., Cavicchi, R., Ganda, O., Hamdy, O., Kirby, R., Murtha, T., Schlossman, D., Shah, S., Sharuk, G., Silva, P., Silver, P., Stockman, M., Sun, J., Weimann, E., Wolpert, H., Aiello, L.M., Jacobson, A., Rand, L., Rosenzwieg, J., Nathan, D.M., Larkin, M.E., Christofi, M., Folino, K., Godine, J., Lou, P., Stevens, C., Anderson, E., Bode, H., Brink, S., Cornish, C., Cros, D., Delahanty, L., deManbey, A., Haggan, C., Lynch, J., McKitrick, C., Norman, D., Moore, D., Ong, M., Taylor, C., Zimbler, D., Crowell, S., Fritz, S., Hansen, K., Gauthier-Kelly, C., Service, F.J., Ziegler, G., Colligan, R., Schmidt, L., French, B., Woodwick, R., Rizza, R., Schwenk, W.F., Haymond, M., Pach, J., Mortenson, J., Zimmerman, B., Lucas, A., Luttrell, L., Lopes-Virella, M., Caulder, S., Pittman, C., Patel, N., Lee, K., Nutaitis, M., Fernandes, J., Hermayer, K., Kwon, S., Blevins, A., Parker, J., Colwell, J., Lee, D., Soule, J., Lindsey, P., Bracey, M., Farr, A., Elsing, S., Thompson, T., Selby, J., Lyons, T., Yacoub-Wasef, S., Szpiech, M., Wood, D., Mayfield, R., Molitch, M., Adelman, D., Colson, S., Jampol, L., Lyon, A., Gill, M., Strugula, Z., Kaminski, L., Mirza, R., Simjanoski, E., Ryan, D., Johnson, C., Wallia, A., Ajroud-Driss, S., Astelford, P., Leloudes, N., Degillio, A., Schaefer, B., Mudaliar, S., Lorenzi, G., Goldbaum, M., Jones, K., Prince, M., Swenson, M., Grant, I., Reed, R., Lyon, R., Kolterman, O., Giotta, M., Clark, T., Friedenberg, G., Sivitz, W.I., Vittetoe, B., Kramer, J., Bayless, M.,

Zeitler, R., Schrott, H., Olson, N., Snetselaar, L., Hoffman, R., MacIndoe, J., Weingeist, T., Fountain, C., Mendley, S., Johnsonbaugh, S., Patronas, M., Carney, M., Salemi, P., Liss, R., Hebdon, M., Counts, D., Donner, T., Gordon, J., Hemady, R., Kowarski, A., Ostrowski, D., Steidl, S., Jones, B., Herman, W.H., Martin, C.L., Pop-Busui, R., Greene, D.A., Stevens, M.J., Burkhart, N., Sandford, T., Floyd, J., Bantle, J., Wimmergren, N., Terry, J., Koozekanani, D., Montezuma, S., Rogness, B., Mech, M., Strand, T., Olson, J., McKenzie, L., Kwong, C., Goetz, F., Warhol, R., Hainsworth, D., Goldstein, D., Hitt, S., Giangiacomo, J., Schade, D.S., Canady, J.L., Burge, M. R., Das, A., Avery, R.B., Ketai, L.H., Chapin, J.E., L Schluter, M., Rich, J., Johannes, C., Hornbeck, D., Schutta, M., Bourne, P.A., Brucker, A., Braunstein, S., Schwartz, S., Maschak-Carey, B.J., Baker, L., Orchard, T., Cimino, L., Songer, T., Doft, B., Olson, S., Becker, D., Rubinstein, D., Bergren, R.L., Fruit, J., Hyre, R., Palmer, C., Silvers, N., Lobes, L., Paczan Rath, P., Conrad, P.W., Yalamanchi, S., Wesche, J., Bratkowksi, M., Arslanian, S., Rinkoff, J., Warnicki, J., Curtin, D., Steinberg, D., Vagstad, G., Harris, R., Steranchak, L., Arch, J., Kelly, K., Ostrosaka, P., Guiliani, M., Good, M., Williams, T., Olsen, K., Campbell, A., Shipe, C., Conwit, R., Finegold, D., Zaucha, M., Drash, A., Morrison, A., Malone, J.I., Bernal, M.L., Pavan, P.R., Grove, N., Tanaka, E.A., McMillan, D., Vaccaro-Kish, J., Babbione, L., Solc, H., DeClue, T.J., Dagogo-Jack, S., Wigley, C., Ricks, H., Kitabchi, A., Chaum, E., Murphy, M.B., Moser, S., Meyer, D., Iannacone, A., Yoser, S., Bryer-Ash, M., Schussler, S., Lambeth, H., Raskin, P., Strowig, S., Basco, M., Cercone, S., Zinman, B., Barnie, A., Devenyi, R., Mandelcorn, M., Brent, M., Rogers, S., Gordon, A., Bakshi, N., Perkins, B., Tuason, L., Perdikaris, F., Ehrlich, R., Daneman, D., Perlman, K., Ferguson, S., Palmer, J., Fahlstrom, R., de Boer, I.H., Kinyoun, J., Van Ottingham, L., Catton, S., Ginsberg, J., McDonald, C., Harth, J., Driscoll, M., Sheidow, T., Mahon, J., Canny, C., Nicolle, D., Colby, P., Dupre, J., Hramiak, I., Rodger, N.W., Jenner, M., Smith, T., Brown, W., May, M., Lipps Hagan, J., Agarwal, A., Adkins, T., Lorenz, R., Feman, S., Survant, L., White, N.H., Levandoski, L., Grand, G., Thomas, M., Joseph, D., Blinder, K., Shah, G., Burgess, D., Boniuk, I., Santiago, J., Tamborlane, W., Gatcomb, P., Stoessel, K., Ramos, P., Fong, K., Ossorio, P., Ahern, J., Gubitosi-Klug, R., Beck, C., Genuth, S., Quin, J., Gaston, P., Palmert, M., Trail, R., Dahms, W., Lachin, J., Cleary, P., Backlund, J., Bebu, I., Braffett, B., Diminick, L., Gao, X., Hsu, W., Klumpp, K., Larsen, M., McGee, P., Sun, W., Villavicencio, S., Anderson, K., Dews, L., Younes, N., Rutledge, B., Chan, K., Rosenberg, D., Petty, B., Determan, A., Kenny, D., Williams, C., Cowie, C., Siebert, C., Steffes, M., Arends, V., Bucksa, J., Nowicki, M., Chavers, B., O'Leary, D., Polak, J., Harrington, A., Funk, L., Crow, R., Gloeb, B., Thomas, S., O'Donnell, C., Soliman, E.Z., Zhang, Z.M., Li, Y., Campbell, C., Keasler, L., Hensley, S., Hu, J., Barr, M., Taylor, T., Prineas, R., Feldman, E.L., Albers, J. W., Low, P., Sommer, C., Nickander, K., Speigelberg, T., Pfiefer, M., Schumer, M., Moran, M., Farquhar, J., Ryan, C., Sandstrom, D., Williams, T., Geckle, M., Cupelli, E., Thoma, F., Burzuk, B., Woodfill, T., Danis, R., Blodi, B., Lawrence, D., Wabers, H., Gangaputra, S., Neill, S., Burger, M., Dingledine, J., Gama, V., Sussman, R., Davis, M., Hubbard, L., Budoff, M., Darabian, S., Rezaeian, P., Wong, N., Fox, M., Oudiz, R., Kim, L., Detrano, R., Cruickshanks, K., Dalton, D., Bainbridge, K., Lima, J., Bluemke, D., Turkbey, E., van der Geest, R.J., Liu, C., Malayeri, A., Jain, A., Miao, C., Chahal, H., Jarboe, R., Nathan, D.M., Monnier, V., Sell, D., Strauch, C., Hazen, S., Pratt, A., Tang, W., Brunzell, J., Purnell, J.,

Natarajan, R., Miao, F., Zhang, L., Chen, Z., Paterson, A., Boright, A., Bull, S., Sun, L., Scherer, S., Lopes-Virella, M., Lyons, T.J., Jenkins, A., Klein, R., Virella, G., Jaffa, A., Carter, R., Stoner, J., Garvey, W.T., Lackland, D., Brabham, M., McGee, D., Zheng, D., Mayfield, R.K., Maynard, J., Wessells, H., Sarma, A., Jacobson, A., Dunn, R., Holt, S., Hotaling, J., Kim, C., Clemens, Q., Brown, J., McVary, K., 2016. Epigenomic profiling reveals an association between persistence of DNA methylation and metabolic memory in the DCCT/EDIC type 1 diabetes cohort. Proc. Natl. Acad. Sci. 113 (21). https://doi.org/10.1073/pnas.1603712113.

Chen, X., Lin, Q., Wen, J., Lin, W., Liang, J., Huang, H., Li, L., Huang, J., Chen, F., Liu, D., Chen, G., 2020. Whole genome bisulfite sequencing of human spermatozoa reveals differentially methylated patterns from type 2 diabetic patients. J. Diabetes Investig. 11 (4), 856–864. https://doi.org/10.1111/jdi.13201.

Cheng, X., Kumar, S., Posfai, J., Pflugrath, J.W., Roberts, R.J., 1993. Crystal structure of the Hhal DNA methyltransferase complexed with S-adenosyl-l-methionine. Cell 74 (2), 299–307. https://doi.org/10.1016/0092-8674(93)90421-L.

Clemens, A.W., Wu, D.Y., Moore, J.R., Christian, D.L., Zhao, G., Gabel, H.W., 2020. MeCP2 represses enhancers through chromosome topology-associated DNA methylation. Mol. Cell 77 (2), 279. https://doi.org/10.1016/j.molcel.2019.10.033.

Dalamaga, M., Kounatidis, D., Tsilingiris, D., Vallianou, N.G., Karampela, I., Psallida, S., Papavassiliou, A.G., 2024. The role of endocrine disruptors bisphenols and phthalates in obesity: current evidence, perspectives and controversies. Int. J. Mol. Sci. 25 (1). https://doi.org/10.3390/ijms25010675. Available from: http://www.mdpi.com/journal/ijms.

Day, S.E., Coletta, R.L., Kim, J.Y., Garcia, L.A., Campbell, L.E., Benjamin, T.R., Roust, L.R., De Filippis, E.A., Mandarino, L.J., Coletta, D.K., 2017. Potential epigenetic biomarkers of obesity-related insulin resistance in human whole-blood. Epigenetics 12 (4), 254–263. https://doi.org/10.1080/15592294.2017.1281501.

Dayeh, T., Volkov, P., Salö, S., Hall, E., Nilsson, E., Olsson, A.H., Kirkpatrick, C. L., Wollheim, C.B., Eliasson, L., Rönn, T., Bacos, K., Ling, C., 2014. Genome-wide DNA methylation analysis of human pancreatic islets from type 2 diabetic and non-diabetic donors identifies candidate genes that influence insulin secretion. PLoS Genet. 10 (3). https://doi.org/10.1371/journal.pgen.1004160. Available from: http://www.plosgenetics.org/article/fetchObject.action?uri=info%3Adoi%2F10.1371%2Fjournal.pgen.1004160&representation=PDF.

de Vos, L., Gevensleben, H., Schröck, A., Franzen, A., Kristiansen, G., Bootz, F., Dietrich, D., 2017. Comparison of quantification algorithms for circulating cell-free DNA methylation biomarkers in blood plasma from cancer patients. Clin. Epigenet. 9 (1). https://doi.org/10.1186/s13148-017-0425-4. Available from: http://www.springer.com/biomed/human+genetics/journal/13148.

Desai, M.A., Webb, H.D., Sinanan, L.M., Scarsdale, J.N., Walavalkar, N.M., Ginder, G.D., Williams, D.C., 2015. An intrinsically disordered region of methyl-CpG binding domain protein 2 (MBD2) recruits the histone deacetylase core of the NuRD complex. Nucleic Acids Res. 43 (6), 3100–3113. https://doi.org/10.1093/nar/gkv168.

Du, J.E., You, Y.A., Kwon, E.J., Kim, S.M., Lee, J., Han, K.H., Kim, Y.J., 2020. Maternal malnutrition affects hepatic metabolism through decreased hepatic taurine levels and changes in hnf4a methylation. Int. J. Mol. Sci. 21 (23), 1–14. https://doi.org/10.3390/ijms21239060.

Du, G., Yan, Y., Gao, J.F., Guo, C.Y., Shen, X., Lei, X.W., 2023. Therapeutic effect of folic acid combined with decitabine on diabetic mice. Int. J. Ophthalmol. 16 (11), 1766–1772. https://doi.org/10.18240/ijo.2023.11.05.

Ejarque, M., Ceperuelo-Mallafré, V., Serena, C., Maymo-Masip, E., Duran, X., Díaz-Ramos, A., Millan-Scheiding, M., Núñez-Álvarez, Y., Núñez-Roa, C., Gama, P., Garcia-Roves, P.M., Peinado, M.A., Gimble, J.M., Zorzano, A., Vendrell, J., Fernández-Veledo, S., 2019. Adipose tissue mitochondrial dysfunction in human obesity is linked to a specific DNA methylation signature in adipose-derived stem cells. Int. J. Obes. 43 (6), 1256–1268. https://doi.org/10.1038/s41366-018-0219-6.

El Henafy, H.M.A., Ibrahim, M.A., Abd El Aziz, S.A., Gouda, E.M., 2020. Oxidative Stress and DNA methylation in male rat pups provoked by the transplacental and translactational exposure to bisphenol A. Environ. Sci. Pollut. Control Ser. 27 (4), 4513–4519. https://doi.org/10.1007/s11356-019-06553-5.

Fadul, S.M., Arshad, A., Mehmood, R., 2023. CRISPR-based epigenome editing: mechanisms and applications. Epigenomics 15 (21), 1137–1155. https://doi.org/10.2217/epi-2023-0281.

Friedman, S., 1979. The effect of 5-azacytidine on E.coli DNA methylase. Biochem. Biophys. Res. Commun. 89 (4), 1328–1333. https://doi.org/10.1016/0006-291x(79)92154-5.

Frommer, M., E McDonald, L., S Millar, D., M Collis, C., Watt, F., W Grigg, G., L Molloy, P., L Paul, C., 1992. A genomic sequencing protocol that yields a positive display of 5-methylcytosine residues in individual DNA strands. Proc. Natl. Acad. Sci. 89 (5), 1827–1831. https://doi.org/10.1073/pnas.89.5.1827.

Galupa, R., Heard, E., 2018. X-chromosome inactivation: a crossroads between chromosome architecture and gene regulation. Annu. Rev. Genet. 52 (1), 535–566. https://doi.org/10.1146/annurev-genet-120116-024611.

Gao, L., Zhang, Y., Liu, J., Li, X., Sang, Y., Zhou, G., Xue, J., Jing, L., Shi, Z., Wei, J., Lu, X., Zhou, X., 2022. Fat mass and obesity-associated gene (FTO) hypermethylation induced by decabromodiphenyl ethane causing cardiac dysfunction via glucolipid metabolism disorder. Ecotoxicol. Environ. Saf. 237, 113534. https://doi.org/10.1016/j.ecoenv.2022.113534.

Genger, R.K., Kovac, K.A., Dennis, E.S., Peacock, W.J., Finnegan, E.J., 1999. Multiple DNA methyltransferase genes in *Arabidopsis thaliana*. Plant Mol. Biol. 41 (2), 269–278. https://doi.org/10.1023/A:1006347010369.

Ghosh, S., Dhar, S., Bhattacharjee, S., Bhattacharjee, P., 2023. Contribution of environmental, genetic and epigenetic factors to obesity-related metabolic syndrome. Nucleus (Karachi) 66 (2), 215–237. https://doi.org/10.1007/s13237-023-00420-y.

Guo, W., Chen, J., Yang, Y., Zhu, J., Wu, J., 2016. Epigenetic programming of Dnmt3a mediated by AP2α is required for granting preadipocyte the ability to differentiate. Cell Death Dis. 7 (12), e2496. https://doi.org/10.1038/cddis.2016.378.

Hagemann, E., Silva, D.T., Davis, J.A., Gibson, L.Y., Prescott, S.L., 2021. Developmental Origins of Health and Disease (DOHaD): the importance of life-course and transgenerational approaches. Paediatr. Respir. Rev. 40, 3–9. https://doi.org/10.1016/j.prrv.2021.05.005.

Hall, E., Dekker Nitert, M., Volkov, P., Malmgren, S., Mulder, H., Bacos, K., Ling, C., 2018. The effects of high glucose exposure on global gene expression and DNA methylation in human pancreatic islets. Mol. Cell. Endocrinol. 472, 57–67. https://doi.org/10.1016/j.mce.2017.11.019.

Hark, A.T., Schoenherr, C.J., Katz, D.J., Ingram, R.S., Levorse, J.M., Tilghman, S. M., 2000. CTCF mediates methylation-sensitive enhancer-blocking activity at the H19/Igf2 locus. Nature 405 (6785), 486–489. https://doi.org/10.1038/35013106.

He, S., Wang, F., Zhang, Y., Chen, J., Liang, L., Li, Y., Zhang, M., Yang, X., Pang, H., Li, Y., Huang, X., Qin, D., Pei, D., Sun, H., Zheng, H., 2019. Hemi-methylated CpG sites connect Dnmt1-knockdown-induced and Tet1-induced DNA demethylation during somatic cell reprogramming. Cell Discov. 5 (1). https://doi.org/10.1038/s41421-018-0074-6.

Heo, J., Lim, J., Lee, S., Jeong, J., Kang, H., Kim, Y.H., Kang, J.W., Yu, H.Y., Jeong, E.M., Kim, K., Kucia, M., Waigel, S.J., Zacharias, W., Chen, Y., Kim, I.-G., Ratajczak, M.Z., Shin, D.-M., 2017. Sirt1 regulates DNA methylation and differentiation potential of embryonic stem cells by antagonizing Dnmt3l. Cell Rep. 18 (8), 1930–1945. https://doi.org/10.1016/j.celrep.2017.01.074.

Honma, K., Kamikubo, M., Mochizuki, K., Goda, T., 2017. Insulin-induced inhibition of gluconeogenesis genes, including glutamic pyruvic transaminase 2, is associated with reduced histone acetylation in a human liver cell line. Metabolism 71, 118–124. https://doi.org/10.1016/j.metabol.2017.03.009.

Hor, K., Dearden, L., Herzstein, E., Ozanne, S., Hardingham, G., Drake, A.J., 2025. Maternal high fat and high sugar diet impacts on key DNA methylation enzymes in offspring brain in a sex-specific manner. J. Neuroendocrinol. 37 (8). https://doi.org/10.1111/jne.70046. Available from: http://onlinelibrary.wiley.com/journal/10.1111/(ISSN)1365-2826.

Horiguchi, M., Turudome, Y., Ushijima, K., 2021. The transplantation resistance of type II diabetes mellitus adipose-derived stem cells is due to G6PC and IGF1 genes related to the foxo signaling pathway. Int. J. Mol. Sci. 22 (12). https://doi.org/10.3390/ijms22126595. Available from: https://www.mdpi.com/1422-0067/22/12/6595/pdf.

Hosseini, H., Teimouri, M., Shabani, M., Koushki, M., Babaei Khorzoughi, R., Namvarjah, F., Izadi, P., Meshkani, R., 2020. Resveratrol alleviates non-alcoholic fatty liver disease through epigenetic modification of the Nrf2 signaling pathway. Int. J. Biochem. Cell Biol. 119. https://doi.org/10.1016/j.biocel.2019.105667. Available from: http://www.elsevier.com/locate/biocel.

Houshmand-Oeregaard, A., Hansen, N.S., Hjort, L., Kelstrup, L., Broholm, C., Mathiesen, E.R., Clausen, T.D., Damm, P., Vaag, A., 2017. Differential adipokine DNA methylation and gene expression in subcutaneous adipose tissue from adult offspring of women with diabetes in pregnancy. Clin. Epigenet. 9 (1). https://doi.org/10.1186/s13148-017-0338-2. Available from: http://www.springer.com/biomed/human+genetics/journal/13148.

Howard, T.D., Mathias, R.A., Seeds, M.C., Herrington, D.M., Hixson, J.E., Shimmin, L.C., Hawkins, G.A., Sellers, M., Ainsworth, H.C., Sergeant, S., Miller, L.R., Chilton, F.H., 2014. DNA methylation in an enhancer region of the FADS cluster is associated with FADS activity in human liver. PLoS One 9 (5). https://doi.org/10.1371/journal.pone.0097510. Available from: http://www.plosone.org/article/fetchObject.action?uri=info%3Adoi%2F10.1371%2Fjournal.pone.0097510&representation=PDF.

Howe, C.G., Cox, B., Fore, R., Jungius, J., Kvist, T., Lent, S., Miles, H.E., Salas, L. A., Rifas-Shiman, S., Starling, A.P., Yousefi, P., Ladd-Acosta, C., Baccarelli, A., Binder, E.B., Chatzi, V.L., Czamara, D., Dabelea, D., DeMeo, D.L., Ghantous, A., Herceg, Z., Kajantie, E., Lahti, J.M.T., Lawlor, D.

A., Litonjua, A., Nawrot, T.S., Nohr, E.A., Oken, E., Pizzi, C., Plusquin, M., Räikkönen, K., Relton, C.L., Sharp, G.C., Sørensen, T.I.A., Sunyer, J., Vrijheid, M., Zhang, W., Hivert, M.F., Breton, C.V., 2020. Maternal gestational diabetes mellitus and newborn DNA Methylation: findings from the pregnancy and childhood epigenetics consortium. Diabetes Care 43 (1), 98–105. https://doi.org/10.2337/dc19-0524.

Hunter, D.J., James, L.S., Hussey, B., Ferguson, R.A., Lindley, M.R., Mastana, S. S., 2023. Impacts of eccentric resistance exercise on DNA methylation of candidate genes for inflammatory cytokines in skeletal muscle and leukocytes of healthy males. Genes 14 (2). https://doi.org/10.3390/genes14020478. Available from: http://www.mdpi.com/journal/genes/.

Indumathi, B., Oruganti, S.S., Sreenu, B., Kutala, V.K., 2022. Association of promoter methylation and expression of inflammatory genes IL-6 and TNF-α with the risk of coronary artery disease in diabetic and obese subjects among Asian Indians. Indian J. Clin. Biochem. 37 (1), 29–39. https://doi.org/10.1007/s12291-020-00932-3.

Ismail, J.N., Ghannam, M., Al Outa, A., Frey, F., Shirinian, M., 2020. Ten-eleven translocation proteins and their role beyond DNA demethylation–what we can learn from the fly. Epigenetics 15 (11), 1139–1150. https://doi.org/10.1080/15592294.2020.1767323.

Jackson, J.P., Lindroth, A.M., Cao, X., Jacobsen, S.E., 2002. Control of CpNpG DNA methylation by the KRYPTONITE histone H3 methyltransferase. Nature 416 (6880), 556–560. https://doi.org/10.1038/nature731.

Jin, L., Wang, D., Zhang, J., Liu, P., Wang, Y., Lin, Y., Liu, C., Han, Z., Long, K., Li, D., Jiang, Y., Li, G., Zhang, Y., Bai, J., Li, X., Li, J., Lu, L., Kong, F., Wang, X., Li, H., Huang, Z., Ma, J., Fan, X., Shen, L., Zhu, L., Jiang, Y., Tang, G., Feng, B., Zeng, B., Ge, L., Li, X., Tang, Q., Zhang, Z., Li, M., 2023. Dynamic chromatin architecture of the porcine adipose tissues with weight gain and loss. Nat. Commun. 14 (1). https://doi.org/10.1038/s41467-023-39191-0.

Johnson, T.B., Coghill, R.D., 1925. Researches on pyrimidines. C111. The discovery of 5-methyl-cytosine in tuberculinic acid, the nucleic acid of the tubercle bacillus. J. Am. Chem. Soc. 47 (11), 2838–2844. https://doi.org/10.1021/ja01688a030.

Jones, P.A., M Taylor, S., Mohandas, T., J Shapiro, L., 1982. Cell cycle-specific reactivation of an inactive X-chromosome locus by 5-azadeoxycytidine. Proc. Natl. Acad. Sci. 79 (4), 1215–1219. https://doi.org/10.1073/pnas.79.4.1215.

Kadakia, R., Zheng, Y., Zhang, Z., Zhang, W., Hou, L., Josefson, J.L., 2017. Maternal pre-pregnancy BMI downregulates neonatal cord blood LEP methylation. Pediatric Obesity 12 (S1), 57–64. https://doi.org/10.1111/ijpo.12204.

Kadayifci, F.Z., Haggard, S., Jeon, S., Ranard, K., Tao, D., Pan, Y.X., 2019. Early-life programming of type 2 diabetes mellitus: understanding the association between epigenetics/genetics and environmental factors. Curr. Genom. 20 (6), 453–463. https://doi.org/10.2174/1389202920666191009110724.

Kameswaran, V., Golson, M.L., Ramos-Rodríguez, M., Ou, K., Wang, Y.J., Zhang, J., Pasquali, L., Kaestner, K.H., 2018. The dysregulation of the DLK1-MEg3 locus in islets from patients with type 2 diabetes is mimicked by targeted epimutation of its promoter with TALE-DNMT constructs. Diabetes 67 (9), 1807–1815. https://doi.org/10.2337/db17-0682.

Kanholm, T., Rentia, U., Hadley, M., Karlow, J.A., Cox, O.L., Diab, N., Bendall, M.L., Dawson, T., McDonald, J.I., Xie, W., Crandall, K.A., Burns, K.

H., Baylin, S.B., Easwaran, H., Chiappinelli, K.B., 2023. Oncogenic transformation drives DNA methylation loss and transcriptional activation at transposable element loci. Cancer Res. 83 (15), 2584–2599. https://doi.org/10.1158/0008-5472.CAN-22-3485.

Karin, M., Shalapour, S., 2022. Regulation of antitumor immunity by inflammation-induced epigenetic alterations. Cell. Mol. Immunol. 19 (1), 59–66. https://doi.org/10.1038/s41423-021-00756-y.

Khan, S., Jena, G., 2015. The role of butyrate, A histone deacetylase inhibitor in diabetes mellitus: experimental evidence for therapeutic intervention. Epigenomics 7 (4), 669–680. https://doi.org/10.2217/epi.15.20.

Kim, Y.C., Seok, S., Zhang, Y., Ma, J., Kong, B., Guo, G., Kemper, B., Kemper, J. K., 2020. Intestinal FGF15/19 physiologically repress hepatic lipogenesis in the late fed-state by activating SHP and DNMT3A. Nat. Commun. 11 (1). https://doi.org/10.1038/s41467-020-19803-9. Available from: http://www.nature.com/ncomms/index.html.

King-Himmelreich, T.S., Schramm, S., Wolters, M.C., Schmetzer, J., Möser, C.V., Knothe, C., Resch, E., Peil, J., Geisslinger, G., Niederberger, E., 2016. The impact of endurance exercise on global and AMPK gene-specific DNA methylation. Biochem. Biophys. Res. Commun. 474 (2), 284–290. https://doi.org/10.1016/j.bbrc.2016.04.078.

Kirchner, H., Sinha, I., Gao, H., Ruby, M.A., Schönke, M., Lindvall, J.M., Barrès, R., Krook, A., Näslund, E., Dahlman-Wright, K., Zierath, J.R., 2016. Altered DNA methylation of glycolytic and lipogenic genes in liver from obese and type 2 diabetic patients. Mol. Metabol. 5 (3), 171–183. https://doi.org/10.1016/j.molmet.2015.12.004.

Klemm, S.L., Shipony, Z., Greenleaf, W.J., 2019. Chromatin accessibility and the regulatory epigenome. Nat. Rev. Genet. 20 (4), 207–220. https://doi.org/10.1038/s41576-018-0089-8.

Krause, C., Geißler, C., Tackenberg, H., El Gammal, A.T., Wolter, S., Spranger, J., Mann, O., Lehnert, H., Kirchner, H., 2020. Multi-layered epigenetic regulation of IRS2 expression in the liver of obese individuals with type 2 diabetes. Diabetologia 63 (10), 2182–2193. https://doi.org/10.1007/s00125-020-05212-6. Available from: link.springer.de/link/service/journals/00125/index.htm.

Kriaucionis, S., Heintz, N., 2009. The nuclear DNA base 5-hydroxymethylcytosine is present in purkinje neurons and the brain. Science 324 (5929), 929–930. https://doi.org/10.1126/science.1169786.

Kruczek, I., Doerfler, W., 1983. Expression of the chloramphenicol acetyltransferase gene in mammalian cells under the control of adenovirus type 12 promoters: effect of promoter methylation on gene expression. Proc. Natl. Acad. Sci. 80 (24), 7586–7590. https://doi.org/10.1073/pnas.80.24.7586.

Kuroda, A., Rauch, T.A., Todorov, I., Ku, H.T., Al-Abdullah, I.H., Kandeel, F., Mullen, Y., Pfeifer, G.P., Ferreri, K., 2009. Insulin gene expression is regulated by DNA methylation. PLoS One 4 (9). https://doi.org/10.1371/journal.pone.0006953. Available from: http://www.plosone.org/article/fetchObjectAttachment.action?uri=info%3Adoi%2F10.1371%2Fjournal.pone.0006953&representation=PDF.

Lacagnina, S., 2020. The developmental origins of health and disease (DOHaD). Am. J. Lifestyle Med. 14 (1), 47–50. https://doi.org/10.1177/1559827619879694.

Laker, R.C., Lillard, T.S., Okutsu, M., Zhang, M., Hoehn, K.L., Connelly, J.J., Yan, Z., 2014. Exercise prevents maternal high-fat diet-induced hypermethylation of the Pgc-1α gene and age-dependent metabolic dysfunction in the offspring. Diabetes 63 (5), 1605–1611. https://doi.org/10.2337/db13-1614.

Lauster, R., Trautner, T.A., Noyer-Weidner, M., 1989. Cytosine-specific type II DNA methyltransferases. A conserved enzyme core with variable target-recognizing domains. J. Mol. Biol. 206 (2), 305–312. https://doi.org/10.1016/0022-2836(89)90480-4.

Lee, J.T., Bartolomei, M.S., 2013. X-inactivation, imprinting, and long noncoding RNAs in health and disease. Cell 152 (6), 1308–1323. https://doi.org/10.1016/j.cell.2013.02.016.

Lee, J.H., Park, S.J., Nakai, K., 2017. Differential landscape of non-CpG methylation in embryonic stem cells and neurons caused by DNMT3s. Sci. Rep. 7 (1). https://doi.org/10.1038/s41598-017-11800-1. Available from: www.nature.com/srep/index.html.

Li, E., Bestor, T.H., Jaenisch, R., 1992. Targeted mutation of the DNA methyltransferase gene results in embryonic lethality. Cell 69 (6), 915–926. https://doi.org/10.1016/0092-8674(92)90611-F.

Li, S., Hursting, S.D., Davis, B.J., McLachlan, J.A., Barrett, J.C., 2003. Academy of Sciences United States Environmental exposure, DNA methylation, and gene regulation: lessons from diethylstilbesterol-induced cancers. Ann. N. Y. Acad. Sci. 983, 161–169. https://doi.org/10.1111/j.1749-6632.2003.tb05971.x.

Li, Y.Y., Tang, D., Du, Y.L., Cao, C.Y., Nie, Y.Q., Cao, J., Zhou, Y.J., 2018. Fatty liver mediated by peroxisome proliferator-activated receptor-α DNA methylation can be reversed by a methylation inhibitor and curcumin. J. Dig. Dis. 19 (7), 421–430. https://doi.org/10.1111/1751-2980.12610. Available from: http://onlinelibrary.wiley.com/journal/10.1111/(ISSN)1751-2980.

Li, Q., Zhang, H., Zou, J., Mai, H., Su, D., Feng, X., Feng, D., 2019. Bisphenol A exposure induces cholesterol synthesis and hepatic steatosis in C57BL/6 mice by down-regulating the DNA methylation levels of SREBP-2. Food Chem. Toxicol. 133, 110786. https://doi.org/10.1016/j.fct.2019.110786.

Li, Y., Pollock, C.A., Saad, S., 2021. Aberrant dna methylation mediates the transgenerational risk of metabolic and chronic disease due to maternal obesity and overnutrition. Genes 12 (11). https://doi.org/10.3390/genes12111653. Available from: https://www.mdpi.com/2073-4425/12/11/1653/pdf.

Li, W., Gao, R., Ding, Y., Chen, X., Liu, X., He, J., Li, F., Long, J., Lu, S., Yang, C., Wang, Y., 2022. Imbalance hepatic metabolism homeostasis in the F1 generation of endometrial DNMT3B conditional knockout female mice. Front. Physiol. 13. https://doi.org/10.3389/fphys.2022.1042449.

Liang, F., Quan, Y., Wu, A., Chen, Y., Xu, R., Zhu, Y., Xiong, J., 2021. Insulin-resistance and depression cohort data mining to identify nutraceutical related DNA methylation biomarker for type 2 diabetes. Genes Dis. 8 (5), 669–676. https://doi.org/10.1016/j.gendis.2020.01.013.

Liu, R., Kim, K.Y., Jung, Y.W., Park, I.H., 2016. Dnmt1 regulates the myogenic lineage specification of muscle stem cells. Sci. Rep. 6. https://doi.org/10.1038/srep35355. Available from: www.nature.com/srep/index.html.

Liu, Y., He, T., Li, Z., Sun, Z., Wang, S., Shen, H., Hou, L., Li, S., Wei, Y., Zhuo, B., Li, S., Zhou, C., Guo, H., Zhang, R., Li, B., 2023. TET2 is recruited by CREB to promote Cebpb, Cebpa, and Pparg transcription by facilitating hydroxymethylation during adipocyte differentiation. iScience 26 (11), 108312. https://doi.org/10.1016/j.isci.2023.108312.

Liu, Q., Li, X., Fan, J., Chen, W., 2025. # 662 the DNA methyltransferase inhibitor 5-azacytidine alleviates podocyte injury by reversing DNA hypermethylation-mediated inhibition of INSR in podocytes of diabetic db/db mice. Nephrol. Dial. Transplant. 40 (Suppl. ment_3), gfaf116–0382.
Łoboś, P., Regulska-Ilow, B., 2021. Link between methyl nutrients and the DNA methylation process in the course of selected diseases in adults. Rocz. Panstw. Zakl. Hig. 72 (2), 123–136. https://doi.org/10.32394/rpzh.2021.0157.
Lochmann, T.L., Thomas, R.R., Bennett, J.P., Taylor, S.M., 2015. Epigenetic modifications of the PGC-1α promoter during exercise induced expression in mice. PLoS One 10 (6). https://doi.org/10.1371/journal.pone.0129647. Available from: http://www.plosone.org/article/fetchObject.action?uri=info:doi/10.1371/journal.pone.0129647&representation=PDF.
Long, H.K., King, H.W., Patient, R.K., Odom, D.T., Klose, R.J., 2016. Protection of CpG islands from DNA methylation is DNA-encoded and evolutionarily conserved. Nucleic Acids Res. 44 (14), 6693–6706. https://doi.org/10.1093/nar/gkw258.
Lyu, S.Y., Xiao, W., Cui, G.Z., Yu, C., Liu, H., Lyu, M., Kuang, Q.Y., Xiao, E.H., Luo, Y.H., 2023. Role and mechanism of DNA methylation and its inhibitors in hepatic fibrosis. Front. Genet. 14. https://doi.org/10.3389/fgene.2023.1124330. Available from: https://www.frontiersin.org/journals/genetics#.
Małodobra-Mazur, M., Cierzniak, A., Kaliszewski, K., Dobosz, T., 2021. PPARG hypermethylation as the first epigenetic modification in newly onset insulin resistance in human adipocytes. Genes 12 (6), 889. https://doi.org/10.3390/genes12060889.
Martínez-Montoro, J.I., Martín-Núñez, G.M., González-Jiménez, A., Garrido-Sánchez, L., Moreno-Indias, I., Tinahones, F.J., 2024. Interactions between the gut microbiome and DNA methylation patterns in blood and visceral adipose tissue in subjects with different metabolic characteristics. J. Transl. Med. 22 (1). https://doi.org/10.1186/s12967-024-05746-y. Available from: https://translational-medicine.biomedcentral.com.
Mattei, A.L., Bailly, N., Meissner, A., 2022. DNA methylation: a historical perspective. Trends Genet. 38 (7), 676–707. https://doi.org/10.1016/j.tig.2022.03.010.
Meissner, A., Mikkelsen, T.S., Gu, H., Wernig, M., Hanna, J., Sivachenko, A., Zhang, X., Bernstein, B.E., Nusbaum, C., Jaffe, D.B., Gnirke, A., Jaenisch, R., Lander, E.S., 2008. Genome-scale DNA methylation maps of pluripotent and differentiated cells. Nature 454 (7205), 766–770. https://doi.org/10.1038/nature07107.
Miguel-Escalada, I., Bonàs-Guarch, S., Cebola, I., Ponsa-Cobas, J., Mendieta-Esteban, J., Atla, G., Javierre, B.M., Rolando, D.M.Y., Farabella, I., Morgan, C. C., García-Hurtado, J., Beucher, A., Morán, I., Pasquali, L., Ramos-Rodríguez, M., Appel, E.V.R., Linneberg, A., Gjesing, A.P., Witte, D.R., Pedersen, O., Grarup, N., Ravassard, P., Torrents, D., Mercader, J.M., Piemonti, L., Berney, T., de Koning, E.J.P., Kerr-Conte, J., Pattou, F., Fedko, I.O., Groop, L., Prokopenko, I., Hansen, T., Marti-Renom, M.A., Fraser, P., Ferrer, J., 2019. Human pancreatic islet three-dimensional chromatin architecture provides insights into the genetics of type 2 diabetes. Nat. Genet. 51 (7), 1137–1148. https://doi.org/10.1038/s41588-019-0457-0.
Miller, O., Shakespeare-Finch, J., Bruenig, D., Mehta, D., 2020. DNA methylation of NR3C1 and FKBP5 is associated with posttraumatic stress disorder, posttraumatic growth, and resilience. Psychol. Trauma, Theory Res. Pract. Pol. 12 (7), 750–755. https://doi.org/10.1037/tra0000574.

Montoya-Williams, D., Quinlan, J., Clukay, C., Rodney, N.C., Kertes, D.A., Mulligan, C.J., 2018. Associations between maternal prenatal stress, methylation changes in IGF1 and IGF2, and birth weight. J. Dev. Origins Health Dis. 9 (2), 215–222. https://doi.org/10.1017/s2040174417000800.

Moore, L.D., Le, T., Fan, G., 2013. DNA methylation and its basic function. Neuropsychopharmacology 38 (1), 23–38. https://doi.org/10.1038/npp.2012.112.

Morrison, A.J., 2020. Chromatin-remodeling links metabolic signaling to gene expression. Mol. Metabol. 38, 100973. https://doi.org/10.1016/j.molmet.2020.100973.

Nerlich, A., Janze, N., Goethe, R., 2021. Analysis of Il36a induction by C/EBPβ via a half-CRE•C/EBP element in murine macrophages in dependence of its CpG methylation level. Gene Immun. 22 (7–8), 313–321. https://doi.org/10.1038/s41435-021-00153-5.

Ng, H.H., Zhang, Y., Hendrich, B., Johnson, C.A., Turner, B.M., Erdjument-Bromage, H., Tempst, P., Reinberg, D., Bird, A., 1999. MBD2 is a transcriptional repressor belonging to the MeCP1 histone deacetylase complex. Nat. Genet. 23 (1), 58–61. https://doi.org/10.1038/12659.

Niwa, O., Yokota, Y., Ishida, H., Sugahara, T., 1983. Independent mechanisms involved in suppression of the moloney leukemia virus genome during differentiation of murine teratocarcinoma cells. Cell 32 (4), 1105–1113. https://doi.org/10.1016/0092-8674(83)90294-5.

Okano, M., Bell, D.W., Haber, D.A., Li, E., 1999. DNA methyltransferases Dnmt3a and Dnmt3b are essential for de novo methylation and mammalian development. Cell 99 (3), 247–257. https://doi.org/10.1016/S0092-8674(00)81656-6.

Osório, J., 2014. Looking at the epigenetic link between obesity and its consequences—the promise of EWAS. Nat. Rev. Endocrinol. 10 (5). https://doi.org/10.1038/nrendo.2014.42, 249–249.

Pacaud, R., Sery, Q., Oliver, L., Vallette, F.M., Tost, J., Cartron, P.F., 2014. DNMT3L interacts with transcription factors to target DNMT3L/DNMT3B to specific DNA sequences: role of the DNMT3L/DNMT3B/p65-NFκB complex in the (de-)methylation of TRAF1. Biochimie 104 (1), 36–49. https://doi.org/10.1016/j.biochi.2014.05.005.

Paluvai, H., Shanmukha, K.D., Tyedmers, J., Backs, J., 2023. Insights into the function of HDAC3 and NCoR1/NCoR2 co-repressor complex in metabolic diseases. Front. Mol. Biosci. 10. https://doi.org/10.3389/fmolb.2023.1190094.

Park, Y.J., Lee, S., Lim, S., Nahmgoong, H., Ji, Y., Young Huh, J., Alfadda, A.A., Kim, S., Kim, J.B., 2021. DNMT1 maintains metabolic fitness of adipocytes through acting as an epigenetic safeguard of mitochondrial dynamics. Proc. Natl. Acad. Sci. 118 (11). https://doi.org/10.1073/pnas.2021073118.

Park, J., Lee, D.H., Ham, S., Oh, J., Noh, J.R., Lee, Y.K., Park, Y.J., Lee, G., Han, S. M., Han, J.S., Kim, Y.Y., Jeon, Y.G., Nahmgoong, H., Shin, K.C., Kim, S.M., Choi, S.H., Lee, C.H., Park, J., Roh, T.Y., Kim, S., Kim, J.B., 2022. Targeted erasure of DNA methylation by TET3 drives adipogenic reprogramming and differentiation. Nat. Metab. 4 (7), 918–931. https://doi.org/10.1038/s42255-022-00597-7.

Parveen, N., Wang, J.K., Bhattacharya, S., Cuala, J., Rajkumar, M.S., Butler, A.E., Wu, X., Shih, H.P., Georgia, S.K., Dhawan, S., 2023. DNA methylation–dependent restriction of tyrosine hydroxylase contributes to pancreatic β-cell heterogeneity. Diabetes 72 (5), 575–589. https://doi.org/10.2337/db22-0506.

Pennacchio, L.A., 2003. Insights from human/mouse genome comparisons. Mamm. Genome 14 (7), 429–436. https://doi.org/10.1007/s00335-002-4001-1.
Popov, D.V., Lysenko, E.A., Makhnovskii, P.A., Kurochkina, N.S., Vinogradova, O.L., 2017. Regulation of PPARGC1A gene expression in trained and untrained human skeletal muscle. Feder. Physiol. Rep. 5 (23). https://doi.org/10.14814/phy2.13543. Available from: http://physoc.onlinelibrary.wiley.com/hub/journal/10.1002/(ISSN)2051-817X/.
Poursafa, P., Kamali, Z., Fraszczyk, E., Boezen, H.M., Vaez, A., Snieder, H., 2022. DNA methylation: a potential mediator between air pollution and metabolic syndrome. Clin. Epigenet. 14 (1). https://doi.org/10.1186/s13148-022-01301-y. Available from: http://www.springer.com/biomed/human+genetics/journal/13148.
Rajagopal, G., Bhaskaran, R.S., Karundevi, B., 2019. Developmental exposure to DEHP alters hepatic glucose uptake and transcriptional regulation of GLUT2 in rat male offspring. Toxicology 413, 56–64. https://doi.org/10.1016/j.tox.2018.12.004.
Remely, M., Ferk, F., Sterneder, S., Setayesh, T., Roth, S., Kepcija, T., Noorizadeh, R., Rebhan, I., Greunz, M., Beckmann, J., Wagner, K.H., Knasmüller, S., Haslberger, A.G., 2017. EGCG prevents high fat diet-induced changes in gut microbiota, decreases of DNA strand breaks, and changes in expression and DNA methylation of Dnmt1 and MLH1 in C57BL/6J male mice. Oxid. Med. Cell. Longev. 2017. https://doi.org/10.1155/2017/3079148. Available from: http://www.hindawi.com/journals/oximed/.
Ren, J., Cheng, Y., Ming, Z.H., Dong, X.Y., Zhou, Y.Z., Ding, G.L., Pang, H.Y., Rahman, T.U., Akbar, R., Huang, H.F., Sheng, J.Z., 2018. Intrauterine hyperglycemia exposure results in intergenerational inheritance via DNA methylation reprogramming on F1 PGCs. Epigenet. Chromat. 11 (1). https://doi.org/10.1186/s13072-018-0192-2. Available from: http://www.epigeneticsandchromatin.com/.
Ribel-Madsen, R., Fraga, M.F., Jacobsen, S., Bork-Jensen, J., Lara, E., Calvanese, V., Fernandez, A.F., Friedrichsen, M., Vind, B.F., Højlund, K., Beck-Nielsen, H., Esteller, M., Allan, V., Poulsen, P., Dahlman, I.A., 2012. Genome-wide analysis of DNA methylation differences in muscle and fat from monozygotic twins discordant for type 2 diabetes. PLoS One 7 (12), e51302. https://doi.org/10.1371/journal.pone.0051302.
Riggs, A.D., 2004. X inactivation, differentiation, and DNA methylation. Cytogenet. Genome Res. 14 (1), 9–25. https://doi.org/10.1159/000130315.
Rui, J., Deng, S., Perdigoto, A.L., Ponath, G., Kursawe, R., Lawlor, N., Sumida, T., Levine-Ritterman, M., Stitzel, M.L., Pitt, D., Lu, J., Herold, K.C., 2021. Tet2 controls the responses of β cells to inflammation in autoimmune diabetes. Nat. Commun. 12 (1). https://doi.org/10.1038/s41467-021-25367-z. Available from: http://www.nature.com/ncomms/index.html.
Sae-Lee, C., de Biasi, J., Robinson, N., Barrow, T.M., Mathers, J.C., Koutsidis, G., Byun, H.M., 2020. DNA methylation patterns of LINE-1 and Alu for pre-symptomatic dementia in type 2 diabetes. PLoS One 15 (6). https://doi.org/10.1371/journal.pone.0234578. Available from: https://journals.plos.org/plosone/article/file?id=10.1371/journal.pone.0234578&type=printable.
Sager, R., Kitchin, R., 1975. Selective Silencing of Eukaryotic DNA: a molecular basis is proposed for programmed inactivation or loss of eukaryotic DNA. Science 189 (4201), 426–433.
Sala, P., De Miranda Torrinhas, R.S.M., Fonseca, D.C., Ravacci, G.R., Waitzberg, D.L., Giannella-Neto, D., 2017. Tissue-specific methylation profile in obese patients with type 2 diabetes before and after Roux-en-Y

gastric bypass. Diabetol. Metab. Syndr. 9 (1). https://doi.org/10.1186/s13098-017-0214-4. Available from: http://www.dmsjournal.com/.

Salmeron-Barcenas, E.G., Zacapala-Gomez, A.E., Torres-Rojas, F.I., Antonio-Vejar, V., Ávila-López, P.A., Banos-Hernandez, C.J., Jimenez-Wences, H., 2023. TET enzymes and 5hmC levels in carcinogenesis and progression of breast cancer: potential therapeutic targets. Int. J. Mol. Sci. 25 (1), 272.

Sanches, P.H.G., de Melo, N.C., Porcari, A.M., de Carvalho, L.M., 2024. Integrating molecular perspectives: strategies for comprehensive multi-omics integrative data analysis and machine learning applications in transcriptomics, proteomics, and metabolomics. Biology 13 (11). https://doi.org/10.3390/biology13110848. Available from: www.mdpi.com/journal/biology.

Saxonov, S., Berg, P., Brutlag, D.L., 2006. A genome-wide analysis of CpG dinucleotides in the human genome distinguishes two distinct classes of promoters. Proc. Natl. Acad. Sci. 103 (5), 1412–1417. https://doi.org/10.1073/pnas.0510310103.

Selvaraji, S., Lim, K.L., Lai, M.K.P., Chen, C., Arumugam, T.V., 2021. Intermittent fasting: a potential modifier of DNA methylation landscape in a chronic cerebral hypoperfusion mouse model of vascular dementia. Alzheimer's Dement. 17, e052516.

Sharples, A.P., Seaborne, R.A., 2019. Exercise and DNA methylation in skeletal muscle. In: Sports, Exercise, and Nutritional Genomics. Academic Press, pp. 211–229.

Shayevitch, R., Askayo, D., Keydar, I., Ast, G., 2018. The importance of DNA methylation of exons on alternative splicing. RNA 24 (10), 1351–1362. https://doi.org/10.1261/rna.064865.117.

Singer, J., Roberts-Ems, J., Riggs, A.D., 1979. Methylation of mouse liver DNA studied by means of the restriction enzymes Msp I and Hpa II. Science 203 (4384), 1019–1021. https://doi.org/10.1126/science.424726.

Stenz, L., Schechter, D.S., Serpa, S.R., Paoloni-Giacobino, A., 2018. Intergenerational transmission of dna methylation signatures associated with early life stress. Curr. Genom. 19 (8), 665–675. https://doi.org/10.2174/1389202919666171229145656.

Świątowy, W.J., Drzewiecka, H., Kliber, M., Sąsiadek, M., Karpiński, P., Pławski, A., Jagodziński, P.P., 2021. Physical activity and DNA methylation in humans. Int. J. Mol. Sci. 22 (23). https://doi.org/10.3390/ijms222312989. Available from: https://www.mdpi.com/1422-0067/22/23/12989/pdf.

Tahiliani, M., Koh, K.P., Shen, Y., Pastor, W.A., Bandukwala, H., Brudno, Y., Agarwal, S., Iyer, L.M., Liu, D.R., Aravind, L., Rao, A., 2009. Conversion of 5-methylcytosine to 5-hydroxymethylcytosine in mammalian DNA by MLL partner TET1. Science 324 (5929), 930–935. https://doi.org/10.1126/science.1170116.

Tajima, S., Suetake, I., Takeshita, K., Nakagawa, A., Kimura, H., Song, J., 2022. Domain Structure of the Dnmt1, Dnmt3a, and Dnmt3b DNA Methyltransferases, 1389. Springer Science and Business Media LLC, pp. 45–68. https://doi.org/10.1007/978-3-031-11454-0_3.

Tamaru, H., Selker, E.U., 2001. A histone H3 methyltransferase controls DNA methylation in Neurospora crassa. Nature 414 (6861), 277–283.

Tran, R.K., Henikoff, J.G., Zilberman, D., Ditt, R.F., Jacobsen, S.E., Henikoff, S., 2005. DNA methylation profiling identifies CG methylation clusters in Arabidopsis genes. Curr. Biol. 15 (2), 154–159. https://doi.org/10.1016/j.cub.2005.01.008.

Vasileva, F., Hristovski, R., Font-Lladó, R., Georgiev, G., Sacot, A., López-Ros, V., Calleja-González, J., Barretina-Ginesta, J., López-Bermejo, A., Prats-Puig, A., 2024. Physical exercise–induced DNA methylation in disease-related genes in healthy adults—a systematic review with bioinformatic analysis. J. Strength Condit Res. 38 (2), 384–393. https://doi.org/10.1519/JSC.0000000000004686.

Vavouri, T., Lehner, B., 2012. Human genes with CpG island promoters have a distinct transcription-associated chromatin organization. Genome Biol. 13 (11). https://doi.org/10.1186/gb-2012-13-11-r110.

Volberg, V., Yousefi, P., Huen, K., Harley, K., Eskenazi, B., Holland, N., 2017. CpG Methylation across the adipogenic PPARγ gene and its relationship with birthweight and child BMI at 9 years. BMC Med. Genet. 18 (1). https://doi.org/10.1186/s12881-016-0365-4.

Vongs, A., Kakutani, T., Martienssen, R.A., Richards, E.J., 1993. *Arabidopsis thaliana* DNA methylation mutants. Science 260 (5116), 1926–1928.

Watson, J.D., Crick, F.H.C., 1953. Molecular structure of nucleic acids: a structure for deoxyribose nucleic acid. Nature 171 (4356), 737–738. https://doi.org/10.1038/171737a0.

Waziry, R., Ryan, C.P., Corcoran, D.L., Huffman, K.M., Kobor, M.S., Kothari, M., Graf, G.H., Kraus, V.B., Kraus, W.E., Lin, D.T.S., Pieper, C.F., Ramaker, M.E., Bhapkar, M., Das, S.K., Ferrucci, L., Hastings, W.J., Kebbe, M., Parker, D.C., Racette, S.B., Shalev, I., Schilling, B., Belsky, D.W., 2023. Effect of long-term caloric restriction on DNA methylation measures of biological aging in healthy adults from the CALERIE trial. Nat. Aging 3 (3), 248–257. https://doi.org/10.1038/s43587-022-00357-y.

Weyman-Vela, Sandoval-Carrillo, Salas-Pacheco, Guerrero-Romero, Salas-Leal, Simental-Mendía, 2025. Methylation levels of the LEP, LEPR, and ADIPOQ genes and their association with metabolically healthy obesity. J. Invest. Med.

Willmer, T., Johnson, R., Louw, J., Pheiffer, C., 2018. Blood-based DNA methylation biomarkers for type 2 diabetes: potential for clinical applications. Front. Endocrinol. 9. https://doi.org/10.3389/fendo.2018.00744.

Wrigglesworth, J., Ancelin, M.L., Ritchie, K., Ryan, J., 2019. Association between DNA methylation of the KITLG gene and cortisol levels under stress: a replication study. Stress 22 (1), 162–168. https://doi.org/10.1080/10253890.2018.1519019.

Wu, J., Liu, Y., 2021. The evaluation for CpG island methylation of FASN and SREBP promoter in Mongolian gerbils NAFLD model. Arch. Med. Sci. 1734–1922. https://doi.org/10.5114/aoms/120001.

Wu, X., Zhang, Y., 2017. TET-mediated active DNA demethylation: mechanism, function and beyond. Nat. Rev. Genet. 18 (9), 517–534. https://doi.org/10.1038/nrg.2017.33.

Wu, Y.L., Lin, Z.J., Li, C.C., Lin, X., Shan, S.K., Guo, B., Zheng, M.H., Li, F., Yuan, L.Q., Li, Z.h., 2023. Epigenetic regulation in metabolic diseases: mechanisms and advances in clinical study. Signal Transduct. Targeted Ther. 8 (1). https://doi.org/10.1038/s41392-023-01333-7. Available from: https://www.nature.com/sigtrans.

Xu, J.W., Ling, S., Liu, J., 2017. Higher-order chromatin regulation of inflammatory gene expression. Mediat. Inflamm. 2017 (1), 7848591.

Yang, B.T., Dayeh, T.A., Volkov, P.A., Kirkpatrick, C.L., Malmgren, S., Jing, X., Renström, E., Wollheim, C.B., Nitert, M.D., Ling, C., 2012. Increased DNA methylation and decreased expression of PDX-1 in pancreatic islets from patients with type 2 diabetes. Mol. Endocrinol. 26 (7), 1203–1212. https://doi.org/10.1210/me.2012-1004Sweden.

Yu, W., Wang, Z., Zhang, K., Chi, Z., Xu, T., Jiang, D., Chen, S., Li, W., Yang, X., Zhang, X., Wu, Y., Wang, Di, 2019. One-carbon metabolism supports S-adenosylmethionine and histone methylation to drive inflammatory macrophages. Mol. Cell 75 (6), 1147. https://doi.org/10.1016/j.molcel.2019.06.039.

Yu, V., Yong, F., Marta, A., Khadayate, S., Osakwe, A., Bhattacharya, S., Varghese, S.S., Chabosseau, P., Tabibi, S.M., Chen, K., Georgiadou, E., Parveen, N., Suleiman, M., Stamoulis, Z., Marselli, L., De Luca, C., Tesi, M., Ostinelli, G., Delgadillo-Silva, L., Wu, X., Hatanaka, Y., Montoya, A., Elliott, J., Patel, B., Demchenko, N., Whilding, C., Hajkova, P., Shliaha, P., Kramer, H., Ali, Y., Marchetti, P., Sladek, R., Dhawan, S., Withers, D.J., Rutter, G.A., Millership, S.J., 2024. Differential CpG methylation at Nnat in the early establishment of beta cell heterogeneity. Diabetologia 67 (6), 1079–1094. https://doi.org/10.1007/s00125-024-06123-6.

Zeng, H., Li, W., Xia, M., Ge, J., Ma, H., Chen, L., Pan, B., Lin, H., Wang, S., Gao, X., 2024. Longitudinal association of peripheral blood DNA methylation with liver fat content: distinguishing between predictors and biomarkers. Lipids Health Dis. 23 (1). https://doi.org/10.1186/s12944-024-02304-9.

Zheng, K., Lyu, Z., Chen, J., Chen, G., 2024. Guodong chen, 5-hydroxymethylcytosine: far beyond the intermediate of DNA demethylation. Int. J. Mol. Sci. 25 (21), 11780. https://doi.org/10.3390/ijms252111780.

Ziller, M.J., Gu, H., Müller, F., Donaghey, J., Tsai, L.T.Y., Kohlbacher, O., De Jager, P.L., Rosen, E.D., Bennett, D.A., Bernstein, B.E., Gnirke, A., Meissner, A., 2013. Charting a dynamic DNA methylation landscape of the human genome. Nature 500 (7463), 477–481. https://doi.org/10.1038/nature12433.

Zimmerman, J., 2022. Methylation Levels of Genes in the Insulin Signaling Pathway Differentially Altered by Saturated and Polyunsaturated Fatty Acids in Adipogenesis. Master's thesis, Saint Louis University.

Further reading

Lihong, L., Xiuyun, Z., Meihui, Z., Tulian, L., Wenjun, L., Yaqin, Y., Xiaoping, L., 2025. Epigenetic modification of Igf2/H19 imprinting control region regulates PGC-1α/PI3K/AKT2 pathway in a rat model of intrauterine growth restriction. Chin. Med. J.

Liu, J., Lang, G., Shi, J., 2021. Epigenetic regulation of PDX-1 in type 2 diabetes mellitus. Diabetes Metab. Syndr. Obes. 431–442.

4

The central role of histone modifications in metabolic dysfunction

1. Introduction

Histone posttranslational modifications, including acetylation, methylation, phosphorylation, ubiquitination, SUMOylation, crotonylation, citrullination, and ADP-ribosylation, serve as fundamental regulators of chromatin architecture and transcriptional activity. They occur primarily on the N-terminal tails of histone proteins (H2A, H2B, H3, and H4), which form the core structure of nucleosomes around which DNA is wrapped. These modifications collectively constitute a highly coordinated regulatory system often referred to as the "histone code" (Jenuwein and Allis, 2001)." This code determines whether chromatin adopts a relaxed, transcriptionally active state (euchromatin) or a tightly condensed, transcriptionally repressive state (heterochromatin). Crucially, the establishment and removal of histone marks are directly influenced by cellular metabolism, as the enzymes responsible for these modifications depend on metabolic intermediates such as acetyl-CoA, S-adenosylmethionine (SAM), NAD^+, ATP, and crotonyl-CoA (Ye and Tu, 2018). Thus, histone modifications not only regulate metabolic gene expression but are themselves regulated by metabolic flux, forming a bidirectional epigenetic–metabolic interface.

The metabolic sensitivity of histone modifications makes them uniquely positioned to mediate the long-term biological effects of nutritional status, obesity, inflammatory signaling, and environmental stressors. For example, excess caloric intake increases acetyl-CoA levels and promotes histone acetylation at lipogenic genes, driving hepatic steatosis and adipocyte hypertrophy (Assante et al., 2022). Conversely, nutrient deprivation elevates NAD^+ levels, activating sirtuin deacetylases that enhance mitochondrial biogenesis, improve insulin sensitivity, and suppress inflammatory pathways (Purhonen et al., 2018). Similarly,

Metabolic Memory. https://doi.org/10.1016/B978-0-443-44591-0.00010-2

disruptions in one-carbon metabolism, which generates SAM, the universal methyl donor for histone methylation, alter histone methylation patterns that regulate insulin secretion, β-cell identity, adipocyte differentiation, and hepatic lipid metabolism (Yu et al., 2019). Environmental factors such as pollutants, endocrine-disrupting chemicals (EDCs), and circadian misalignment further contribute to histone modification changes that exacerbate metabolic dysfunction (Plunk and Richards, 2020).

Given the central role of histone modifications in metabolic regulation, understanding their biological functions is crucial for deciphering the epigenetic origins of metabolic diseases. Histone modifications act as integrative molecular sensors, translating physiological and environmental cues into stable or dynamic transcriptional programs (Plunk and Richards, 2020). In pancreatic β-cells, histone marks maintain the expression of genes essential for insulin synthesis and secretion, and their dysregulation contributes to β-cell dedifferentiation and exhaustion in T2DM (Chakrabarti et al., 2003). In skeletal muscle, histone modifications govern glucose transport, insulin signaling, mitochondrial biogenesis, and oxidative phosphorylation, processes that become impaired in obesity and insulin resistance (Huang et al., 2025). In the liver, histone marks regulate gluconeogenesis, fatty acid oxidation, lipogenesis and inflammatory signaling while their dysregulation underlies excessive hepatic glucose production and the progression from simple steatosis to NASH and fibrosis (Shi and Qi, 2023). Adipose tissue is similarly affected, where aberrant histone marks disrupt adipogenesis, promote chronic inflammation, and impair lipid storage, reinforcing systemic metabolic dysfunction (Castellano-Castillo et al., 2019). These processes illustrate how epigenetic alterations contribute to disease pathogenesis even in the absence of genetic mutations.

Histone modifications also play a critical role in intergenerational metabolic programming. During pregnancy, the placenta and developing fetus are especially sensitive to metabolic and inflammatory cues (Gao et al., 2025). In gestational diabetes mellitus (GDM), maternal hyperglycemia induces changes in histone acetylation and methylation in placental and fetal tissues, altering nutrient transport, pancreatic development, adipogenesis, and neural appetite regulatory circuits (Yi et al., 2024). These epigenetic marks persist after birth, predisposing offspring to obesity, insulin resistance, and type 2 diabetes later in life, a phenomenon known as intergenerational metabolic memory (Crisóstomo et al., 2021). This highlights how maternal metabolic health exerts long-lasting effects on the next generation through epigenetic mechanisms.

Beyond the direct effects of diet and metabolism, environmental exposures significantly contribute to the epigenetic regulation of metabolic health. Pollutants, EDCs, heavy metals, microplastics, and air particulate matter induce oxidative stress and inflammation, reshaping chromatin landscapes in metabolic tissues (Lehle et al., 2024; Feng et al., 2026). These external agents can increase repressive histone marks at insulin-sensitizing genes, promote acetylation at inflammatory enhancers, and alter histone phosphorylation patterns involved in stress responses (Pedrotti et al., 2019). Circadian disruption, commonly experienced in shift work or irregular sleep patterns, further affects the rhythmic activity of histone acetyltransferases (HATs) and deacetylases, destabilizing daily oscillations of metabolic gene expression and contributing to obesity, fatty liver disease, and metabolic syndrome (González-Suárez and Aguilar-Arnal, 2024). Together, these findings emphasize the profound influence of environmental and lifestyle factors on epigenome stability and metabolic resilience.

Importantly, the reversibility of histone modifications has made them attractive therapeutic targets. Epigenetic therapies have the potential to restore normal gene expression patterns, improve insulin sensitivity, enhance mitochondrial function, and reduce inflammation. HDAC inhibitors, for example, enhance insulin secretion, suppress inflammatory signaling, and ameliorate hepatic steatosis (Yamato, 2018). Sirtuin activators promote fatty acid oxidation, improve mitochondrial biogenesis, and reduce chronic inflammation associated with obesity and diabetes (Palabiyik and Palabiyik, 2025). Drugs targeting histone methyltransferases or demethylases offer potential benefits for reversing fibrosis, restoring β-cell identity, and improving mitochondrial function in metabolic tissues (Backe et al., 2018). Dietary interventions, nutrient supplementation, and lifestyle modifications similarly influence histone modifications and offer accessible strategies to modulate epigenetic states (Asif et al., 2020). However, given the global impact of many chromatin regulators, therapeutic approaches must be developed with caution, emphasizing tissue-specificity and minimizing off-target effects.

As research advances, it is becoming increasingly clear that histone modifications not only reflect metabolic states but actively shape them. They serve as a molecular memory system, capturing the effects of metabolic stressors and transmitting them across cell divisions and, in some cases, across generations (Yu et al., 2012). This intricate interplay between chromatin and metabolism underscores the importance of epigenetics in understanding metabolic diseases and highlights the potential of epigenetic-based interventions in precision medicine.

This chapter provides a comprehensive exploration of the major histone modifications and their regulatory roles in metabolic diseases. We examine the biochemical pathways that generate histone marks, their enzymatic writers and erasers, and the metabolic intermediates that shape these modifications. We discuss their specific roles in T2DM, obesity, NAFLD, cardiovascular dysfunction, and gestational diabetes, and explore how diet, micronutrients, and environmental exposures modulate chromatin landscapes. Finally, we highlight emerging therapeutic strategies targeting histone modifications and their potential to transform the prevention and treatment of metabolic disorders. By elucidating the epigenetic mechanisms underpinning metabolic health and disease, this chapter aims to contribute to a deeper understanding of metabolic disease pathophysiology and to inform future therapeutic innovation.

2. Overview of histone modifications

Histone proteins, H2A, H2B, H3, and H4, assemble into octamers to form nucleosomes, around which approximately 147 base pairs of DNA are wrapped. The N-terminal tails of these histones extend outward from the nucleosome core and serve as accessible platforms for a wide variety of posttranslational modifications (PTMs) (Fig. 4.1). These modifications collectively contribute to the formation of a "histone code" that influences chromatin structure and determines whether DNA adopts an open (euchromatin) or compact (heterochromatin) configuration (Jenuwein and Allis, 2001). The functional outcome of these modifications directly impacts gene accessibility and transcriptional activity. Importantly, histone modifications are deeply interconnected with cellular metabolism because they rely on metabolic intermediates such as acetyl-CoA, S-adenosylmethionine (SAM), ATP, and NAD^+. This biochemical dependency links chromatin structure and gene regulation to nutrient availability, mitochondrial function, hormonal signals, and metabolic stress (Ye and Tu, 2018). Table 4.1 summarizes major histone posttranslational modifications and highlights how their regulatory enzymes and metabolic cofactors link chromatin structure to gene expression in metabolic tissues. It illustrates how dysregulation of these epigenetic marks contributes to insulin resistance, inflammation, altered lipid metabolism, and the persistence of metabolic disease states.

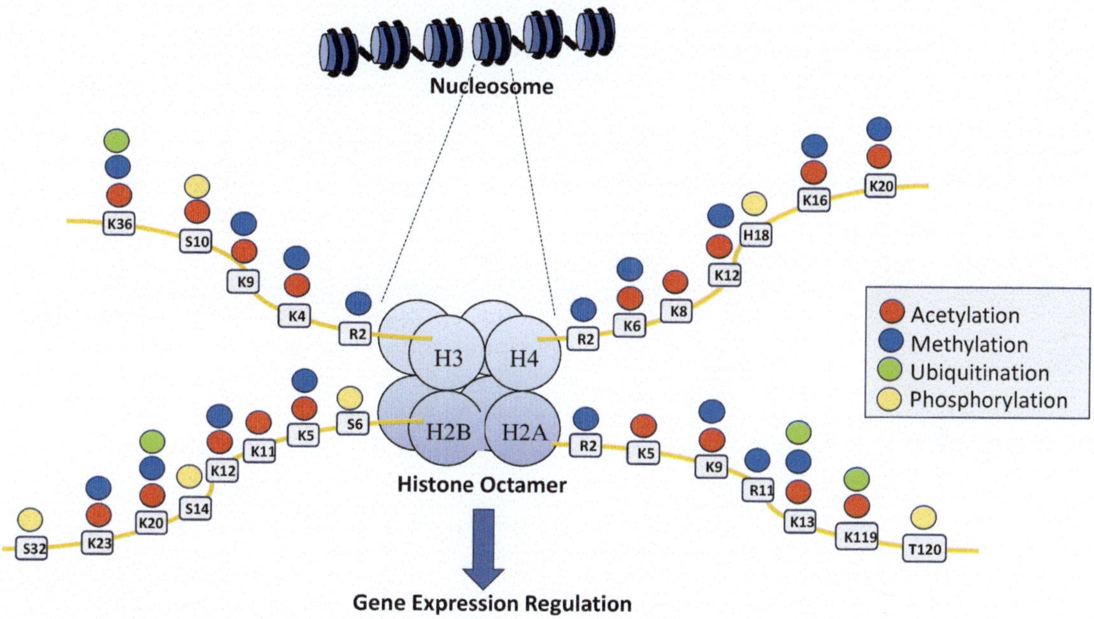

Figure 4.1 Major post-translational modifications on histone tails and their regulatory roles. Schematic representation of the nucleosome core showing histones H2A, H2B, H3, and H4 with their N-terminal tails decorated by key posttranslational modifications. Colored circles indicate acetylation, methylation, ubiquitination, and phosphorylation at specific amino acid residues. These histone modifications dynamically regulate chromatin structure and gene expression by modulating DNA accessibility and transcriptional activity.

2.1 Histone acetylation

Histone acetylation involves the enzymatic transfer of an acetyl group to lysine residues on histone tails. This reaction is catalyzed by HATs, including major families such as GNAT (e.g., GCN5, PCAF), MYST (e.g., Tip60, MOF), and p300/CBP. Acetylation neutralizes the positive charge of lysine residues, thereby weakening DNA–histone interactions and creating a more open chromatin state that favors transcription factor binding and RNA polymerase II recruitment. In contrast, histone deacetylases (HDACs), comprising Class I, II, III (Sirtuins), and IV enzymes, remove acetyl groups and restore chromatin to a condensed structure, leading to transcriptional repression (Shahbazian and Grunstein, 2007).

The regulation of histone acetylation is tightly linked to metabolism. Cellular acetyl-CoA levels directly determine the extent of histone acetylation. High glucose availability increases cytosolic acetyl-CoA via ATP-citrate lyase (ACL), driving global H3 and H4 acetylation in hepatocytes and adipocytes (Bradshaw,

Table 4.1 Histone modifications in metabolic regulation and disease.

Histone modification	Key enzymes/ cofactors	Mechanism and functional role	Metabolic/disease associations	References
Histone acetylation	HATs: GNAT (GCN5, PCAF), MYST (Tip60, MOF), p300/ CBP; HDACs: Class I–IV (including Sirtuins)	Acetylation of lysine residues neutralizes positive charge, weakens DNA–histone interactions, promotes open chromatin and transcription; deacetylation causes chromatin condensation and repression	Increased H3/H4 acetylation with high acetyl-CoA; p300/CBP activation of PPARγ, SREBP-1c; reduced SIRT1 activity in obesity/diabetes leads to hyperacetylation of inflammatory and lipogenic genes	Shahbazian and Grunstein (2007), Bradshaw (2021), Pedroso et al. (2020), Jukarainen et al. (2016), Kim et al. (2022), Bing Zhou et al. (2020)
Disease-specific acetylation marks	p300/CBP, HDACs, Sirtuins	H3K27ac enhances enhancer activity; H4K16ac promotes transcriptional activation; reduced H3K9ac limits gene expression	H3K27ac at *PCK1/G6PC* enhancers → increased hepatic gluconeogenesis; H4K16ac → fatty liver; reduced H3K9ac → decreased GLUT4 and insulin resistance	Ma et al. (2022), Pessoa Rodrigues et al. (2021), Klymenko et al. (2020)
Histone methylation	HMTs: SETD2, MLL1/2, EZH2; KDMs (demethylases); SAM as methyl donor	Addition/removal of methyl groups on lysine/arginine residues; does not alter charge but recruits effector proteins to activate or repress transcription	Active marks: H3K4me3, H3K36me3; Repressive marks: H3K9me2/3, H3K27me3; dysregulation affects insulin secretion, lipid metabolism, and mitochondrial genes	Mosammaparast and Shi (2010), Li et al. (2023), Kolasinska-Zwierz et al. (2009), Castellano-Castillo et al. (2021), Padeken et al. (2022), Meng et al. (2020)
Disease-specific methylation marks	EZH2 (PRC2), KDM6A/B	Altered methylation represses metabolic gene programs and mitochondrial function	Increased H3K9me2 suppresses fatty acid oxidation in NAFLD; loss of H3K4me3 at *Pdx1* reduces insulin transcription; elevated H3K27me3 impairs skeletal muscle oxidative capacity	Pinney et al. (2011), Mushtaq et al. (2023), Monné et al. (2022), Boila et al. (2023)

Table 4.1 Histone modifications in metabolic regulation and disease.—*continued*

Histone modification	Key enzymes/ cofactors	Mechanism and functional role	Metabolic/disease associations	References
Histone phosphorylation	Kinases (AMPK-linked pathways)	Phosphorylation on Ser/ Thr/Tyr residues regulates stress response, transcriptional activation, cell cycle, and DNA repair	H3S10 phosphorylation activates immediate-early genes in response to insulin and growth factors	Bungard et al. (2010), Healy et al. (2012), Gong et al. (2025)
Histone ubiquitination	E3 ubiquitin ligases	H2Bub1 promotes H3K4/H3K79 methylation (active transcription); H2Aub is repressive	H2Aub linked to inflammatory signaling and insulin resistance	Marsh et al. (2020), Kadakol et al. (2017)
SUMOylation	SUMO-conjugating enzymes	Generally represses transcription by stabilizing repressive chromatin	Elevated during lipotoxicity and oxidative stress in metabolic disorders	Ryu and Hochstrasser (2021), Zou et al. (2024)
Crotonylation	Crotonyl-CoA	Marks active chromatin; associated with metabolic flexibility	Enriched during fasting; links fatty acid oxidation to gene activation	Sabari (2016)
Citrullination	PAD enzymes	Converts arginine to citrulline, altering chromatin structure	Promotes inflammation, contributing to metabolic disease	Osca-Verdegal et al. (2022)
ADP-ribosylation	PARP enzymes	Stress-responsive modification influencing DNA repair and transcription	Excessive PARP activation causes mitochondrial dysfunction and β-cell exhaustion	Lee et al. (2022), Yao et al. (2024)

2021). During fasting, a reduction in acetyl-CoA lowers histone acetylation, resulting in decreased expression of lipogenic genes (Pedroso et al., 2020). NAD^+-dependent Sirtuins (SIRT1, SIRT3, SIRT6) couple cellular energy status to epigenetic control; in obesity and diabetes, reduced NAD^+ levels impair SIRT1 activity, leading to hyperacetylation of inflammatory and lipogenic genes (Jukarainen et al., 2016). Key HATs such as p300/CBP activate PPARγ, SREBP-1c, and pro-inflammatory cytokines, linking acetylation to adipogenesis and metabolic inflammation (Kim et al., 2022; Feiye Zhou et al., 2020).

Several acetylation patterns have been directly implicated in metabolic diseases. Increased H3K27ac at enhancers of gluconeogenic genes such as PCK1 and G6PC contributes to elevated hepatic glucose output in type 2 diabetes (Ma et al., 2022). Enhanced H4K16ac promotes the activation of lipogenic transcription factors, facilitating the development of fatty liver (Pessoa Rodrigues et al., 2021). Conversely, reduced H3K9ac in skeletal muscle is associated with decreased GLUT4 expression, diminishing insulin-stimulated glucose uptake (Klymenko et al., 2020).

2.2 Histone methylation

Histone methylation entails the addition of one, two, or three methyl groups to lysine or arginine residues. This modification is catalyzed by histone methyltransferases (HMTs), many of which contain a SET domain, such as SETD2, MLL1/2, and EZH2 (Li et al., 2023). Histone demethylases (KDMs) remove these methyl groups, allowing for dynamic regulation of gene expression (Mosammaparast and Shi, 2010). In contrast to acetylation, methylation does not alter the charge of the histone tail; instead, it functions by recruiting specific effector proteins that interpret methylation marks and direct downstream transcriptional outcomes.

Depending on the specific residue and degree of methylation, histone methylation can either activate or repress gene expression. Active marks include H3K4me3, which is enriched at promoters of genes involved in processes such as insulin secretion, and H3K36me3, which labels actively transcribed gene bodies and influences RNA splicing (Kolasinska-Zwierz et al., 2009; Castellano-Castillo et al., 2021). Repressive marks include H3K9me2/3, associated with heterochromatin and transcriptional silencing of metabolic genes, and H3K27me3, catalyzed by the EZH2 methyltransferase within the Polycomb

Repressive Complex 2 (PRC2), which suppresses developmentally regulated genes (Padeken et al., 2022; Meng et al., 2020).

Histone methylation is metabolically sensitive because it requires SAM as a methyl donor. SAM levels depend on one-carbon metabolism, which is influenced by dietary methionine, folate, and vitamin B12 (Mentch and Locasale, 2016). Mitochondrial function also affects the methionine cycle, and disruptions such as those seen in obesity or insulin resistance lower SAM levels and cause epigenetic dysregulation (Monné et al., 2022). In metabolic diseases, increased H3K9me2 in the liver suppresses fatty acid oxidation genes and contributes to non-alcoholic fatty liver disease (NAFLD) (Mushtaq et al., 2023). Loss of H3K4me3 at the Pdx1 locus reduces insulin gene transcription in type 2 diabetes (Pinney et al., 2011). Elevated H3K27me3 at mitochondrial genes diminishes oxidative capacity in skeletal muscle, while altered KDM6A/B activity affects H3K27 demethylation and contributes to obesity by modifying adipocyte differentiation pathways (Boila et al., 2023).

2.3 Additional histone modifications

In addition to acetylation and methylation, several other histone PTMs play vital roles in metabolic homeostasis. Histone phosphorylation occurs on serine, threonine, or tyrosine residues and is commonly associated with stress signaling, AMPK activation, cell cycle regulation, and DNA repair (Bungard et al., 2010; Gong et al., 2025). For instance, H3S10 phosphorylation enhances the transcription of immediate-early genes in response to insulin and growth factors (Healy et al., 2012). Histone ubiquitination, particularly H2B ubiquitination (H2Bub1), supports H3K4 and H3K79 methylation and thus functions as a key integrator of multiple PTMs (Marsh et al., 2020). Conversely, H2A ubiquitination (H2Aub) is primarily repressive and has been linked to inflammatory pathways associated with insulin resistance (Kadakol et al., 2017).

SUMOylation involves the attachment of SUMO proteins to histones or metabolic transcription factors, generally leading to transcriptional repression (Ryu and Hochstrasser, 2021). This modification is elevated under conditions of lipotoxicity and oxidative stress, contributing to the epigenetic dysregulation observed in metabolic disorders (Zou et al., 2024). Crotonylation, which requires crotonyl-CoA produced during fatty acid oxidation, marks active chromatin regions such as H3K18cr and H3K9cr and is enriched during fasting, suggesting a role in metabolic flexibility (Sabari, 2016). Citrullination, catalyzed by PAD enzymes, converts arginine to citrulline and is strongly associated with inflammation, a central driver of metabolic disease (Osca-Verdegal et al., 2022). ADP-ribosylation, mediated by PARP enzymes, increases under oxidative stress and contributes to mitochondrial dysfunction and β-cell exhaustion through excessive PARP activation (Lee et al., 2022).

Histone modifications therefore, form an intricate and dynamic epigenetic network that allows metabolic tissues to integrate signals from nutrient status, hormonal cues, mitochondrial activity, and environmental stress. Because these modifications depend on key metabolic intermediates such as acetyl-CoA, SAM, NAD^+, and ATP, they are uniquely sensitive to disturbances in metabolic homeostasis. In chronic metabolic diseases, these histone marks become dysregulated, leading to persistent alterations in gene expression that contribute to insulin resistance, inflammation, impaired lipid metabolism, and long-term metabolic dysfunction (Yao et al., 2024).

3. Histone modifications in type 2 diabetes mellitus

T2DM arises from a combination of insulin resistance and progressive impairment of pancreatic β-cell function. Histone modifications critically shape gene expression in all tissues involved in glucose homeostasis (Fig. 4.2).

3.1 In pancreatic β-cells

Pancreatic β-cells rely on a finely tuned epigenetic landscape to maintain their identity and ensure proper insulin synthesis and secretion. Histone acetylation is a key regulator of β-cell adaptation and function (Kim and Kulkarni, 2020). This modification is controlled by HATs and HDACs, which add or remove acetyl groups from lysine residues. Acetylation neutralizes the positive charge on histones, loosening DNA–histone interactions and increasing chromatin accessibility. It also creates docking sites for reader proteins, facilitating transcription factor binding and downstream gene expression changes (Akbari and Hassan-Zadeh, 2020). Altered histone acetylation patterns are linked to islet development, β-cell dysfunction, and T2DM. For example, reduced H3K27ac, an active enhancer mark, is observed in intrauterine growth retardation (IUGR) in rats (Lien et al., 2020) and high-fat diet induced obese mice (Nammo et al., 2018).

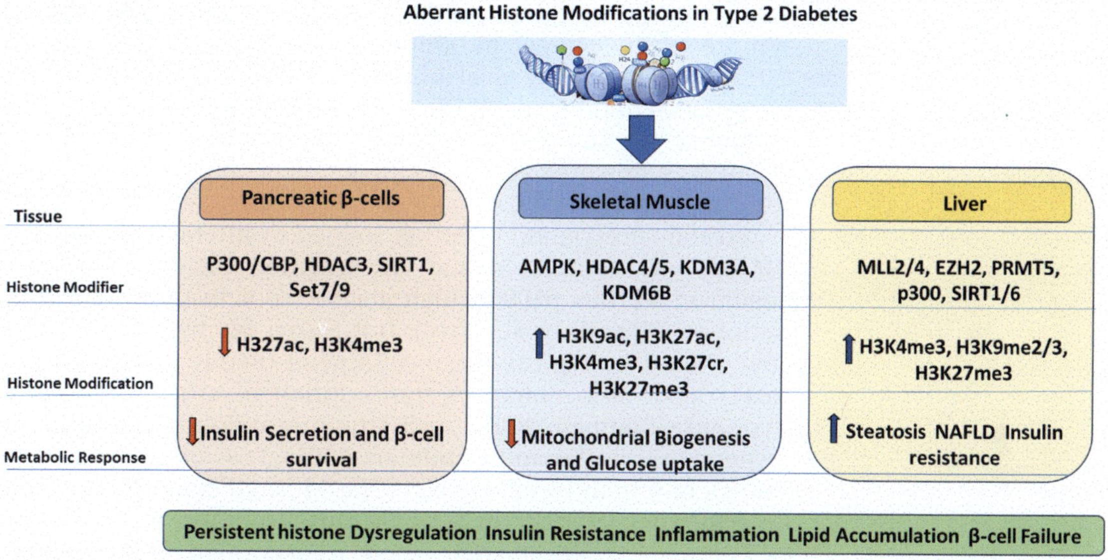

Figure 4.2 Tissue-specific histone modifications driving metabolic dysfunction in type 2 diabetes mellitus. This schematic illustrates tissue-specific histone-modifying enzymes and epigenetic marks in pancreatic β-cells, skeletal muscle, and liver that regulate gene expression in glucose and lipid metabolism. Dysregulation of these histone modifications contributes to impaired insulin secretion, reduced glucose uptake, mitochondrial dysfunction, hepatic steatosis, and insulin resistance, leading to persistent metabolic disease. Where p300/CBP – histone acetyltransferase p300/CREB-binding protein, HDAC3, HDAC4/5 – histone deacetylases (class I and II), SIRT1, SIRT6 – NAD^+-dependent sirtuin deacetylases, Set7/9 (SETD7) – histone lysine methyltransferase for H3K4, AMPK – AMP-activated protein kinase, KDM3A – lysine demethylase 3A (H3K9 demethylase), KDM6B (JMJD3) – lysine demethylase 6B (H3K27 demethylase), MLL2/4 – Mixed lineage leukemia methyltransferases (H3K4 methylation), EZH2 – enhancer of zeste homolog 2 (H3K27 methyltransferase), PRMT5 – protein arginine methyltransferase 5, H3K27ac – histone H3 lysine 27 acetylation, H3K9ac – histone H3 lysine 9 acetylation, H3K4me3 – histone H3 lysine 4 trimethylation, H3K9me2/3 – histone H3 lysine 9 di/trimethylation, H3K27me3 – histone H3 lysine 27 trimethylation, H3K27cr – histone H3 lysine 27 crotonylation, NAFLD – non-alcoholic fatty liver disease.

HDAC inhibitors have been widely used to test the functional impact of acetylation. Studies in embryonic rat pancreas show that HDAC inhibition decreases exocrine differentiation while increasing Ngn3+ endocrine progenitors (Haumaitre et al., 2008, 2014), demonstrating that acetylation status influences final endocrine cell numbers. HDACs are also implicated in diabetes pathogenesis (Makkar et al., 2020), with selective inhibitors enhancing insulin secretion and β-cell mass (Rafehi et al., 2017; Lundh et al., 2015). Pan-class I HDAC inhibitors such as SAHA and TSA reduce β-cell apoptosis and improve insulin secretion, partly through increasing histone H4 polyacetylation and bromodomain protein recruitment (Slaughter et al., 2021). However, toxicity limits their therapeutic potential. HDAC3 has emerged as a more selective target, as both genetic deletion (Remsberg et al., 2017) and pharmacological inhibition (BRD3308) improve insulin secretion (Lundh et al., 2015). Class II HDACs (HDAC4/5/9) also influence β- and δ-cell numbers (Lenoir et al., 2011), and HDAC6 is downregulated in db/db islets (Inoue et al., 2021), although their specific epigenetic mechanisms remain unclear.

Histone acetylation is further shaped by interactions between HAT/HDAC complexes and transcription factors. PDX1, for instance, recruits p300 at high glucose to activate insulin transcription (Spaeth et al., 2016), but associates with HDAC1/2 at low glucose to repress the insulin gene (Reddy and Natarajan, 2011). p300 also enhances transcription of other β-cell genes (Vo and Goodman, 2001), including pro-apoptotic Txnip under hyperglycemia (Vo and Goodman, 2001). Loss of p300 has been shown to impair β-cell survival (Cha-Molstad et al., 2009).

Other deacetylases such as Sirtuins also affect β-cell biology. SIRT1 deacetylates histones and transcription factors (Wang et al., 2014), enhances glucose-stimulated insulin secretion (Banks et al., 2008; Sun et al., 2007), and is disrupted under inflammatory stress (Javeed et al., 2021).

Histone methylation is another critical layer of β-cell gene regulation. H3K4me3 marks active promoters, and loss of methyltransferase Set7/9 reduces expression of key β-cell genes such as Pdx1, impairing GSIS (Deering et al., 2009; Maganti et al., 2015). Arginine methylation also contributes to β-cell function, as PRMT5 deletion reduces insulin secretion and impairs glucose tolerance (Ma et al., 2020). Disrupted H3K4 methylation in TrxG-deficient models destabilizes β-cell identity and function (Vanderkruk et al., 2021).

3.2 In skeletal muscle

Specific histone modifications play critical roles in regulating key metabolic genes in skeletal muscle, particularly PGC-1α and GLUT4 (McGee et al., 2009). Endurance exercise and chronic training increase activating histone acetylation marks, notably H3K9ac and H3K27ac, at promoters and enhancers of PGC-1α and other mitochondrial genes, thereby promoting PGC-1α transcription, mitochondrial biogenesis, and a shift toward oxidative (slow-twitch) muscle fibers (McGee et al., 2009; Barrès et al., 2012). These changes are mediated by exercise-activated signaling pathways, including AMPK, ROS, and CaMK, which facilitate chromatin opening and recruitment of HATs to PGC-1α regulatory regions. Acute exercise also elevates H3K4me3 at the PGC-1α promoter, a hallmark of active transcription that correlates with rapid increases in PGC-1α mRNA and enhanced expression of oxidative metabolism genes (Barrès et al., 2012). At the enhancer level, H3K27ac marks broadly regulate metabolic gene programs and are dynamically modulated by exercise, while aging and lipid overload can disrupt these enhancer signatures, potentially contributing to maladaptive metabolic responses (McGee et al., 2008). In contrast, HDACs such as HDAC4 and HDAC5 repress GLUT4 expression by deacetylating chromatin and corepressing MEF2. exercise-induced nuclear export or pharmacological inhibition of these HDACs relieves repression, resulting in increased GLUT4 expression and enhanced insulin-stimulated glucose uptake in muscle cells (Ramachandran et al., 2019; Galmozzi et al., 2013).

Beyond acetylation, emerging evidence indicates that non-acetyl histone acyl marks, such as H3K27 crotonylation, regulate GLUT4 transcription in metabolic disease, linking nutrient-derived acyl-CoA availability to chromatin remodeling and glucose transport (Liao et al., 2022). Histone methylation enzymes, including lysine demethylases and methyltransferases such as KDM3A, further modulate skeletal muscle metabolism by shaping PGC-1α-dependent transcriptional programs and influencing mitochondrial biogenesis and oxidative capacity (Qian et al., 2019; Wang et al., 2025). Manipulation of these enzymes can shift muscle fiber composition and protect against diet-induced metabolic dysfunction in preclinical models. Additionally, coordinated dynamics between activating methylation marks (H3K4me1/3) and repressive marks (H3K27me3) at promoters and enhancers govern fiber-type gene expression, with temporal resolution of repressive marks being essential for exercise-induced metabolic adaptation (Li et al., 2024). Collectively, these findings highlight that activating histone marks consistently promote oxidative and mitochondrial gene expression, whereas deacetylation or repressive methylation suppress these programs.

3.3 In the liver

The liver plays a critical role in maintaining glucose balance through the regulation of gluconeogenesis, glycogen storage, and lipid metabolism. Epigenetic dysregulation in hepatocytes is a defining feature of type 2 diabetes and NAFLD. Histone methylation plays a critical role in NAFLD development by regulating lipid metabolism, insulin sensitivity, and fibrosis. Early studies identified H3K4 methyltransferases MLL2 and MLL4 as metabolic regulators, where *Mll2* mutations induced insulin resistance (Goldsworthy et al., 2013), and HFD-enhanced MLL4–PPARγ2 interactions increased H3K4 methylation and transcription of steatotic genes (Kim et al., 2019). In hepatic stellate cells, the H3K4 methyltransferase ASH1 activates fibrogenic genes (*α-SMA, Col1, TIMP1, TGF-β1*), promoting fibrosis progression (Perugorria et al., 2012). Arginine methylation by PRMT5 further contributes to steatosis by repressing PPARα and mitochondrial biogenesis, while its inhibition enhances fatty acid oxidation and delays fatty liver development (Zhang et al., 2023).

Repressive methylation marks also modulate disease progression. EZH2/PRC2-mediated H3K27me3 exhibits stage-dependent effects—reduced in early NAFLD but contributing to hepatocellular carcinoma by silencing tumor-suppressive microRNAs (Xu et al., 2020). H3K9 methyltransferases, particularly SUV39H2, promote steatosis and NASH by repressing SIRT1, whereas *Suv39h2* deletion alleviates liver injury (Shao et al., 2017). Histone demethylases exert isoform-specific effects: PHF2 protects against insulin resistance and inflammation (Bricambert et al., 2018), whereas KDM7A, KDM4B, and JMJD1C promote steatosis by activating lipogenic genes and integrating nutrient signalin (Kim et al., 2021; Viscarra et al., 2020). Conversely, JMJD3/KDM6B, acting with SIRT1, enhances fatty acid oxidation and autophagy during fasting and protects against hepatic steatosis (Seok et al., 2018).

Histone acetylation and deacetylation dynamically regulate hepatic metabolic programs. Insulin and nutrient signaling increase histone acetylation at lipogenic gene promoters (*FASN, CD36*) via p300/CBP and nuclear receptors, promoting steatosis (Ruiqing Zhou et al., 2020). In contrast, SIRT1 and SIRT6 suppress lipogenesis, enhance fatty acid oxidation, and limit inflammation; hepatic loss of either exacerbates NAFLD, while pharmacological activation is protective (Ka et al., 2017; Hou et al., 2022). Class I/II HDACs further modulate lipid metabolism and fibrosis through chromatin and transcription factor deacetylation, with HDAC inhibitors showing antifibrotic effects in preclinical models (Wang et al., 2018)

Emerging histone modifications also contribute to NAFLD pathogenesis. H2BK120 ubiquitination suppresses pro-fibrotic cytokine expression (Lifang Chen et al., 2021), while H3S10 phosphorylation, coordinated with acetylation and methylation, enhances ChREBP-driven FASN transcription and hepatic steatosis (Cai et al., 2018). Collectively, these findings highlight histone-modifying enzymes as promising but context-dependent therapeutic targets in NAFLD.

4. Histone modifications in obesity

Obesity is characterized by chronic nutrient excess, hormonal imbalance, and persistent low-grade inflammation, all of which reshape the epigenetic landscape of metabolic tissues. Histone modifications act as molecular sensors that convert nutritional, hormonal, and inflammatory signals into stable transcriptional programs (Thaker, 2017; Keating and El-Osta, 2015). Alterations in activating and repressive histone marks influence adipogenesis, inflammation, lipid metabolism, and insulin sensitivity, thereby reinforcing obesity as a disease with strong epigenetic underpinnings (Zhang et al., 2012).

4.1 Adipogenesis and adipocyte function

Adipocyte differentiation requires permissive chromatin states enriched in activating histone marks such as H3K4me3, H3K27ac, and H3K9ac at key adipogenic genes, including PPARγ, C/EBPα, and aP2. These marks are deposited by HATs (e.g., p300/CBP) and MLL-family methyltransferases during normal adipogenesis (Zhang et al., 2012). In precursor cells, antiadipogenic genes such as Pref-1 are maintained in a repressed state through elevated H3K27me3, which is removed upon differentiation (Zhang et al., 2012),

In obesity, chronic overnutrition disrupts this tightly regulated epigenetic program. Altered availability of metabolites such as acetyl-CoA and S-adenosylmethionine leads to aberrant histone acetylation and methylation, impairing adipocyte differentiation. This favors hypertrophic adipocyte expansion rather than healthy hyperplasia, resulting in cells that are insulin resistant, hypoxic, and prone to lipotoxicity (Zhang et al., 2012). Consequently, dysfunctional adipocytes fail to buffer excess lipids, promoting free fatty acid spillover and systemic insulin resistance.

4.2 Inflammatory pathways

Obesity-associated adipose tissue inflammation is driven by epigenetic remodeling at inflammatory gene loci. High-fat diets induce enhancer activation marked by H3K27ac and H3K4me1 at pro-inflammatory genes such as TNF-α, IL-6, and MCP-1, particularly at sites bound by transcription factors including NF-κB, STAT3, and AP-1 (Wang et al., 2021; Hu et al., 2024). These changes are tissue and strainspecific and may persist even after dietary reversal, indicating epigenetic memory in metabolic tissues (Wang et al., 2021; Kain et al., 2025).

A key regulator of inflammatory chromatin states is SIRT1, an NAD^+-dependent deacetylase that suppresses inflammatory transcription. In obesity, reduced NAD^+ availability lowers SIRT1 activity, leading to increased H3K9ac and acetylation of NF-κB p65 at inflammatory promoters, thereby sustaining cytokine expression (Choi et al., 2013). This establishes a feed-forward loop linking inflammation, adipocyte dysfunction, and insulin resistance.

4.3 Lipid metabolism and energy homeostasis

Histone modifications also control lipid synthesis and energy metabolism. Obesity increases activating histone marks such as H3K27ac, H3K36me3, and H3K4me1 at lipogenic genes including FASN, ACC, and SCD1, promoting de novo lipogenesis and triglyceride accumulation (Keating and El-Osta, 2015; Zhe Wang et al., 2021). Conversely, oxidative and mitochondrial genes exhibit reduced activating marks and increased repressive methylation, impairing metabolic flexibility.

Sirtuins play a central protective role in this context. SIRT6, which deacetylates H3K9ac, promotes fatty acid oxidation and suppresses glycolytic and lipogenic programs. Reduced SIRT6 activity in obesity leads to increased acetylation at lipogenic genes and decreased expression of oxidative regulators such as PPARα, CPT1, and ACOX1, thereby exacerbating lipid accumulation and insulin resistance (Gasmi et al., 2021). Additional alterations in histone methylation, including increased H3K9me2 and reduced H3K4me3 at mitochondrial genes, further disrupt energy homeostasis (Jinpeng Wang et al., 2021).

4.3.1 Emerging and systemic epigenetic effects

Beyond classical histone marks, obesity is associated with oxidative stress–driven histone carbonylation. Lipid peroxidation products such as 4-hydroxynonenal (4-HNE) modify histones in adipose tissue, serving as redox-sensitive epigenomic markers of metabolic stress (Hauck et al., 2020). Moreover, obesity-induced histone modifications extend beyond metabolic tissues; reduced H3K4me2, increased DNA damage, and transcriptional dysregulation in oocytes and early embryos link maternal obesity to impaired embryonic development and potential transgenerational effects (Pan et al., 2021).

These findings demonstrate that histone modifications integrate nutrient excess, inflammation, and metabolic stress into stable transcriptional states that drive adipocyte dysfunction, insulin resistance, and systemic metabolic disease, highlighting epigenetic enzymes as promising but context-dependent therapeutic targets in obesity.

5. Histone modifications in NAFLD/MAFLD

NAFLD, now termed metabolic-associated fatty liver disease (MAFLD), encompasses a spectrum from simple steatosis to NASH, fibrosis, cirrhosis, and hepatocellular carcinoma. It is closely associated with obesity, insulin resistance, and type 2 diabetes. Accumulating evidence demonstrates that histone modifications, particularly acetylation and methylation, play a central role in regulating hepatic lipid metabolism, oxidative stress responses, inflammation, and fibrogenesis, thereby driving disease initiation and progression. Nutrient overload and chronic metabolic stress remodel the hepatic epigenome, resulting in persistent transcriptional dysregulation.

5.1 Histone modifications and dysregulation of lipid metabolism

Hepatic steatosis, the earliest hallmark of NAFLD, is driven by epigenetic activation of lipogenic gene programs. Activating histone marks such as H3K27ac and H3K4me3 are enriched at promoters and enhancers of key lipogenic genes, including SREBP-1c, ACC, FASN, and SCD1, leading to increased de novo lipogenesis (Du et al., 2017; Rohrbach et al., 2019). Recruitment of HATs p300/CBP and H3K4 methyltransferases of the MLL/COMPASS complex further amplifies transcriptional activation under conditions of nutrient excess (Kim et al., 2016).

Obesity and insulin resistance increase hepatic acetyl-CoA availability, globally enhancing histone acetylation and reinforcing lipogenic transcription (Cai et al., 2018). In parallel, repressive histone marks such as H3K9me2 and H3K27me3 are selectively reduced at lipogenic loci through the action of histone demethylases (e.g., JMJD2B, PHF2), increasing chromatin accessibility and sustaining lipid accumulation (Kim et al., 2020; Bricambert et al., 2018). These coordinated histone changes shift hepatic metabolism toward lipid synthesis and storage, establishing metabolic memory in NAFLD.

5.2 Histone modifications in oxidative stress and mitochondrial dysfunction

Progression from steatosis to NASH is marked by oxidative stress and mitochondrial dysfunction. Epigenetic repression of antioxidant and mitochondrial genes is a critical contributor to this transition. Reduced H3K9ac and H3K27ac at promoters of antioxidant genes such as NRF2, SOD2, GPX1, and CAT limits transcriptional activation, weakening cellular defenses against reactive oxygen species (ROS) (Sun et al., 2015; Manne et al., 2018).

Concurrently, increased deposition of repressive marks including H3K9me3 and H3K27me3 occurs at genes regulating mitochondrial biogenesis and oxidative phosphorylation, notably PGC-1α and TFAM (Becares et al., 2019; Siersbæk et al., 2017). These changes impair mitochondrial integrity, reduce ATP production, and exacerbate lipid-induced hepatocellular injury. Thus, histone modifications act as a molecular link between metabolic stress, oxidative damage, and inflammatory progression in NAFLD.

5.3 Histone modifications in fibrosis and disease progression

Advanced NAFLD is characterized by hepatic stellate cell (HSC) activation and progressive fibrosis. Epigenomic reprogramming in HSCs is dominated by increased H3K27ac at enhancers and promoters of profibrotic genes, including COL1A1, COL3A1, ACTA2 (α-SMA), and TGF-β1, promoting extracellular matrix deposition (Ding et al., 2015; Perugorria et al., 2012). Chromatin readers such as BRD4, together with p300, are highly enriched at these regulatory regions, sustaining fibrogenic transcription (Ding et al., 2015; Gao et al., 2021).

Simultaneously, loss of repressive histone marks (H3K9me3, H4K20me3, H3K27me3) derepresses fibrotic pathways and reinforces myofibroblast trans-differentiation (Zeybel et al., 2017). Increased acetyl-CoA availability during metabolic stress further fuels histone acetylation in HSCs, creating a feed-forward loop that perpetuates fibrosis. Pharmacological inhibition of histone acetylation readers or writers (e.g., BRD4 or p300 inhibitors) has shown antifibrotic effects in experimental NAFLD/NASH models, highlighting the therapeutic relevance of histone-based regulation (Zhang et al., 2021).

These histone-driven epigenetic changes not only amplify fibrosis but also influence clinical outcomes by making fibrotic pathways self-perpetuating. Even after metabolic improvement, persistent histone alterations within HSCs form an epigenetic memory, making fibrosis difficult to reverse and contributing to chronic liver disease progression.

6. Histone modifications in cardiovascular and metabolic syndrome

Metabolic syndrome is defined by central obesity, insulin resistance, dyslipidemia, hypertension, and chronic low-grade inflammation, all creates a systemic metabolic environment that markedly increases the risk of atherosclerosis, vascular remodeling, heart failure, and ischemic heart disease. Histone modifications function as key epigenetic mediators that translate metabolic and inflammatory stress into persistent transcriptional reprogramming in endothelial cells, vascular smooth muscle cells (VSMCs), cardiomyocytes, and immune cells.

6.1 Endothelial dysfunction and atherogenesis

Endothelial dysfunction is a hallmark of early atherosclerosis and a critical link between metabolic syndrome and cardiovascular disease. Metabolic stressors such as hyperglycemia, dyslipidemia, and oxidative stress alter histone acetylation and methylation at endothelial gene loci. Reduced H3K27ac at the eNOS (NOS3) promoter diminishes nitric oxide (NO) production, impairing vasodilation and promoting early atherogenesis (He et al., 2019). Concurrently, increased repressive marks (H3K9me2, H3K27me3) at antiinflammatory genes such as KLF2, IL-10, and HO-1 suppress endothelial protective programs, enhancing leukocyte adhesion and vascular inflammation (Haskard et al., 2013).

Inflammatory stimuli activate HATs p300 and HAT1, increasing acetylation at the Nox5 promoter and driving superoxide production, thereby exacerbating oxidative stress and plaque development (Vlad et al., 2019). This positions epigenetic regulation of Nox5 as a therapeutic target beyond conventional ROS scavenging.

HDACs exert context-dependent effects in atherosclerosis. SIRT1, an NAD^+-dependent deacetylase, suppresses macrophage LOX-1 expression, limiting oxidized LDL uptake and foam cell formation, thereby slowing plaque progression (Chan et al., 2018). In contrast, HDAC5 represses KLF2, leading to reduced eNOS expression and endothelial dysfunction (18). Pharmacological HDAC inhibition with SAHA (vorinostat) enhances histone acetylation, activates KLF2, suppresses VCAM1, and reduces monocyte adhesion, demonstrating protective effects in early-stage atherosclerosis (Xu et al., 2017; Liu et al., 2008). Additionally,

HDAC3 limits inflammatory signaling and endothelial-to-mesenchymal transition (EndMT); its selective inhibition attenuates plaque formation in $ApoE^{-/-}$ mice (Zhe Wang et al., 2021; Shanshan Chen et al., 2021).

Histone methylation further modulates vascular pathology. The H3K9 methyltransferase SUV39H1 promotes VSMC proliferation by depositing H3K9me3 at cell-cycle inhibitors such as p21, contributing to neointimal hyperplasia (Zhang et al., 2019). In obesity, reduced SUV39H1 expression alters H3K9 methylation/acetylation balance at the p66Shc promoter, increasing mitochondrial ROS and endothelial dysfunction, thereby accelerating atherosclerosis (Masi et al., 2021). These findings highlight SUV39H1 as a key epigenetic link between obesity and vascular disease.

Aging-related atherosclerosis involves mitochondrial epigenetic regulation. Activation of AMPK (e.g., by metformin) increases DOT1L-mediated H3K79me3 at SIRT1 and SIRT3 promoters, enhancing mitochondrial biogenesis, reducing oxidative stress, and protecting against age-associated plaque formation (Karnewar et al., 2018). Advanced plaques also exhibit distinct histone methylation signatures, including increased H3K4 methylation and reduced H3K9/H3K27 methylation in smooth muscle and inflammatory cells, correlating with disease severity and potential biomarker utility (Greiβel et al., 2016).

6.2 Cardiac metabolic stress and remodeling

The heart is highly sensitive to metabolic overload associated with obesity, insulin resistance, and hypertension. Under these conditions, HATs **p300/CBP** are activated, increasing **H3K9ac and H3K27ac** at promoters of hypertrophic and fibrotic genes such as **ANP, BNP, β-MHC**, and extracellular matrix regulators. This acetylation-driven transcriptional activation promotes pathological cardiac hypertrophy and remodeling.

Reduced activity of NAD^{+}-dependent deacetylases **SIRT1 and SIRT3**, commonly observed in metabolic syndrome and diabetes, further exacerbates histone hyperacetylation and mitochondrial dysfunction. Loss of SIRT3 increases acetylation of mitochondrial proteins, elevates oxidative stress, and impairs cardiac metabolic flexibility. Class I HDACs (**HDAC1/3**) promote fibrosis and maladaptive remodeling, whereas class IIa HDACs restrain cardiac hypertrophy by repressing transcription factors such as **MEF2 and GATA4** (Chelladurai et al., 2021; Han et al., 2022). Sirtuins (**SIRT1/3**) exert cardioprotective effects by improving mitochondrial metabolism, calcium handling, autophagy, and redox balance (Gorski et al., 2019).

Pharmacological HDAC inhibition has demonstrated partial reversal of hypertrophic gene programs, reduced fibrosis, and improved cardiac function, underscoring the therapeutic potential of targeting histone acetylation in cardiometabolic disease. Emerging histone modifications, including **lactylation and crotonylation**, further regulate post-myocardial infarction repair, angiogenesis, and metabolic adaptation, highlighting new epigenetic avenues for cardiovascular therapy (Wang et al., 2022; Liu et al., 2017).

7. Histone modifications in gestational diabetes mellitus (GDM)

GDM induces significant metabolic and inflammatory stress during pregnancy, leading to profound epigenetic remodeling in both maternal and fetal tissues (Kerr et al., 2018). Histone modifications play a critical role in regulating placental function, fetal nutrient exposure, and developmental programming of metabolic pathways (Mesa et al., 2020). Because pregnancy is a period of heightened epigenetic plasticity, disruptions in histone marks during GDM can have long-lasting effects that extend into childhood and adulthood, increasing susceptibility to obesity, insulin resistance, and type 2 diabetes (T2DM) (Mansfield, 2017). These changes represent a key mechanism underlying *intergenerational metabolic memory*, wherein maternal metabolic environment shapes future disease risk in offspring.

7.1 Placental epigenetic remodeling in GDM

The placenta serves as a metabolically responsive interface between mother and fetus, and its chromatin architecture is highly sensitive to maternal hyperglycemia. In GDM, placental epigenetic remodeling is evident at the level of histone modifications. Hepp et al. demonstrated that both syncytiotrophoblast and extravillous trophoblast cells from GDM pregnancies exhibit significantly reduced H3K9 acetylation, while H3K4 trimethylation remains unchanged, indicating selective impairment of activating histone marks rather than global chromatin disruption (Hepp et al., 2018). Given the established association between vitamin D deficiency and GDM (Soheilykhah et al., 2010), in vitro supplementation with calcitriol was tested but failed to restore

H3K9 acetylation, suggesting limited reversibility of placental histone acetylation defects once GDM is established (Hepp et al., 2018).

Such reductions in activating histone marks may compromise transcriptional control of genes involved in glucose transport, oxidative stress defense, and placental metabolic homeostasis. This dysregulation likely contributes to excessive glucose transfer to the fetus, increased oxidative stress, and altered placental function, thereby influencing fetal growth trajectories and increasing the risk of macrosomia or metabolic instability (Jiang et al., 2022).

7.2 Fetal programming and long-term effects

Epigenetic alterations induced by the hyperglycemic intrauterine environment extend beyond the placenta and may persist systemically, contributing to long-term metabolic programming. Michalczyk et al. reported that women with GDM who later progressed to type 2 diabetes exhibited ~80% lower H3K4me2 and ~50% lower H3K27me2 levels in peripheral blood leukocytes postpartum compared with women whose glucose tolerance normalized after pregnancy (Michalczyk et al., 2016). These findings indicate that GDM is associated with durable disruptions in histone methylation patterns linked to transcriptional plasticity and metabolic resilience.

Although direct fetal tissue data remain limited, such persistent maternal epigenetic signatures support the concept that fetal tissues exposed to GDM undergo parallel histone-mediated programming (Bhadsavle and Golding, 2022). These changes may predispose offspring to impaired insulin sensitivity, altered β-cell development, increased adiposity, and chronic inflammation later in life, reinforcing the developmental origins of metabolic disease.

8. Nutritional and environmental influences

Histone modifications are highly responsive to external cues, making them a major interface between the environment and the genome. Diet, micronutrient status, circadian rhythms, and exposure to pollutants or endocrine disruptors all influence the supply of metabolic cofactors likes acetyl-CoA, SAM, NAD^+, and ATP, that are essential for histone-modifying enzymes. Because of this metabolic epigenetic coupling, even subtle lifestyle and environmental changes can reshape chromatin structure and gene expression, modulating susceptibility to insulin resistance, obesity, dyslipidemia, and related metabolic disorders.

8.1 Diet and metabolic inputs

Diet is one of the most fundamental regulators of the epigenome, as nutrients provide the biochemical substrates required for DNA methylation and histone modifications. It is estimated that more than 60% of disease-related mortality is attributable to dietary patterns rather than genetic or environmental factors alone (Palou, 2006). Nutritional status during critical developmental windows, particularly pregnancy, profoundly influences epigenetic programming, with malnutrition and micronutrient deficiencies linked to low birth weight, preterm delivery, and increased risk of metabolic, cardiovascular, and neurodevelopmental disorders in offspring (Lukaszewski et al., 2013). Low birth weight itself is strongly associated with later-life susceptibility to diabetes, obesity, and cardiovascular disease, reflecting disrupted epigenetic regulation of developmental genes via altered DNA methylation and histone modification patterns (Haggarty et al., 2013).

8.1.1 Epigenetic nutrients and histone regulation

Certain micronutrients, termed *epi-nutrients*, exert a disproportionate influence on chromatin structure due to their direct involvement in one-carbon metabolism and histone modification pathways. These include methionine (a precursor of S-adenosylmethionine, SAM), folate, vitamins B6, B12, and B2, choline, betaine, biotin, and minerals such as magnesium and zinc (Oommen et al., 2005; Rush et al., 2014). Adequate availability of these nutrients sustains activating histone marks such as H3K4me3 and balanced repression via H3K27me3, thereby supporting insulin signaling, lipid metabolism, and genomic stability. Deficiencies reduce SAM availability, impair histone methylation, and are associated with insulin resistance, neural tube defects, neurodevelopmental disorders, and metabolic disease (LaSalle, 2013; Rush et al., 2014).

8.1.1.1 One-carbon metabolism and developmental programming

The importance of maternal one-carbon metabolism was first demonstrated in the Agouti mouse model, where maternal epinutrient deficiency resulted in locus-specific DNA hypomethylation and persistent phenotypic changes in offspring (Kim et al.,

2009). In humans, folate deficiency during pregnancy is associated with neural tube defects, poor birth outcomes, hyperglycemia, and transgenerational metabolic dysfunction (Krishnaveni et al., 2014; Stover, 2012). In adults, impaired folate metabolism leads to hyperhomocysteinemia, reduced histone methylation, and increased risk of cardiovascular disease, diabetes, and neurodegeneration (Fiorito et al., 2014).

Choline and betaine further support histone methylation by facilitating remethylation of homocysteine to methionine. Adequate maternal choline intake improves offspring cognitive function and protects against hippocampal dysfunction, while deficiency promotes epigenetic instability and fatty liver disease (Corbin and Zeisel, 2012)].

8.1.1.2 Bioactive compounds and epigenetic plasticity

Beyond essential nutrients, bioactive dietary compounds (*epi-bioactives*) can modulate histone-modifying enzymes. Polyphenols such as resveratrol, curcumin, epigallocatechin gallate (EGCG), quercetin, sulforaphane, and genistein regulate HATs, HDACs, and histone methyltransferases, thereby reducing inflammation, oxidative stress, and metabolic dysfunction in liver, adipose tissue, and pancreatic β-cells (Guerrero-Bosagna and Skinner, 2014). Dietary patterns such as caloric restriction and the Mediterranean diet are similarly associated with improved chromatin stability, attenuation of age-related histone alterations, and reduced cardiometabolic risk (Tollefsbol, 2013).

8.2 Environmental exposures

Environmental stressors, ranging from air pollutants to EDCs, have strong epigenetic impacts that influence metabolic health. Particulate matter (PM2.5), heavy metals such as cadmium, and persistent organic pollutants increase oxidative stress and inflammation, leading to widespread changes in histone acetylation and methylation patterns in metabolic tissues (Afthab et al., 2024; Zhou et al., 2020). For example, exposure to pollutants often increases repressive marks such as H3K9me2 on insulin-signaling genes, predisposing individuals to insulin resistance.

Endocrine disruptors such as bisphenol A (BPA), phthalates, and pesticides can mimic or interfere with hormonal signaling, altering histone marks at genes regulating adipogenesis, appetite control, and glucose metabolism (Kirtana and Seetharaman, 2022). Prenatal exposure to EDCs has been associated with increased H3K4me3 and H3K9ac at pro-adipogenic genes in fetal tissues, contributing to childhood obesity risk.

Additionally, circadian rhythm disruption, caused by shift work, irregular sleep cycles, or chronic light exposure at night, impairs the rhythmic activity of HATs and deacetylases that regulate metabolic gene oscillation (da Silveira et al., 2024). This leads to misalignment between metabolic needs and gene expression patterns, increasing the risk for obesity, fatty liver disease, and type 2 diabetes.

9. Therapeutic targeting of histone modifications

Unlike conventional drugs that target single enzymes or pathways, epigenetic interventions can rewind maladaptive chromatin states and restore healthy gene expression patterns. However, the global nature of histone modifiers requires cautious application, as widespread chromatin remodeling can affect essential cellular functions. Future clinical success will likely depend on targeted, tissue-specific epigenetic modulation.

9.1 HDAC inhibitors

HDAC inhibitors increase histone acetylation, promoting a more open chromatin structure and transcriptional activation of metabolic genes. In obesity and type 2 diabetes, HDAC inhibition reduces chronic inflammation by suppressing NF-κB activity and shifting macrophages toward an antiinflammatory M2 phenotype (Suchitra et al., 2023). In pancreatic β-cells, HDAC inhibitors enhance insulin gene expression, improve glucose-stimulated insulin secretion, and protect against lipotoxicity-induced apoptosis (Suchitra et al., 2023). In the liver, HDAC inhibition reduces SREBP-1c–mediated lipogenesis and improves steatosis (Shin et al., 2021). Compounds such as valproate, sodium butyrate, and newer class-selective HDAC inhibitors have shown significant metabolic benefits in preclinical models, highlighting their therapeutic potential.

9.2 Sirtuin activators

Sirtuins (SIRT1–7) are NAD^+-dependent HDACs that function as metabolic sensors, linking nutrient status to chromatin remodeling. Activators of SIRT1 and SIRT6, including resveratrol, nicotinamide riboside (NR), nicotinamide mononucleotide (NMN), and synthetic SIRT1 agonists, have demonstrated strong metabolic benefits (Vachharajani et al., 2016). These compounds promote mitochondrial biogenesis through PGC-1α activation, enhance fatty acid oxidation, suppress hepatic gluconeogenesis, and reduce inflammatory signaling in adipose tissue and macrophages. SIRT6 activation improves glucose homeostasis by repressing glycolytic genes and enhancing DNA repair and genomic stability (Roichman et al., 2021). Because sirtuins also regulate circadian metabolic rhythms, their activation helps realign disrupted metabolic cycles associated with obesity, aging, and sleep disturbances (Zhuang et al., 2024).

9.3 Methylation modulators

Drugs that modify histone methylation, either by inhibiting histone methyltransferases (HMTs) or demethylases (KDMs), represent a newer therapeutic avenue. Inhibitors of EZH2, the enzyme responsible for adding the repressive mark H3K27me3, have shown potential in reducing hepatic and pancreatic fibrosis by suppressing pro-fibrotic gene programs (Yiheng Zhang et al., 2023). LSD1 (KDM1A) inhibitors reverse pathological demethylation of H3K4 and H3K9, restoring expression of genes involved in mitochondrial function, β-cell identity, and lipid oxidation (Bailey et al., 2020). In NAFLD and NASH models, methylation-targeting agents reduce extracellular matrix deposition, improve lipid clearance, and correct insulin resistance. Targeting methylation pathways may offer distinct advantages for diseases such as metabolic syndrome, where chronic inflammation, fibrosis, and impaired oxidative metabolism play major roles (Swathi et al., 2025).

10. Conclusion

Histone modifications provide a dynamic and reversible mechanism through which the environment shapes metabolic physiology. Their dysregulation lies at the core of insulin resistance, mitochondrial impairment, chronic inflammation, lipid accumulation, and fibrosis, the hallmarks of metabolic diseases. Understanding these epigenetic processes offers critical insights into disease origins, progression, and intergenerational transmission. Moreover, the therapeutic modulation of histone marks, through dietary, pharmacological, and lifestyle interventions, holds promise for transforming patient outcomes and paving the way toward personalized epigenetic medicine.

References

Afthab, M.uhammed, Hambo, S., Kim, H., Ali, A., Harb, H., 2024. Particulate matter-induced epigenetic modifications and lung complications. Eur. Respir. Rev. 33 (174), 240129. https://doi.org/10.1183/16000617.0129-2024.

Akbari, M., Hassan-Zadeh, V., 2020. The inflammatory effect of epigenetic factors and modifications in type 2 diabetes. Inflammopharmacology 28 (2), 345–362. https://doi.org/10.1007/s10787-019-00663-9.

Asif, S., Morrow, N.M., Mulvihill, E.E., Kim, K.H., 2020. Understanding dietary intervention-mediated epigenetic modifications in metabolic diseases. Front. Genet. 11. https://doi.org/10.3389/fgene.2020.590369.

Assante, G., Chandrasekaran, S., Ng, S., Tourna, A., Chung, C.H., Isse, K.A., Banks, J.L., Soffientini, U., Filippi, C., Dhawan, A., Liu, M., Rozen, S.G., Hoare, M., Campbell, P., Ballard, J.W.O., Turner, N., Morris, M.J., Chokshi, S., Youngson, N.A., 2022. Acetyl-CoA metabolism drives epigenome change and contributes to carcinogenesis risk in fatty liver disease. Genome Med. 14 (1). https://doi.org/10.1186/s13073-022-01071-5.

Backe, M.B., Andersson, J.L., Bacos, K., Christensen, D.P., Hansen, J.B., Dorosz, J.J., Gajhede, M., Dahlby, T., Bysani, M., Kristensen, L.H., Ling, C., Olsen, L., Mandrup-Poulsen, T., 2018. Lysine demethylase inhibition protects pancreatic β cells from apoptosis and improves β-cell function. Mol. Cell. Endocrinol. 460, 47–56. https://doi.org/10.1016/j.mce.2017.07.001.

Bailey, C.P., Figueroa, M., Gangadharan, A., Lee, D.A., Chandra, J., 2020. Scaffolding LSD1 inhibitors impair NK cell metabolism and cytotoxic function through depletion of glutathione. Front. Immunol. 11. https://doi.org/10.3389/fimmu.2020.02196.

Banks, A.S., Kon, N., Knight, C., Matsumoto, M., Gutiérrez-Juárez, R., Rossetti, L., Gu, W., Accili, D., 2008. SirT1 gain of function increases energy efficiency and prevents diabetes in mice. Cell Metab. 8 (4), 333–341. https://doi.org/10.1016/j.cmet.2008.08.014.

Barrès, R., Yan, J., Egan, B., Treebak, J.T., Rasmussen, M., Fritz, T., Caidahl, K., Krook, A., O'Gorman, D.J., Zierath, J.R., 2012. Acute exercise remodels promoter methylation in human skeletal muscle. Cell Metab. 15 (3), 405–411. https://doi.org/10.1016/j.cmet.2012.01.001.

Becares, N., Gage, M.C., Voisin, M., Shrestha, E., Martin-Gutierrez, L., Liang, N., Louie, R., Pourcet, B., Pello, O.M., Luong, T.V., Goñi, S., Pichardo-Almarza, C., Røberg-Larsen, H., Diaz-Zuccarini, V., Steffensen, K.R., O'Brien, A., Garabedian, M.J., Rombouts, K., Treuter, E., Pineda-Torra, I., 2019. Impaired LXRα phosphorylation attenuates progression of fatty liver disease. Cell Rep. 26 (4), 984. https://doi.org/10.1016/j.celrep.2018.12.094.

Bhadsavle, S.S., Golding, M.C., 2022. Paternal epigenetic influences on placental health and their impacts on offspring development and disease. Front. Genet. 13. https://doi.org/10.3389/fgene.2022.1068408.

Boila, L.D., Ghosh, S., Bandyopadhyay, S.K., Jin, L., Murison, A., Zeng, A.G.X., Shaikh, W., Bhowmik, S., Muddineni, S.S.N.A., Biswas, M., Sinha, S., Chatterjee, S.S., Mbong, N., Gan, O.I., Bose, A., Chakraborty, S., Arruda, A., Kennedy, J.A., Mitchell, A., Lechman, E.R., Banerjee, D., Milyavsky, M., Minden, M.D., Dick, J.E., Sengupta, A., 2023. KDM6 demethylases integrate DNA repair gene regulation and loss of KDM6A sensitizes human acute myeloid leukemia to PARP and BCL2 inhibition. Leukemia 37 (4), 751–764. https://doi.org/10.1038/s41375-023-01833-z.

Bradshaw, P.C., 2021. Acetyl-coa metabolism and histone acetylation in the regulation of aging and lifespan. Antioxidants 10 (4). https://doi.org/10.3390/antiox10040572.

Bricambert, J., Alves-Guerra, M.C., Esteves, P., Prip-Buus, C., Bertrand-Michel, J., Guillou, H., Chang, C.J., Vander Wal, M.N., Canonne-Hergaux, F., Mathurin, P., Raverdy, V., Pattou, F., Girard, J., Postic, C., Dentin, R., 2018. The histone demethylase Phf2 acts as a molecular checkpoint to prevent NAFLD progression during obesity. Nat. Commun. 9 (1). https://doi.org/10.1038/s41467-018-04361-y.

Bungard, D., Fuerth, B.J., Zeng, P.Y., Faubert, B., Maas, N.L., Viollet, B., Carling, D., Thompson, C.B., Jones, R.G., Berger, S.L., 2010. Signaling kinase AMPK activates stress-promoted transcription via histone H2B phosphorylation. Science 329 (5996), 1201–1205. https://doi.org/10.1126/science.1191241.

Cai, C., Yu, H., Huang, G., Du, X., Yu, X., Zhou, Y., Shen, W., 2018. Histone modifications in fatty acid synthase modulated by carbohydrate responsive element binding protein are associated with non-alcoholic fatty liver disease. Int. J. Mol. Med. 42 (3), 1215–1228. https://doi.org/10.3892/ijmm.2018.3702.

Castellano-Castillo, D., Denechaud, P.-D., Fajas, L., Moreno-Indias, I., Oliva-Olivera, W., Tinahones, F., Queipo-Ortuño, M.I., Cardona, F., Kaser, S., 2019. Human adipose tissue H3K4me3 histone mark in adipogenic, lipid metabolism and inflammatory genes is positively associated with BMI and HOMA-IR. PLoS One 14 (4), e0215083. https://doi.org/10.1371/journal.pone.0215083.

Castellano-Castillo, D., Ramos-Molina, B., Oliva-Olivera, W., Ocaña-Wilhelmi, L., Queipo-Ortuño, M.I., Cardona, F., 2021. Genome profiling of h3k4me3 histone modification in human adipose tissue during obesity and insulin resistance. Biomedicines 9 (10). https://doi.org/10.3390/biomedicines9101363.

Cha-Molstad, H., Saxena, G., Chen, J., Shalev, A., 2009. Glucose-stimulated expression of Txnip is mediated by carbohydrate response element-binding protein, p300, and histone H4 acetylation in pancreatic beta cells. J. Biol. Chem. 284 (25), 16898–16905. https://doi.org/10.1074/jbc.m109.010504.

Chakrabarti, S.K., Francis, J., Ziesmann, S.M., Garmey, J.C., Mirmira, R.G., 2003. Covalent histone modifications underlie the developmental regulation of insulin gene transcription in pancreatic β cells. J. Biol. Chem. 278 (26), 23617–23623. https://doi.org/10.1074/jbc.M303423200.

Chan, S.H., Hung, C.H., Shih, J.Y., Chu, P.M., Cheng, Y.H., Lin, H.C., Hsieh, P.L., Tsai, K.L., 2018. Exercise intervention attenuates hyperhomocysteinemia-induced aortic endothelial oxidative injury by regulating SIRT1 through mitigating NADPH oxidase/LOX-1 signaling. Redox Biol. 14, 116–125. https://doi.org/10.1016/j.redox.2017.08.016.

Chelladurai, P., Boucherat, O., Stenmark, K., Kracht, M., Seeger, W., Bauer, U. M., Bonnet, S., Pullamsetti, S.S., 2021. Targeting histone acetylation in pulmonary hypertension and right ventricular hypertrophy. Br. J. Pharmacol. 178 (1), 54–71. https://doi.org/10.1111/bph.14932.

Chen, L., Shang, C., Wang, B., Wang, G., Jin, Z., Yao, F., Yue, Z., Bai, L., Wang, R., Zhao, S., Liu, E., Wang, W., 2021. HDAC3 inhibitor suppresses endothelial-to-mesenchymal transition via modulating inflammatory response in atherosclerosis. Biochem. Pharmacol. 192, 114716. https://doi.org/10.1016/j.bcp.2021.114716.

Chen, S., Dai, X., Li, H., Gong, Y., Zhao, Y., Huang, H., 2021. Overexpression of ring finger protein 20 inhibits the progression of liver fibrosis via mediation of histone H2B lysine 120 ubiquitination. Hum. Cell 34 (3), 759–770. https://doi.org/10.1007/s13577-021-00498-z.

Choi, S. E., Fu, T., Seok, S., Kim, D. H., Yu, E., Lee, K. W., et al., 2013. Elevated microRNA-34a in obesity reduces NAD+ levels and SIRT1 activity by directly targeting NAMPT. Aging Cell, 12 (6), 1062–1072.

Corbin, K.D., Zeisel, S.H., 2012. Choline metabolism provides novel insights into nonalcoholic fatty liver disease and its progression. Curr. Opin. Gastroenterol. 28 (2), 159–165. https://doi.org/10.1097/MOG.0b013e32834e7b4b.

Crisóstomo, L., Jarak, I., Rato, L.P., Raposo, J.F., Batterham, R.L., Oliveira, P.F., Alves, M.G., 2021. Inheritable testicular metabolic memory of high-fat diet causes transgenerational sperm defects in mice. Sci. Rep. 11 (1). https://doi.org/10.1038/s41598-021-88981-3.

da Silveira, E.J.D., Barros, C.C.D.S., Bottino, M.C., Castilho, R.M., Squarize, C., 2024. The rhythms of histones in regeneration: the epigenetic modifications determined by clock genes. Exp. Dermatol. 33 (1). https://doi.org/10.1111/exd.15005.

Deering, T.G., Ogihara, T., Trace, A.P., Maier, B., Mirmira, R.G., 2009. Methyltransferase set7/9 maintains transcription and euchromatin structure at islet-enriched genes. Diabetes 58 (1), 185–193. https://doi.org/10.2337/db08-1150.

Ding, N., Hah, N., Yu, R.T., Sherman, M.H., Benner, C., Leblanc, M., He, M., Liddle, C., Downes, M., Evans, R.M., 2015. BRD4 is a novel therapeutic target for liver fibrosis. Proc. Natl. Acad. Sci. U. S. A. 112 (51), 15713–15718. https://doi.org/10.1073/pnas.1522163112.

Du, X., Cai, C., Yao, J., Zhou, Y., Yu, H., Shen, W., 2017. Histone modifications in FASN modulated by sterol regulatory element-binding protein 1c and carbohydrate responsive-element binding protein under insulin stimulation are related to NAFLD. Biochem. Biophys. Res. Commun. 483 (1), 409–417. https://doi.org/10.1016/j.bbrc.2016.12.129.

Feng, T., Gu, S.Y., Shi, L.F., Gu, Y.H., Yuan, B.F., 2026. Mass spectrometry analysis reveals changes in patterns and correlations of nucleic acid epigenetic modifications in mouse tissues exposed to polystyrene microplastics. Chin. Chem. Lett. 37 (3). https://doi.org/10.1016/j.cclet.2025.111546.

Fiorito, G., Guarrera, S., Valle, C., Ricceri, F., Russo, A., Grioni, S., Mattiello, A., Di Gaetano, C., Rosa, F., Modica, F., Iacoviello, L., Frasca, G., Tumino, R., Krogh, V., Panico, S., Vineis, P., Sacerdote, C., Matullo, G., 2014. B-vitamins intake, DNA-methylation of One Carbon Metabolism and homocysteine pathway genes and myocardial infarction risk: the EPICOR study. Nutr. Metabol. Cardiovasc. Dis. 24 (5), 483–488. https://doi.org/10.1016/j.numecd.2013.10.026.

Galmozzi, A., Mitro, N., Ferrari, A., Gers, E., Gilardi, F., Godio, C., Cermenati, G., Gualerzi, A., Donetti, E., Rotili, D., Valente, S., Guerrini, U., Caruso, D., Mai, A., Saez, E., De Fabiani, E., Crestani, M., 2013. Inhibition of class I histone deacetylases unveils a mitochondrial signature and enhances oxidative metabolism in skeletal muscle and adipose tissue. Diabetes 62 (3), 732–742. https://doi.org/10.2337/db12-0548.

Gao, J., Wei, B., Liu, M., Hirsova, P., Sehrawat, T.S., Cao, S., Hu, X., Xue, F., Yaqoob, U., Kang, N., Cui, H., Pomerantz, W.C.K., Kostallari, E., Shah, V.H., 2021. Endothelial p300 promotes portal hypertension and hepatic fibrosis through C-C motif chemokine ligand 2–mediated angiocrine signaling. Hepatology 73 (6), 2468–2483. https://doi.org/10.1002/hep.31617.

Gao, Y., Yu, X., Wang, Y., Wang, H., Wang, Y.L., Shyh-Chang, N., 2025. Metabolic control of feto–placental development and pregnancy outcomes. Nat. Rev. Endocrinol. https://doi.org/10.1038/s41574-025-01206-9.

Gasmi, A., Noor, S., Menzel, A., Dosa, A., Pivina, L., Bjørklund, G., 2021. Obesity and insulin resistance: associations with chronic inflammation, genetic and epigenetic factors. Curr. Med. Chem. 28 (4), 800–826. https://doi.org/10.2174/0929867327666200824112056.

Goldsworthy, M., Absalom, N.L., Schröter, D., Matthews, H.C., Bogani, D., Moir, L., Long, A., Church, C., Hugill, A., Anstee, Q.M., Goldin, R., Thursz, M., Hollfelder, F., Cox, R.D., 2013. Mutations in Mll2, an H3K4 methyltransferase, result in insulin resistance and impaired glucose tolerance in mice. PLoS One 8 (6). https://doi.org/10.1371/journal.pone.0061870.

Gong, P., Guo, Z., Wang, S., Gao, S., Cao, Q., 2025. Histone phosphorylation in DNA damage response. Int. J. Mol. Sci. 26 (6), 2405. https://doi.org/10.3390/ijms26062405.

González-Suárez, M., Aguilar-Arnal, L., 2024. Histone methylation: at the crossroad between circadian rhythms in transcription and metabolism. Front. Genet. 15. https://doi.org/10.3389/fgene.2024.1343030.

Gorski, P.A., Jang, S.P., Jeong, D., Lee, A., Lee, P., Oh, J.G., Chepurko, V., Yang, D.K., Kwak, T.H., Eom, S.H., Park, Z.Y., Yoo, Y.J., Kim, D.H., Kook, H., Sunagawa, Y., Morimoto, T., Hasegawa, K., Sadoshima, J., Vangheluwe, P., Hajjar, R.J., Park, W.J., Kho, C., 2019. Role of SIRT1 in modulating acetylation of the Sarco-Endoplasmic Reticulum Ca2+-ATPase in heart failure. Circ. Res. 124 (9), e63. https://doi.org/10.1161/CIRCRESAHA.118.313865.

Greißel, A., Culmes, M., Burgkart, R., Zimmermann, A., Eckstein, H.H., Zernecke, A., Pelisek, J., 2016. Histone acetylation and methylation significantly change with severity of atherosclerosis in human carotid plaques. Cardiovasc. Pathol. 25 (2), 79–86. https://doi.org/10.1016/j.carpath.2015.11.001.

Guerrero-Bosagna, C.M., Skinner, M.K., 2014. Environmental epigenetics and phytoestrogen/phytochemical exposures. J. Steroid Biochem. Mol. Biol. 139, 270–276. https://doi.org/10.1016/j.jsbmb.2012.12.011.

Haggarty, P., Hoad, G., Horgan, G.W., Campbell, D.M., 2013. DNA methyltransferase candidate polymorphisms, imprinting methylation, and birth outcome. PLoS One 8 (7). https://doi.org/10.1371/journal.pone.0068896.

Han, Y., Nie, J., Wang, D.W., Ni, L., 2022. Mechanism of histone deacetylases in cardiac hypertrophy and its therapeutic inhibitors. Front. Cardiovasc. Med. 9. https://doi.org/10.3389/fcvm.2022.931475.

Haskard, D.O., Boyle, J.J., Evans, P.C., Mason, J.C., Randi, A.M., 2013. Cytoprotective signaling and gene expression in endothelial cells and macrophages-lessons for atherosclerosis. Microcirculation 20 (3), 203–216. https://doi.org/10.1111/micc.12020.

Hauck, A.K., Zhou, T., Upadhyay, A., Sun, Y., O'connor, M.B., Chen, Y., Bernlohr, D.A., 2020. Histone carbonylation is a redox-regulated epigenomic mark that accumulates with obesity and aging. Antioxidants 9 (12), 1–13. https://doi.org/10.3390/antiox9121210.

Haumaitre, C., Lenoir, O., Scharfmann, R., 2008. Histone deacetylase inhibitors modify pancreatic cell fate determination and amplify endocrine progenitors. Mol. Cell Biol. 28 (20), 6373–6383. https://doi.org/10.1128/mcb.00413-08.

Haumaitre, C., Lenoir, O., Scharfmann, R., 2014. Directing cell differentiation with small-molecule histone deacetylase inhibitors: the example of promoting pancreatic endocrine cells. Cell Cycle 8 (4), 536–544. https://doi.org/10.4161/cc.8.4.7610.

He, M., Huang, T.-S., Li, S., Hong, H.-C., Chen, Z., Martin, M., Zhou, X., Huang, H.-Y., Su, S.-H., Zhang, J., Wang, W.-T., Kang, J., Huang, H.-D., Zhang, J., Chien, S., Shyy, J.Y.-J., 2019. Atheroprotective flow upregulates ITPR3 (inositol 1,4,5-trisphosphate receptor 3) in vascular endothelium via KLF4 (Krüppel-Like factor 4)-mediated histone modifications. Arterioscler. Thromb. Vasc. Biol. 39 (5), 902–914. https://doi.org/10.1161/atvbaha.118.312301.

Healy, S., Khan, P., He, S., Davie, J.R., 2012. Histone H3 phosphorylation, immediate-early gene expression, and the nucleosomal response: a historical perspective. Biochem. Cell. Biol. 90 (1), 39–54. https://doi.org/10.1139/o11-092.

Hepp, P., Hutter, S., Knabl, J., Hofmann, S., Kuhn, C., Mahner, S., Jeschke, U., 2018. Histone H3 lysine 9 acetylation is downregulated in GDM placentas and calcitriol supplementation enhanced this effect. Int. J. Mol. Sci. 19 (12), 4061. https://doi.org/10.3390/ijms19124061.

Hou, T., Tian, Y., Cao, Z., Zhang, J., Feng, T., Tao, W., Sun, H., Wen, H., Lu, X., Zhu, Q., Li, M., Lu, X., Liu, B., Zhao, Y., Yang, Y., Zhu, W.-G., 2022. Cytoplasmic SIRT6-mediated ACSL5 deacetylation impedes nonalcoholic fatty liver disease by facilitating hepatic fatty acid oxidation. Mol. Cell 82 (21), 4099. https://doi.org/10.1016/j.molcel.2022.09.018.

Hu, J., Li, G., He, X., Gao, X., Pan, D., Dong, X., Hu, X., 2024. Brd4 modulates metabolic endotoxemia-induced inflammation by regulating colonic macrophage infiltration in high-fat diet-fed mice. Commun. Biol. 7 (1), 1708.

Huang, Z., Hu, L., Liu, Z., Wang, S., 2025. The functions and regulatory mechanisms of histone modifications in skeletal muscle development and disease. Int. J. Mol. Sci. 26 (8), 3644. https://doi.org/10.3390/ijms26083644.

Inoue, H., Asahara, S.I., Sugiura, Y., Kawada, Y., Imai, A., Hara, C., Kanno, A., Kimura-Koyanagi, M., Kido, Y., 2021. Histone deacetylase 6 regulates insulin signaling in pancreatic β cells. Biochem. Biophys. Res. Commun. 534, 896–901. https://doi.org/10.1016/j.bbrc.2020.10.078.

Javeed, N., Brown, M.R., Rakshit, K., Her, T., Sen, S.K., Matveyenko, A.V., 2021. Proinflammatory cytokine interleukin 1β disrupts β-cell circadian clock function and regulation of insulin secretion. Endocrinology (United States) 162 (1), 1–14. https://doi.org/10.1210/endocr/bqaa084.

Jenuwein, T., Allis, C.D., 2001. Translating the histone code. Science 293 (5532), 1074–1080. https://doi.org/10.1126/science.1063127.

Jiang, Y., Zhu, H., Chen, Z., Yu, Y.C., Guo, X.H., Chen, Y., Yang, M.M., Chen, B. W., Sagnelli, M., Xu, D., Zhao, B.H., Luo, Q., 2022. Hepatic IGF2/H19 epigenetic alteration induced glucose intolerance in gestational diabetes mellitus offspring via FoxO1 mediation. Front. Endocrinol. 13. https://doi.org/10.3389/fendo.2022.844707.

Jukarainen, S., Heinonen, S., Rämö, J.T., Rinnankoski-Tuikka, R., Rappou, E., Tummers, M., Muniandy, M., Hakkarainen, A., Lundbom, J., Lundbom, N., Kaprio, J., Rissanen, A., Pirinen, E., Pietiläinen, K.H., 2016. Obesity is associated with low nad+/sirt pathway expression in adipose tissue of BMI-discordant monozygotic twins. J. Clin. Endocrinol. Metab. 101 (1), 275–283. https://doi.org/10.1210/jc.2015-3095.

Ka, S.O., Bang, I.H., Bae, E.J., Park, B.H., 2017. Hepatocyte-specific sirtuin 6 deletion predisposes to nonalcoholic steatohepatitis by up-regulation of Bach1, an Nrf2 repressor. FASEB (Fed. Am. Soc. Exp. Biol.) J. 31 (9), 3999–4010. https://doi.org/10.1096/fj.201700098RR.

Kadakol, A., Malek, V., Goru, S.K., Pandey, A., Sharma, N., Gaikwad, A.B., 2017. Esculetin ameliorates insulin resistance and type 2 diabetic nephropathy through reversal of histone H3 acetylation and H2A lysine 119 monoubiquitination. J. Funct.Foods 35, 256–266. https://doi.org/10.1016/j.jff.2017.05.051.

Kain, V., Upadhyay, G., Marimuthu, M., Ma, Y., Yeatman, T.J., Halade, G.V., 2025. Reversing an obesogenic diet to control diet partially rescues pro-inflammatory lipid-immune memory in splenocardiac aging. J. Cardiovasc. Aging 5 (3).

Karnewar, S., Neeli, P.K., Panuganti, D., Kotagiri, S., Mallappa, S., Jain, N., Jerald, M.K., Kotamraju, S., 2018. Metformin regulates mitochondrial biogenesis and senescence through AMPK mediated H3K79 methylation: relevance in age-associated vascular dysfunction. Biochim. Biophys. Acta (BBA) - Mol. Basis Dis. 1864 (4), 1115–1128. https://doi.org/10.1016/j.bbadis.2018.01.018.

Keating, S.T., El-Osta, A., 2015. Epigenetics and metabolism. Circ. Res. 116 (4), 715–736. https://doi.org/10.1161/CIRCRESAHA.116.303936.

Kerr, B., Leiva, A., Farías, M., Contreras-Duarte, S., Toledo, F., Stolzenbach, F., Silva, L., Sobrevia, L., 2018. Foetoplacental epigenetic changes associated with maternal metabolic dysfunction. Placenta 69, 146–152. https://doi.org/10.1016/j.placenta.2018.04.006.

Kim, H., Kulkarni, R.N., 2020. Epigenetics in β-cell adaptation and type 2 diabetes. Curr. Opin. Pharmacol. 55, 125–131. https://doi.org/10.1016/j.coph.2020.10.008.

Kim, K.c., Friso, S., Choi, S.W., 2009. DNA methylation, an epigenetic mechanism connecting folate to healthy embryonic development and aging. JNB (J. Nutr. Biochem.) 20 (12), 917–926. https://doi.org/10.1016/j.jnutbio.2009.06.008.

Kim, D.H., Kim, J., Kwon, J.S., Sandhu, J., Tontonoz, P., Lee, S.K., Lee, S., Lee, J. W., 2016. Critical roles of the histone methyltransferase MLL4/KMT2D in murine hepatic steatosis directed by ABL1 and PPARγ2. Cell Rep. 17 (6), 1671–1682. https://doi.org/10.1016/j.celrep.2016.10.023.

Kim, J., Lee, B., Kim, D.H., Yeon, J.G., Lee, J., Park, Y., Lee, Y., Lee, S.K., Lee, S., Lee, J.W., 2019. UBE3A suppresses overnutrition-induced expression of the steatosis target genes of MLL4 by degrading MLL4. Hepatology 69 (3), 1122–1134. https://doi.org/10.1002/hep.30284.

Kim, J.H., Jung, D.Y., Kim, H.R., Jung, M.H., 2020. Histone h3k9 demethylase jmjd2b plays a role in lxrα-dependent lipogenesis. Int. J. Mol. Sci. 21 (21), 1–17. https://doi.org/10.3390/ijms21218313.

Kim, J.H., Nagappan, A., Jung, D.Y., Suh, N., Jung, M.H., 2021. Histone demethylase kdm7a contributes to the development of hepatic steatosis by targeting diacylglycerol acyltransferase 2. Int. J. Mol. Sci. 22 (20). https://doi.org/10.3390/ijms222011085.

Kim, H.J., Lee, J., Chung, M.Y., Park, S.H., Park, J.H., Choi, H.K., Hwang, J.T., 2022. Tamarixetin abrogates adipogenesis through inhibiting p300/CBP-associated factor acetyltransferase activity in 3T3-L1 preadipocyte cells. J. Med. Food 25 (3), 272–280. https://doi.org/10.1089/jmf.2021.K.0126.

Kirtana, A., Seetharaman, B., 2022. Comprehending the role of endocrine disruptors in inducing epigenetic toxicity. Endocr. Metab. Immune Disord. - Drug Targets 22 (11), 1059–1072. https://doi.org/10.2174/1871530322666220411082656.

Klymenko, O., Brecklinghaus, T., Dille, M., Springer, C., de Wendt, C., Altenhofen, D., Binsch, C., Knebel, B., Scheller, J., Hardt, C., Herwig, R., Chadt, A., Pfluger, P.T., Al-Hasani, H., Kabra, D.G., 2020. Histone deacetylase 5 regulates interleukin 6 secretion and insulin action in skeletal muscle. Mol. Metabol. 42, 101062. https://doi.org/10.1016/j.molmet.2020.101062.

Kolasinska-Zwierz, P., Down, T., Latorre, I., Liu, T., Liu, X.S., Ahringer, J., 2009. Differential chromatin marking of introns and expressed exons by H3K36me3. Nat. Genet. 41 (3), 376–381. https://doi.org/10.1038/ng.322.

Krishnaveni, G.V., Veena, S.R., Karat, S.C., Yajnik, C.S., Fall, C.H.D., 2014. Association between maternal folate concentrations during pregnancy and insulin resistance in Indian children. Diabetologia 57 (1), 110–121. https://doi.org/10.1007/s00125-013-3086-7.

LaSalle, J.M., 2013. Autism genes keep turning up chromatin. OA Autism 1 (2). https://doi.org/10.13172/2052-7810-1-2-610.

Lee, J.H., Hussain, M., Kim, E.W., Cheng, S.J., Leung, A.K.L., Fakouri, N.B., Croteau, D.L., Bohr, V.A., 2022. Mitochondrial PARP1 regulates NAD+-dependent poly ADP-ribosylation of mitochondrial nucleoids. Exp. Mol. Med. 54 (12), 2135–2147. https://doi.org/10.1038/s12276-022-00894-x.

Lehle, J.D., Lin, Y.H., Gomez, A., Chavez, L., McCarrey, J.R., 2024. An in vitro approach reveals molecular mechanisms underlying endocrine disruptor-induced epimutagenesis. eLife. https://doi.org/10.7554/eLife.93975.4.

Lenoir, O., Flosseau, K., Ma, F.X., Blondeau, B., Mai, A., Bassel-Duby, R., Ravassard, P., Olson, E.N., Haumaitre, C., Scharfmann, R., 2011. Specific control of pancreatic endocrine β- and δ-cell mass by class IIa histone deacetylases HDAC4, HDAC5, and HDAC9. Diabetes 60 (11), 2861–2871. https://doi.org/10.2337/db11-0440France.

Li, Y., Ge, K., Li, T., Cai, R., Chen, Y., 2023. The engagement of histone lysine methyltransferases with nucleosomes: structural basis, regulatory mechanisms, and therapeutic implications. Protein Cell 14 (3), 165–179. https://doi.org/10.1093/procel/pwac032.

Li, J., Zhang, S., Li, C., Zhang, X., Shan, Y., Zhang, Z., Bo, H., Zhang, Y., 2024. Endurance exercise-induced histone methylation modification involved in skeletal muscle fiber type transition and mitochondrial biogenesis. Sci. Rep. 14 (1). https://doi.org/10.1038/s41598-024-72088-6.

Liao, W., Xu, N., Zhang, H., Liao, W., Wang, Y., Wang, S., Zhang, S., Jiang, Y., Xie, W., Zhang, Y., 2022. Persistent high glucose induced EPB41L4A-AS1 inhibits glucose uptake via GCN5 mediating crotonylation and acetylation of histones and non-histones. Clin. Transl. Med. 12 (2). https://doi.org/10.1002/ctm2.699.

Lien, Y.C., Wang, P.Z., Lu, X.M., Simmons, R.A., 2020. Altered transcription factor binding and gene bivalency in islets of intrauterine growth retarded rats. Cells 9 (6). https://doi.org/10.3390/cells9061435.

Liu, M., Kluger, M.S., D'Alessio, A., García-Cardeña, G., Pober, J.S., 2008. Regulation of arterial-venous differences in tumor necrosis factor responsiveness of endothelial cells by anatomic context. Am. J. Pathol. 172 (4), 1088–1099. https://doi.org/10.2353/ajpath.2008.070603.

Liu, S., Yu, H., Liu, Y., Liu, X., Zhang, Y., Bu, C., Yuan, S., Chen, Z., Xie, G., Li, W., Xu, B., Yang, J., He, L., Tong, J., Xiong, Y., Sun, L., Liu, X., Han, C., Cheng, Z., Liang, J., Shang, Y., 2017. Chromodomain protein CDYL acts as a crotonyl-CoA hydratase to regulate histone crotonylation and spermatogenesis. Mol. Cell 67 (5), 853. https://doi.org/10.1016/j.molcel.2017.07.011.

Lukaszewski, M.A., Eberlé, D., Vieau, D., Breton, C., 2013. Nutritional manipulations in the perinatal period program adipose tissue in offspring. Am. J. Physiol. Endocrinol. Metab. 305 (10), E1195. https://doi.org/10.1152/ajpendo.00231.2013.

Lundh, M., Galbo, T., Poulsen, S.S., Mandrup-Poulsen, T., 2015. Histone deacetylase 3 inhibition improves glycaemia and insulin secretion in obese diabetic rats. Diabetes Obes. Metabol. 17 (7), 703–707. https://doi.org/10.1111/dom.12470.

Ma, J., He, X., Cao, Y., O'Dwyer, K., Szigety, K.M., Wu, Y., Gurung, B., Feng, Z., Katona, B.W., Hua, X., 2020. Islet-specific Prmt5 excision leads to reduced insulin expression and glucose intolerance in mice. J. Endocrinol. 244 (1), 41–52. https://doi.org/10.1530/JOE-19-0268.

Ma, J., You, D., Chen, S., Fang, N., Yi, X., Wang, Y., Lu, X., Li, X., Zhu, M., Xue, M., Tang, Y., Wei, X., Huang, J., Zhu, Y., 2022. Epigenetic association study uncovered H3K27 acetylation enhancers and dysregulated genes in high-fat-diet-induced nonalcoholic fatty liver disease in rats. Epigenomics 14 (23), 1523–1540. https://doi.org/10.2217/epi-2022-0362.

Maganti, A.V., Maier, B., Tersey, S.A., Sampley, M.L., Mosley, A.L., Özcan, S., Pachaiyappan, B., Woster, P.M., Hunter, C.S., Stein, R., Mirmira, R.G., 2015. Transcriptional activity of the islet β cell factor Pdx1 Is augmented by lysine methylation catalyzed by the methyltransferase Set7/9. J. Biol. Chem. 290 (15), 9812–9822. https://doi.org/10.1074/jbc.M114.616219.

Makkar, R., Behl, T., Arora, S., 2020. Role of HDAC inhibitors in diabetes mellitus. Curr. Res. Transl. Med. 68 (2), 45–50. https://doi.org/10.1016/j.retram.2019.08.001.

Manne, V., Handa, P., Kowdley, K.V., 2018. Pathophysiology of nonalcoholic fatty liver disease/nonalcoholic steatohepatitis. Clin. Liver Dis. 22 (1), 23–37. https://doi.org/10.1016/j.cld.2017.08.007.

Mansfield, B., 2017. Folded futurity: epigenetic plasticity, temporality, and new thresholds of fetal life. Sci. Cult. 26 (3), 355–379. https://doi.org/10.1080/09505431.2017.1294575.

Marsh, D.J., Ma, Y., Dickson, K.A., 2020. Histone monoubiquitination in chromatin remodelling: focus on the histone h2b interactome and cancer. Cancers 12 (11), 1–24. https://doi.org/10.3390/cancers12113462.

Masi, S., Ambrosini, S., Mohammed, S.A., Sciarretta, S., Lüscher, T.F., Paneni, F., Costantino, S., 2021. Epigenetic remodeling in obesity-related vascular disease. Antioxidants Redox Signal. 34 (15), 1165–1199. https://doi.org/10.1089/ars.2020.8040.

McGee, S.L., Van Denderen, B.J.W., Howlett, K.F., Mollica, J., Schertzer, J.D., Kemp, B.E., Hargreaves, M., 2008. AMP-activated protein kinase regulates GLUT4 transcription by phosphorylating histone deacetylase 5. Diabetes 57 (4), 860–867. https://doi.org/10.2337/db07-0843Australia.

McGee, S.L., Fairlie, E., Garnham, A.P., Hargreaves, M., 2009. Exercise-induced histone modifications in human skeletal muscle. J. Physiol. (Paris) 587 (24), 5951–5958. https://doi.org/10.1113/jphysiol.2009.181065.

Meng, T.G., Zhou, Q., Ma, X.S., Liu, X.Y., Meng, Q.R., Huang, X.J., Liu, H.L., Lei, W.L., Zhao, Z.H., Ouyang, Y.C., Hou, Y., Schatten, H., Ou, X.H., Wang, Z. B., Gao, S.R., Sun, Q.Y., 2020. PRC2 and EHMT1 regulate H3K27me2 and H3K27me3 establishment across the zygote genome. Nat. Commun. 11 (1). https://doi.org/10.1038/s41467-020-20242-9.

Mentch, S.J., Locasale, J.W., 2016. One-carbon metabolism and epigenetics: understanding the specificity. Ann. N. Y. Acad. Sci. 1363 (1), 91–98. https://doi.org/10.1111/nyas.12956.

Mesa, A.M., Rosenfeld, C.S., Tuteja, G., Medrano, T.I., Cooke, P.S., 2020. The roles of the histone protein modifier ezh2 in the uterus and placenta. Epigenomes 4 (3). https://doi.org/10.3390/epigenomes4030020.
Michalczyk, A.A., Dunbar, J.A., Janus, E.D., Best, J.D., Ebeling, P.R., Ackland, M. J., Asproloupos, D., Ackland, M.L., 2016. Epigenetic markers to predict conversion from gestational diabetes to type 2 diabetes. J. Clin. Endocrinol. Metab. 101 (6), 2396–2404. https://doi.org/10.1210/jc.2015-4206.
Monné, M., Marobbio, C.M.T., Agrimi, G., Palmieri, L., Palmieri, F., 2022. Mitochondrial transport and metabolism of the major methyl donor and versatile cofactor S-adenosylmethionine, and related diseases: a review. IUBMB Life 74 (7), 573–591. https://doi.org/10.1002/iub.2658.
Mosammaparast, N., Shi, Y., 2010. Reversal of histone methylation: biochemical and molecular mechanisms of histone demethylases. Annu. Rev. Biochem. 79 (1), 155–179. https://doi.org/10.1146/annurev.biochem.78.070907.103946.
Mushtaq, A., Ul Ashraf, N., Altaf, M., 2023. The mTORC1–G9a–H3K9me2 axis negatively regulates autophagy in fatty acid–induced hepatocellular lipotoxicity. J. Biol. Chem. 299 (3), 102937. https://doi.org/10.1016/j.jbc.2023.102937.
Nammo, T., Udagawa, H., Funahashi, N., Kawaguchi, M., Uebanso, T., Hiramoto, M., Nishimura, W., Yasuda, K., 2018. Genome-wide profiling of histone H3K27 acetylation featured fatty acid signalling in pancreatic beta cells in diet-induced obesity in mice. Diabetologia 61 (12), 2608–2620. https://doi.org/10.1007/s00125-018-4735-7.
Oommen, A.M., Griffin, J.B., Sarath, G., Zempleni, J., 2005. Roles for nutrients in epigenetic events. JNB (J. Nutr. Biochem.) 16 (2), 74–77. https://doi.org/10.1016/j.jnutbio.2004.08.004.
Osca-Verdegal, R., Beltrán-García, J., Paes, A.B., Nacher-Sendra, E., Novella, S., Hermenegildo, C., Carbonell, N., García-Giménez, J.L., Pallardó, F.V., 2022. Histone citrullination mediates a protective role in endothelium and modulates inflammation. Cells 11 (24). https://doi.org/10.3390/cells11244070.
Padeken, J., Methot, S.P., Gasser, S.M., 2022. Establishment of H3K9-methylated heterochromatin and its functions in tissue differentiation and maintenance. Nat. Rev. Mol. Cell Biol. 23 (9), 623–640. https://doi.org/10.1038/s41580-022-00483-w.
Palabiyik, A.A., Palabiyik, E., 2025. Pharmacological approaches to enhance mitochondrial biogenesis: focus on PGC-1A, AMPK, and SIRT1 in cellular health. Mol. Biol. Rep. 52 (1). https://doi.org/10.1007/s11033-025-10368-8.
Palou, A., 2006. New challenges in basic and applied nutrition. Rev. Med. Univ. Navarra 50 (4), 62–70.
Pan, M.H., Zhu, C.C., Ju, J.Q., Xu, Y., Luo, S.M., Sun, S.C., Ou, X.H., 2021. Single-cell transcriptome analysis reveals that maternal obesity affects DNA repair, histone methylation, and autophagy level in mouse embryos. J. Cell. Physiol. 236 (7), 4944–4953. https://doi.org/10.1002/jcp.30201.
Pedroso, J.A.B., Wasinski, F., Donato, J., 2020. Prolonged fasting induces long-lasting metabolic consequences in mice. J. Nutr. Biochem. 84, 108457. https://doi.org/10.1016/j.jnutbio.2020.108457.
Pedrotti, S., Caccia, R., Neguembor, M.V., Garcia-Manteiga, J.M., Ferri, G., De Palma, C., Canu, T., Giovarelli, M., Marra, P., Fiocchi, A., Molineris, I., Raso, M., Sanvito, F., Doglioni, C., Esposito, A., Clementi, E., Gabellini, D., 2019. The Suv420h histone methyltransferases regulate PPAR-γ and energy expenditure in response to environmental stimuli. Sci. Adv. 5 (4). https://doi.org/10.1126/sciadv.aav1472.

Perugorria, M.J., Wilson, C.L., Zeybel, M., Walsh, M., Amin, S., Robinson, S., White, S.A., Burt, A.D., Oakley, F., Tsukamoto, H., Mann, D.A., Mann, J., 2012. Histone methyltransferase ASH1 orchestrates fibrogenic gene transcription during myofibroblast transdifferentiation. Hepatology 56 (3), 1129–1139. https://doi.org/10.1002/hep.25754.

Pessoa Rodrigues, C., Chatterjee, A., Wiese, M., Stehle, T., Szymanski, W., Shvedunova, M., Akhtar, A., 2021. Histone H4 lysine 16 acetylation controls central carbon metabolism and diet-induced obesity in mice. Nat. Commun. 12 (1). https://doi.org/10.1038/s41467-021-26277-w.

Pinney, S.E., Jaeckle Santos, L.J., Han, Y., Stoffers, D.A., Simmons, R.A., 2011. Exendin-4 increases histone acetylase activity and reverses epigenetic modifications that silence Pdx1 in the intrauterine growth retarded rat. Diabetologia 54 (10), 2606–2614. https://doi.org/10.1007/s00125-011-2250-1.

Plunk, E.C., Richards, S.M., 2020. Epigenetic modifications due to environment, ageing, nutrition, and endocrine disrupting chemicals and their effects on the endocrine system. Int. J. Endocrinol. 2020. https://doi.org/10.1155/2020/9251980.

Purhonen, J., Rajendran, J., Tegelberg, S., Smolander, O.P., Pirinen, E., Kallijärvi, J., Fellman, V., 2018. NAD+ repletion produces no therapeutic effect in mice with respiratory chain complex III deficiency and chronic energy deprivation. FASEB (Fed. Am. Soc. Exp. Biol.) J. 32 (11), 5913–5926. https://doi.org/10.1096/fj.201800090R.

Qian, X., Li, X., Shi, Z., Bai, X., Xia, Y., Zheng, Y., Xu, D., Chen, F., You, Y., Fang, J., Hu, Z., Zhou, Q., Lu, Z., 2019. KDM3A senses oxygen availability to regulate PGC-1α-mediated mitochondrial biogenesis. Mol. Cell 76 (6), 885. https://doi.org/10.1016/j.molcel.2019.09.019.

Rafehi, H., Kaspi, A., Ziemann, M., Okabe, J., Karagiannis, T.C., El-Osta, A., 2017. Systems approach to the pharmacological actions of HDAC inhibitors reveals EP300 activities and convergent mechanisms of regulation in diabetes. Epigenetics 12 (11), 991–1003. https://doi.org/10.1080/15592294.2017.1371892.

Ramachandran, K., Senagolage, M.D., Sommars, M.A., Futtner, C.R., Omura, Y., Allred, A.L., Barish, G.D., 2019. Dynamic enhancers control skeletal muscle identity and reprogramming. PLoS Biol. 17 (10). https://doi.org/10.1371/journal.pbio.3000467.

Reddy, M.A., Natarajan, R., 2011. Epigenetic mechanisms in diabetic vascular complications. Cardiovasc. Res. 90 (3), 421–429. https://doi.org/10.1093/cvr/cvr024.

Remsberg, J.R., Ediger, B.N., Ho, W.Y., Damle, M., Li, Z., Teng, C., Lanzillotta, C., Stoffers, D.A., Lazar, M.A., 2017. Deletion of histone deacetylase 3 in adult beta cells improves glucose tolerance via increased insulin secretion. Mol. Metabol. 6 (1), 30–37. https://doi.org/10.1016/j.molmet.2016.11.007.

Rohrbach, T.D., Asgharpour, A., Maczis, M.A., Montefusco, D., Cowart, L.A., Bedossa, P., Sanyal, A.J., Spiegel, S., 2019. FTY720/fingolimod decreases hepatic steatosis and expression of fatty acid synthase in diet-induced nonalcoholic fatty liver disease in mice. JLR (J. Lipid Res.) 60 (7), 1311–1322. https://doi.org/10.1194/jlr.M093799.

Roichman, A., Elhanati, S., Aon, M.A., Abramovich, I., Di Francesco, A., Shahar, Y., Avivi, M.Y., Shurgi, M., Rubinstein, A., Wiesner, Y., Shuchami, A., Petrover, Z., Lebenthal-Loinger, I., Yaron, O., Lyashkov, A., Ubaida-Mohien, C., Kanfi, Y., Lerrer, B., Fernández-Marcos, P.J., Serrano, M., Gottlieb, E., de Cabo, R., Cohen, H.Y., 2021. Restoration of energy homeostasis by SIRT6 extends healthy lifespan. Nat. Commun. 12 (1). https://doi.org/10.1038/s41467-021-23545-7.

Rush, E.C., Katre, P., Yajnik, C.S., 2014. Vitamin B12: one carbon metabolism, fetal growth and programming for chronic disease. Eur. J. Clin. Nutr. 68 (1), 2–7. https://doi.org/10.1038/ejcn.2013.232.

Ryu, H.Y., Hochstrasser, M., 2021. Histone sumoylation and chromatin dynamics. Nucleic Acids Res. 49 (11), 6043–6052. https://doi.org/10.1093/nar/gkab280.

Sabari, B.R., 2016. Metabolic Regulation of Gene Expression through Differential Histone Acylation: The Regulation and Function of Histone Crotonylation.

Seok, S., Kim, Y.C., Byun, S., Choi, S., Xiao, Z., Iwamori, N., Zhang, Y., Wang, C., Ma, J., Ge, K., Kemper, B., Kemper, J.K., 2018. Fasting-induced JMJD3 histone demethylase epigenetically activates mitochondrial fatty acid ß-oxidation. J. Clin. Investig. 128 (7), 3144–3159. https://doi.org/10.1172/JCI97736.

Shahbazian, M.D., Grunstein, M., 2007. Functions of Site-Specific histone acetylation and deacetylation. Annu. Rev. Biochem. 76, 75–100. https://doi.org/10.1146/annurev.biochem.76.052705.162114.

Shao, J., Li, L., Xu, H., Yang, L., Bian, Y., Fang, M., Xu, Y., 2017. Suv39h2 deficiency ameliorates diet-induced steatosis in mice. Biochem. Biophys. Res. Commun. 485 (3), 658–664. https://doi.org/10.1016/j.bbrc.2017.02.093.

Shi, Y., Qi, W., 2023. Histone modifications in NAFLD: mechanisms and potential therapy. Int. J. Mol. Sci. 24 (19), 14653. https://doi.org/10.3390/ijms241914653.

Shin, H.S., Lee, Y., Shin, M.H., Cho, S.I., Zouboulis, C.C., Kim, M.K., Lee, D.H., Chung, J.H., 2021. Histone deacetylase 1 reduces lipogenesis by suppressing srebp1 transcription in human sebocyte cell line sz95. Int. J. Mol. Sci. 22 (9). https://doi.org/10.3390/ijms22094477.

Siersbæk, M., Varticovski, L., Yang, S., Baek, S., Nielsen, R., Mandrup, S., Hager, G.L., Chung, J.H., Grøntved, L., 2017. High fat diet-induced changes of mouse hepatic transcription and enhancer activity can be reversed by subsequent weight loss. Sci. Rep. 7 (1). https://doi.org/10.1038/srep40220.

Slaughter, M.J., Shanle, E.K., Khan, A., Chua, K.F., Hong, T., Boxer, L.D., Allis, C. D., Josefowicz, S.Z., Garcia, B.A., Rothbart, S.B., Strahl, B.D., Davis, I.J., 2021. HDAC inhibition results in widespread alteration of the histone acetylation landscape and BRD4 targeting to gene bodies. Cell Rep. 34 (3). https://doi.org/10.1016/j.celrep.2020.108638.

Soheilykhah, S., Mojibian, M., Rashidi, M., Rahimi-Saghand, S., Jafari, F., 2010. Maternal vitamin D status in gestational diabetes mellitus. Nutr. Clin. Pract. 25 (5), 524–527. https://doi.org/10.1177/0884533610379851.

Spaeth, J.M., Walker, E.M., Stein, R., 2016. Impact of Pdx1-associated chromatin modifiers on islet β-cells . Diabetes. Obes. Metabol. 18 (S1), 123–127. https://doi.org/10.1111/dom.12730.

Stover, P.J., 2012. Polymorphisms in 1-carbon metabolism, epigenetics and folate-related pathologies. Lifestyle Genom. 4 (5), 293–305. https://doi.org/10.1159/000334586.

Suchitra, M., Praveen Kumar, K., Katagi, M.S., Venkateswarlu, G., Sree Mahalakshmi, P., 2023. HDAC inhibitors: a novel approach to hyperglycaemia management and treatment. Health Sci. Rev. 9, 100137. https://doi.org/10.1016/j.hsr.2023.100137.

Sun, C., Zhang, F., Ge, X., Yan, T., Chen, X., Shi, X., Zhai, Q., 2007. SIRT1 improves insulin sensitivity under insulin-resistant conditions by repressing PTP1B. Cell Metab. 6 (4), 307–319. https://doi.org/10.1016/j.cmet.2007.08.014.

Sun, C., Fan, J.G., Qiao, L., 2015. Potential epigenetic mechanism in non-alcoholic fatty liver disease. Int. J. Mol. Sci. 16 (3), 5161–5179. https://doi.org/10.3390/ijms16035161.

Swathi, N.L., Shakhatreh, Z., Tahir, A., Singh, J., Sulaiman, S., Athul, H., Sadhankar, A., Patel, P., Patel, R., Nashwan, A.J., 2025. Epigenetic mechanisms in the transfer of metabolic disorders: a comprehensive review. Cureus 17 (3). https://doi.org/10.7759/cureus.80418.

Thaker, V.V., 2017. Genetic and epigenetic causes of obesity. Adolesc. Med. 28 (2), 379–405.

Tollefsbol, T.O., 2013. Dietary epigenetics in cancer and aging. Adv. Nutr. Cancer 257–267.

Vachharajani, V.T., Liu, T., Wang, X., Hoth, J.J., Yoza, B.K., McCall, C.E., 2016. Sirtuins link inflammation and metabolism. J. Immunol. Res. 2016. https://doi.org/10.1155/2016/8167273.

Vanderkruk, B., Maeshima, N., Pasula, D.J., An, M., Suresh, P., Daniel, A., Hoffman, B.G., 2021. H3K4 methylation in β-cells prevents transcriptional downregulation and variance associated with type 2 diabetes. bioRxiv 2021–01.

Viscarra, J.A., Wang, Y., Nguyen, H.P., Choi, Y.G., Sul, H.S., 2020. Histone demethylase JMJD1C is phosphorylated by mTOR to activate de novo lipogenesis. Nat. Commun. 11 (1). https://doi.org/10.1038/s41467-020-14617-1.

Vlad, M.L., Manea, S.A., Lazar, A.G., Raicu, M., Muresian, H., Simionescu, M., Manea, A., 2019. Histone acetyltransferase-dependent pathways mediate upregulation of NADPH oxidase 5 in human macrophages under inflammatory conditions: a potential mechanism of reactive oxygen species overproduction in atherosclerosis. Oxid. Med. Cell. Longev. 2019 (1), 3201062.

Vo, N., Goodman, R.H., 2001. CREB-Binding protein and p300 in transcriptional regulation. J. Biol. Chem. 276 (17), 13505–13508. https://doi.org/10.1074/jbc.r000025200.

Wang, B., Yang, Q., Sun, Y.Y., Xing, Y.F., Wang, Y.B., Lu, X.T., Bai, W.W., Liu, X. Q., Zhao, Y.X., 2014. Resveratrol-enhanced autophagic flux ameliorates myocardial oxidative stress injury in diabetic mice. J. Cell Mol. Med. 18 (8), 1599–1611. https://doi.org/10.1111/jcmm.12312.

Wang, Y., Zhao, L., Jiao, F.Z., Zhang, W.B., Chen, Q., Gong, Z.J., 2018. Histone deacetylase inhibitor suberoylanilide hydroxamic acid alleviates liver fibrosis by suppressing the transforming growth factor-β1 signal pathway. Hepatobiliary Pancreat. Dis. Int. 17 (5), 423–429. https://doi.org/10.1016/j.hbpd.2018.09.013.

Wang, J., Xu, X., Li, P., Zhang, B., Zhang, J., 2021. HDAC3 protects against atherosclerosis through inhibition of inflammation via the microRNA-19b/PPARγ/NF-κB axis. Atherosclerosis 323, 1–12. https://doi.org/10.1016/j.atherosclerosis.2021.02.013.

Wang, Z., Zhu, M., Wang, M., Gao, Y., Zhang, C., Liu, S., Qu, S., Liu, Z., Zhang, C., 2021. Integrated multiomic analysis reveals the high-fat diet induced activation of the MAPK signaling and inflammation associated metabolic cascades via histone modification in adipose tissues. Front. Genet. 12, 650863. https://doi.org/10.3389/fgene.2021.650863.

Wang, N., Wang, W., Wang, X., Mang, G., Chen, J., Yan, X., Tong, Z., Yang, Q., Wang, M., Chen, L., Sun, P., Yang, Y., Cui, J., Yang, M., Zhang, Y., Wang, D., Wu, J., Zhang, M., Yu, B., 2022. Histone lactylation boosts reparative gene activation post–myocardial infarction. Circ. Res. 131 (11), 893–908. https://doi.org/10.1161/circresaha.122.320488.

Wang, Y., Xie, H., Liu, Q., Wang, N., Luo, X., Sun, F., Zhu, J., Dong, R., Wang, Y., Gao, J., Gao, Z., Huang, T., Liu, X., Yu, Q., Wang, T., Yang, L., Song, D., Liu, S., Zhang, S., Yin, H., Wen, K., Wang, C.-Y., 2025. Kdm2a inhibition in skeletal muscle improves metabolic flexibility in obesity. Nat. Metab. 7 (2), 383–400. https://doi.org/10.1038/s42255-024-01210-9.

Xu, Y., Xu, S., Liu, P., Koroleva, M., Zhang, S., Si, S., Jin, Z.G., 2017. Suberanilohydroxamic acid as a pharmacological Kruppel-like factor 2 activator that represses vascular inflammation and atherosclerosis. J. Am. Heart Assoc. 6 (12). https://doi.org/10.1161/JAHA.117.007134.

Wang, Z., Zhu, M., Wang, M., Gao, Y., Zhang, C., Liu, S., Zhang, C., 2021. Integrated multiomic analysis reveals the high-fat diet induced activation of the MAPK signaling and inflammation associated metabolic cascades via histone modification in adipose tissues. Front. Genet. 12, 650863.

Xu, L., Lin, J., Deng, W., Luo, W., Huang, Y., Liu, C.Q., Zhang, F.P., Qin, Y.F., Wong, P.P., Liu, C., 2020. EZH2 facilitates BMI1-dependent hepatocarcinogenesis through epigenetically silencing microRNA-200c. Oncogenesis 9 (11). https://doi.org/10.1038/s41389-020-00284-w.

Yamato, E., 2018. High dose of histone deacetylase inhibitors affects insulin secretory mechanism of pancreatic beta cell line. Endocr. Regul. 52 (1), 21–26. https://doi.org/10.2478/enr-2018-0004.

Yao, W., Hu, X., Wang, X., 2024. Crossing epigenetic frontiers: the intersection of novel histone modifications and diseases. Signal Transduct. Targeted Ther. 9 (1). https://doi.org/10.1038/s41392-024-01918-w.

Ye, C., Tu, B.P., 2018. Sink into the epigenome: histones as repositories that influence cellular metabolism. Trends Endocrinol. Metabol. 29 (9), 626–637. https://doi.org/10.1016/j.tem.2018.06.002.

Yi, Y., Wang, T., Xu, W., Zhang, S.-H., 2024. Epigenetic modifications of placenta in women with gestational diabetes mellitus and their offspring. World J. Diabetes 15 (3), 378–391. https://doi.org/10.4239/wjd.v15.i3.378.

Yu, X.Y., Geng, Y.J., Liang, J.L., Zhang, S., Lei, H.P., Zhong, S.L., Lin, Q.X., Shan, Z.X., Lin, S.G., Li, Y., 2012. High levels of glucose induce "metabolic memory" in cardiomyocyte via epigenetic histone H3 lysine 9 methylation. Mol. Biol. Rep. 39 (9), 8891–8898. https://doi.org/10.1007/s11033-012-1756-z.

Yu, W., Wang, Z., Zhang, K., Chi, Z., Xu, T., Jiang, D., Chen, S., Li, W., Yang, X., Zhang, X., Wu, Y., Wang, Di, 2019. One-carbon metabolism supports S-adenosylmethionine and histone methylation to drive inflammatory macrophages. Mol. Cell 75 (6), 1147. https://doi.org/10.1016/j.molcel.2019.06.039.

Zeybel, M., Luli, S., Sabater, L., Hardy, T., Oakley, F., Leslie, J., Page, A., Moran Salvador, E., Sharkey, V., Tsukamoto, H., Chu, D.C.K., Singh, U.S., Ponzoni, M., Perri, P., Di Paolo, D., Mendivil, E.J., Mann, J., Mann, D.A., 2017. A proof-of-concept for epigenetic therapy of tissue fibrosis: inhibition of liver fibrosis progression by 3-deazaneplanocin A. Mol. Ther. 25 (1), 218–231. https://doi.org/10.1016/j.ymthe.2016.10.004.

Zhang, Q., Ramlee, M.K., Brunmeir, R., Villanueva, C.J., Halperin, D., Xu, F., 2012. Dynamic and distinct histone modifications modulate the expression of key adipogenesis regulatory genes. Cell Cycle 11 (23), 4310–4322. https://doi.org/10.4161/cc.22224.

Zhang, J., Chen, J., Yang, J., Xu, C., Qi, H., Wu, H., Cai, W., Guo, Q., Gao, W., He, C., Yang, C., Yang, J., 2019. Suv39h1 downregulation inhibits neointimal hyperplasia after vascular injury. Atherosclerosis 288, 76–84. https://doi.org/10.1016/j.atherosclerosis.2019.06.909.

Zhang, H., Ma, Y., Cheng, X., Wu, D., Huang, X., Chen, B., Ren, Y., Jiang, W., Tang, X., Bai, T., Chen, Y., Zhao, Y., Zhang, C., Xiao, X., Liu, J., Deng, Y., Ye, T., Chen, L., Liu, H.-M., Friedman, S.L., Chen, L., Ding, B.-S., Cao, Z., 2021. Targeting epigenetically maladapted vascular niche alleviates liver fibrosis in nonalcoholic steatohepatitis. Sci. Transl. Med. 13 (614). https://doi.org/10.1126/scitranslmed.abd1206.

Zhang, Q., Wu, Y.X., Yu, X.Q., Zhang, B.Y., Ma, L.Y., 2023. EZH2 serves as a promising therapeutic target for fibrosis. Bioorg. Chem. 137. https://doi.org/10.1016/j.bioorg.2023.106578.

Zhang, Y., Verwilligen, R.A.F., Van Eck, M., Hoekstra, M., 2023. PRMT5 inhibition induces pro-inflammatory macrophage polarization and increased hepatic triglyceride levels without affecting atherosclerosis in mice. J. Cell Mol. Med. 27 (8), 1056–1068. https://doi.org/10.1111/jcmm.17676.

Zhou, B., Jia, L., Zhang, Z., Xiang, L., Yuan, Y., Zheng, P., Liu, B., Ren, X., Bian, H., Xie, L., Li, Y., Lu, J., Zhang, H., Lu, Y., 2020. The nuclear orphan receptor NR2F6 promotes hepatic steatosis through upregulation of fatty acid transporter CD36. Adv. Sci. 7 (21). https://doi.org/10.1002/advs.202002273.

Zhou, F., Liu, Q., Zhang, L., Zhu, Q., Wang, S., Zhu, K., Deng, R., Liu, Y., Yuan, G., Wang, X., Zhou, L., 2020. Selective inhibition of CBP/p300 HAT by A-485 results in suppression of lipogenesis and hepatic gluconeogenesis. Cell Death Dis. 11 (9). https://doi.org/10.1038/s41419-020-02960-6.

Zhou, R., Zhao, J., Li, D., Chen, Y., Xiao, Y., Fan, A., Chen, X.-T., Wang, H.-L., 2020. Combined exposure of lead and cadmium leads to the aggravated neurotoxicity through regulating the expression of histone deacetylase 2. Chemosphere 252, 126589. https://doi.org/10.1016/j.chemosphere.2020.126589.

Zhuang, Y., Zhang, Y., Liu, C., Zhong, Y., 2024. Interplay between the circadian clock and sirtuins. Int. J. Mol. Sci. 25 (21), 11469. https://doi.org/10.3390/ijms252111469.

Zou, D., Liao, J., Xiao, M., Liu, L., Dai, D., Xu, M., 2024. Impaired SUMOylation of FoxA1 promotes nonalcoholic fatty liver disease through down-regulation of Sirt6. Cell Death Dis. 15 (9). https://doi.org/10.1038/s41419-024-07054-1.

5

MicroRNAs in metabolic syndrome and diabetes

1. Introduction

miRNAs are increasingly recognized as key epigenetic regulators that modulate gene expression without altering the underlying DNA sequence. Acting predominantly at the post transcriptional level, miRNAs fine-tune cellular phenotypes by binding to complementary sequences in target mRNAs, leading to translational repression or mRNA degradation (Yao et al., 2019). Beyond this classical role, miRNAs actively participate in epigenetic regulation networks by targeting genes that encode epigenetic modifiers, including DNA methyltransferases (DNMTs), histone acetyltransferases (HATs), histone deacetylases (HDACs), and chromatin-remodeling complexes (Humphries et al., 2019). Conversely, the expression of miRNAs themselves is regulated by epigenetic mechanisms such as DNA methylation and histone modifications at miRNA gene promoters, creating a dynamic feedback loop between miRNAs and the epigenome (Kurozumi et al., 2017). Through this bidirectional interaction, miRNAs contribute to the establishment and maintenance of stable gene expression patterns, cellular memory, and phenotypic plasticity. Dysregulation of miRNA-mediated epigenetic control has been implicated in metabolic disorders, cancer, and inflammatory diseases, underscoring their role as both mediators and markers of epigenetic modifications.

miRNAs are small (19–22 nucleotides), non-coding, single-stranded RNA molecules that regulate gene expression at the post transcriptional level in eukaryotic cells (Wronska, 2023). Since their discovery in *Caenorhabditis elegans* in 1993, miRNAs have been identified across multiple species, including flies, mice, and humans (Weiss and Ito, 2018). miRNAs are transcribed by RNA polymerase II and processed by Drosha and Dicer enzymes to generate mature miRNAs (O'Brien et al., 2018). Functionally, miRNAs suppress gene expression by binding to the 3′ untranslated region (3′-UTR) of target mRNAs, leading to

Metabolic Memory. https://doi.org/10.1016/B978-0-443-44591-0.00006-0

translational repression or mRNA degradation. Approximately 30% of protein-coding genes are regulated by miRNAs (Sekar et al., 2016). A single miRNA can target multiple genes, enabling miRNAs to regulate diverse physiological and pathological processes (Alarcón et al., 2015).

miRNAs are involved in cell differentiation, proliferation, apoptosis, and tumorigenesis, thereby influencing diseases such as T2DM, cancer, atherosclerosis, and CVD (Tang et al., 2019). They also regulate insulin homeostasis, and their dysregulation can contribute to metabolic imbalance (Azimzadeh et al., 2015). Importantly, miRNAs are detectable in extracellular fluids such as serum, plasma, saliva, urine, and milk. Their stability and reproducibility in healthy individuals make them promising non-invasive biomarkers for disease diagnosis and prognosis (Chen et al., 2012).

Advances in miRNA biology have reshaped the classical understanding of gene regulation and highlighted miRNAs as potential therapeutic targets with minimal side effects. Recent studies have identified miR-146a and miR-200 as antiinflammatory regulators in diabetic nephropathy (Bhatt et al., 2016), while their pro-inflammatory roles in vascular smooth muscle cells have been linked to diabetic vascular complications (Reddy et al., 2012). Population-based studies have established miRNAs such as miR-126 as diagnostic biomarkers for T2DM and impaired glucose tolerance (IGT) (Rezk et al., 2016), while dysregulation of miR-199a-3p, miR-199b-3p, miR-4454, and miR-519d has been associated with obesity and adipocyte hypertrophy (Ouyang et al., 2017; Martinelli et al., 2010). Additional studies have identified distinct miRNA signatures in metabolically unhealthy obese individuals and cardiometabolic disorders across diverse populations (Mir et al., 2022; Masoudi et al., 2022; Brandão-Lima et al., 2023). Emerging therapeutic strategies, including miRNA-loaded edible plant-derived nanoparticles, offer innovative and safe approaches for treating obesity and metabolic diseases (Campolo et al., 2022).

This book chapter summarizes current evidence on the regulatory roles of miRNAs in the pathogenesis of metabolic syndrome, highlighting their potential as diagnostic biomarkers and therapeutic targets.

2. miRNA biogenesis and function

MicroRNAs (miRNAs) are evolutionarily conserved regulatory molecules found in all multicellular organisms, including humans and plants, highlighting their essential role in normal cellular function. Complete disruption of miRNA processing is lethal, underscoring their biological importance (Bartel, 2009). miRNAs are short, non-coding RNA molecules of approximately 19–22 nucleotides that regulate gene expression at the post transcriptional level. The human genome encodes more than 1100 miRNAs, which collectively regulate over 60% of protein-coding genes in mammals (Friedman et al., 2009). miRNAs exert their regulatory effects by binding to complementary target sequences on messenger RNAs (mRNAs), resulting in translational repression, deadenylation, mRNA cleavage, or degradation (Yekta et al., 2004).

miRNA biogenesis is a highly regulated, multi-step process involving several enzymes localized in both the nucleus and cytoplasm (Mastropasqua et al., 2014). Tight spatial and temporal control of miRNA synthesis is critical, as dysregulation at any stage of this process has been linked to numerous human diseases (Caus et al., 2021). In animals, the canonical pathway represents the primary mechanism of miRNA production and begins with transcription by RNA polymerase II or III (Ha and Kim, 2014). Although alternative non-canonical pathways that bypass Drosha or Dicer processing have been described, these pathways generate only about 1% of conserved miRNAs and are often associated with specific pathological conditions (Stavast and Erkeland, 2019).

In the canonical pathway, miRNA synthesis initiates in the nucleus with the transcription of primary miRNA (pri-miRNA) transcripts by RNA polymerase II (Fig. 5.1). These pri-miRNAs are subsequently processed by the Drosha enzyme into precursor miRNAs (pre-miRNAs), which possess a characteristic stem–loop structure. The pre-miRNAs are then transported from the nucleus to the cytoplasm by the Exportin-5/Ran-GTP complex. In the cytoplasm, the RNase III enzyme Dicer, together with its cofactor TRBP, cleaves the pre-miRNA to generate a double-stranded miRNA duplex. One strand of this duplex, known as the guide strand, is incorporated into the RNA-induced silencing complex (RISC) containing the Argonaute protein, while the passenger strand is typically degraded. The mature miRNA-RISC complex then binds to complementary sequences on target mRNAs, leading to post transcriptional regulation of gene expression (Ha and Kim, 2014).

miRNAs have been established as key regulators of a wide range of developmental and physiological processes, including metabolism, cell proliferation, apoptosis, developmental timing, and neuronal cell fate determination (Zamore and Haley, 2005; Croce and Calin, 2005). Increasing evidence indicates that altered

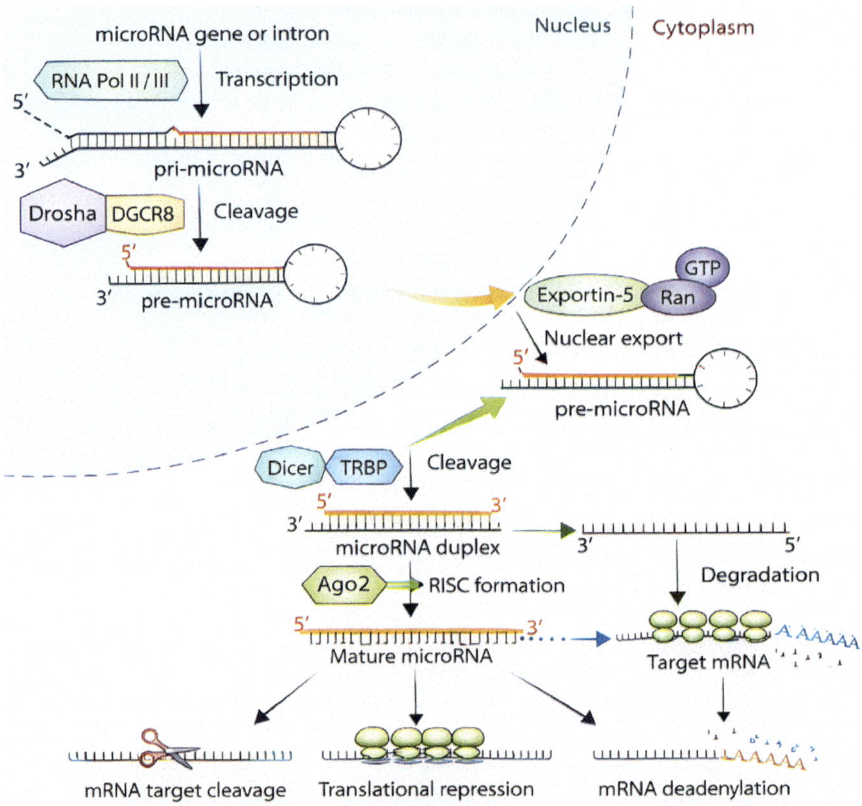

Figure 5.1 Schematic representation of canonical microRNA biogenesis and mechanism of gene regulation. This figure illustrates the canonical pathway of microRNA (miRNA) biogenesis, starting from transcription of primary miRNA (pri-miRNA) in the nucleus to the formation of mature miRNA in the cytoplasm. The mature miRNA, incorporated into the RNA-induced silencing complex (RISC), regulates gene expression through mRNA cleavage, translational repression, or mRNA deadenylation. *Abbreviations*: DGCR8, DiGeorge Syndrome Critical Region 8 (Drosha cofactor), Ran-GTP, Ras-related nuclear protein bound to GTP, TRBP, TAR RNA-Binding Protein, Ago2, Argonaute-2, core component of RISC, RISC, RNA-Induced Silencing Complex, mRNA, Messenger RNA.

miRNA expression profiles are associated with diverse pathological conditions such as viral hepatitis, cancer, metabolic disorders, and myocardial infarction. In disease states, certain miRNAs are downregulated while others are overexpressed, resulting in distinct disease-specific miRNA signatures (Naveed et al., 2017). In eukaryotic organisms, miRNAs play a critical role in controlling developmental pathways and maintaining cellular homeostasis. Due to their ability to regulate cell proliferation and differentiation, miRNAs have emerged as promising therapeutic targets in cancer (Menon et al., 2022). In some cancers, miRNAs act as oncogenes and are referred to as "oncomiRs" because their overexpression contributes to tumor development and progression (Otmani et al., 2024). With rapid advances in miRNA research, these molecules are expected to have significant potential in the diagnosis and treatment of a wide range of diseases in the near future.

3. Role of miRNAs in metabolic-associated disorders

Metabolic syndrome comprises a cluster of metabolic abnormalities, including central obesity, hypertriglyceridemia, reduced high-density lipoprotein (HDL) cholesterol, hypertension, hyperglycemia, and a pro-inflammatory and prothrombotic state. miRNAs play essential roles in regulating metabolic pathways such as glucose homeostasis, lipid metabolism, cholesterol balance, and fatty acid oxidation (Rahman et al., 2024). Obesity and type 2 diabetes mellitus (T2DM) are characterized by increased secretion of inflammatory and pro-inflammatory cytokines and adipokines from adipocytes and infiltrating macrophages in adipose tissue (Sliwinska et al., 2017). Notably, specific miRNAs have been identified as potential biomarkers capable of distinguishing between obesity and T2DM (Hutny et al., 2022). These findings have been validated in both human studies and animal models of obesity and insulin resistance. For example, elevated expression of the pro-inflammatory cytokine interleukin-6 (IL-6) has been associated with reduced levels of miR-132 and miR-155 in adipocytes from obese individuals (Hulsmans et al., 2011). Increased IL-6 expression has also been observed in the circulation and hepatocytes of patients with non-alcoholic fatty liver disease (NAFLD) (Dogru et al., 2008; Wieckowska et al., 2008). Additionally, adipocyte differentiation suppresses the expression of miR-155, miR-130, and miR-1100, which are involved in macrophage infiltration and inflammatory responses (Marques-Rocha et al., 2015).

An increasing number of studies highlight miRNAs as clinically relevant tools, particularly emphasizing circulating miRNAs as diagnostic and prognostic biomarkers in cancer and other disorders (Keller and Meese, 2016; Matsuzaki and Ochiya, 2017). A substantial body of literature has also examined the role of miRNAs in obesity and metabolic diseases, which are major global health challenges (Deiuliis, 2016). Emerging evidence suggests that miRNA expression levels can be modulated by lifestyle factors and dietary habits (Slattery et al., 2017) and are responsive to nutritional interventions (Palmer et al., 2014).

4. miRNA mediated regulation of adipogenesis and inflammation in obesity

Obesity and its related disorders constitute a major global public health challenge, with a continuously rising prevalence that significantly contributes to worldwide morbidity, mortality, and socioeconomic burden (Heneghan et al., 2010). Obesity is defined as excessive accumulation of fat and energy within adipose tissue (Cummings and Schwartz, 2003), arising from sedentary lifestyles, high caloric intake, and genetic susceptibility (Thanikachalam et al., 2018). This pathological state disrupts the normal function of adipose tissue, which is responsible for the tightly regulated storage and release of lipids. Chronic energy surplus leads to adipocyte dysfunction, altered adipokine and hormone secretion, and ectopic lipid deposition in peripheral organs such as the liver, pancreas, skeletal muscle, and kidneys, thereby promoting lipotoxicity, chronic low-grade inflammation, and systemic metabolic disturbances (Unger, 2003). Obesity-associated inflammation is characterized by elevated production of inflammatory cytokines and proteins that interfere with adipokine signaling and lipolytic enzyme activity (Jung and Choi, 2014). Consequently, dysfunctional adipose tissue markedly increases the risk of metabolic complications, including insulin resistance (IR), cardiovascular disease (CVD), and type 2 diabetes mellitus (T2DM) (Hilton et al., 2013).

A comprehensive understanding of adipogenesis, comprising lineage commitment, clonal expansion, and terminal differentiation, is essential for developing effective therapeutic strategies against obesity (Ali et al., 2013). This process is orchestrated by transcription factors such as PPARγ, C/EBPα/β, and SREBP1, with miRNAs emerging as critical modulators that fine-tune adipocyte differentiation and metabolic outcomes in obesity (Lin et al., 2009). The regulatory role of microRNAs (miRNAs) in adipose tissue metabolism was first demonstrated in *Drosophila*, where miR-14 suppressed fat metabolism by targeting the p38 and MAPK signaling pathways (Xu et al., 2003). Since then, large-scale omics studies have established strong associations between altered miRNA expression profiles in metabolic organs, such as adipose tissue, liver, and pancreas; and the development of obesity and metabolic disorders (Dumortier et al., 2013). Accumulating evidence highlights miRNAs as critical regulators of adipogenesis, lipid metabolism, and insulin signaling (Xie et al., 2009). These small non-coding RNAs influence diverse physiological and pathological processes, including cell proliferation, differentiation, apoptosis, hematopoiesis, and limb morphogenesis, as well as metabolic pathways governing insulin secretion, oxidative stress, and lipid synthesis (Aranda et al., 2013).

Multiple miRNAs regulate lipid metabolism across metabolic organs (Table 5.1). In the liver, miR-1 targets liver X receptor alpha (LXRα) and fatty acid synthase (FASN), activating lipogenic genes such as FAS, ChREBP, SREBP, and ACC1 and thereby promoting de novo fatty acid synthesis (Wang and Tontonoz, 2018). Similarly, miR-122 plays a central role in hepatic lipid metabolism by regulating PMVK, HMGCR, CCNG1, and ADAM17, contributing to hepatic steatosis and modulation of circulating triglyceride and cholesterol levels (Fernández-Hernando et al., 2013). Its isoform, miR-122-5p, activates lipogenic gene transcription via LXRα signaling in adipose tissue (Wang and Tontonoz, 2018). In muscle and adipose tissue, the let-7 family targets IGF-1R, INSR, IRS2, and HMGA2, leading to reduced fat mass, impaired glucose-stimulated insulin secretion (GSIS), and increased glucose intolerance (Frost and Olson, 2011). miR-7 regulates insulin sensitivity in the liver by targeting HMGA2, E2F6, and CDC34 (Zhu et al., 2011). Adipogenesis is tightly controlled by several miRNAs: miR-15a regulates adipocyte differentiation by targeting DLK1 (Andersen et al., 2010), while miR-17-5p promotes clonal expansion of adipocytes and contributes to insulin resistance through RBL2 suppression (Klöting et al., 2009). The miR-17–92 cluster further enhances adipocyte development and triglyceride synthesis by targeting RB2 and p130 (Peng et al., 2014).

Fatty acid metabolism is regulated by miR-19b-1, which targets ACSL1 to facilitate conversion of long-chain fatty acids into acyl-CoA (Li et al., 2011), and by miR-26a, which promotes acetyl-CoA production through ACSL4 regulation (Cruz-Gil et al., 2018). In contrast, miR-27a/b inhibits adipocyte differentiation by targeting PPARG, ANGPTL3, GPAM, C/EBPα, and ABCA1 (Paul et al., 2021), while miR-130 suppresses adipogenesis via PPARG inhibition (Lee et al., 2011). Cholesterol metabolism and mitochondrial function are influenced by miR-24, which targets FASN, PGC1α, and HMGCR, and by miR-106b, which facilitates HDL biogenesis through ABCA1 regulation (Wang et al., 2018).

Inflammatory and insulin signaling pathways are modulated by miR-29a/b, which prevents Akt phosphorylation and impairs insulin-stimulated glucose uptake by targeting INSIG1, CAV2, FOXO1/3, and COL4A1 across multiple metabolic tissues

Table 5.1 miRNA-Mediated regulation of adipogenesis, lipid metabolism, and inflammation in obesity.

miRNA	Major target genes	Functional role	Target organ/ tissue	References
miR-1	LXRα, FASN	Activates lipogenic gene transcription (FAS, ChREBP, SREBP, ACC1); promotes de novo fatty acid synthesis	Liver	Wang and Tontonoz (2018)
miR-122	PMVK, HMGCR, CCNG1, ADAM17	Regulates hepatic steatosis; controls circulating triglycerides and cholesterol	Liver	Fernández-Hernando et al. (2013)
miR-122-5p	LXRα	Activates lipogenic gene transcription	Adipose tissue	Wang and Tontonoz (2018)
let-7 family	IGF-1R, INSR, IRS2, HMGA2	Decreases fat mass; impairs GSIS; promotes glucose intolerance	Muscle, adipose tissue	Frost and Olson (2011)
miR-7	HMGA2, E2F6, CDC34	Modulates insulin sensitivity	Liver	Zhu et al. (2011)
miR-15a	DLK1	Regulates adipocyte differentiation	Adipose tissue	Andersen et al. (2010)
miR-17-5p	RBL2	Promotes adipocyte clonal expansion; induces insulin resistance	Adipose tissue	Klöting et al. (2009)
miR-17–92 cluster	RB2, p130	Enhances adipocyte development and triglyceride synthesis	Adipocytes	Peng et al. (2014)
miR-19b-1	ACSL1	Converts long-chain fatty acids into acyl-CoA	Adipose tissue	Li et al. (2011)
miR-26a	ACSL4	Promotes acetyl-CoA production from fatty acids	Adipose tissue	Cruz-Gil et al. (2018)
miR-27a/b	PPARG, ANGPTL3, GPAM, C/EBPα, ABCA1	Inhibits adipocyte differentiation	Adipose tissue	Paul et al. (2021)
miR-130	PPARG	Suppresses adipogenesis	Adipose tissue	Lee et al. (2011)
miR-24	FASN, PGC1α, HMGCR	Regulates cholesterol synthesis, mitochondrial biogenesis, energy metabolism	Adipose tissue	Wang et al. (2018)
miR-106b	ABCA1	Facilitates HDL biogenesis	Adipose tissue	Kim et al. (2015)

miR-29a/b	INSIG1, CAV2, FOXO1/3, COL4A1	Inhibits Akt phosphorylation; impairs insulin-stimulated glucose uptake	Kidney, liver, muscle, adipose tissue	Thanikachalam et al. (2018)
miR-31	C/EBPα	Regulates adipogenesis	Adipose tissue	McGregor and Choi (2011)
miR-31-5p	OLR-1	Activates pro-inflammatory signaling and angiogenesis via oxidized LDL	Adipose tissue	Ruiz-Roso et al. (2020)
miR-21	TGFBR2	Modulates adipogenesis	Mesenchymal stem cells	Gerin et al. (2010)
miR-33a/b	ABCA1, CPT1A, HADHB, IRS2, PRKAA1	Inhibits insulin signaling and fatty acid oxidation	Liver, macrophages, β-cells	Kim et al. (2015)
miR-34	ACSL1, SIRT1, VAMP2	Regulates fatty acid activation and metabolic homeostasis	Adipose tissue, liver, pancreas	Cruz-Gil et al. (2018)
miR-103/107	CAV1, DICER, PDK1, WNT3A	Promotes insulin resistance; impairs adipocyte differentiation	Liver, adipose tissue	Fernández-Hernando et al. (2013)
miR-132	CREB	Activates inflammatory pathways; enhances adipocyte proliferation; induces insulin resistance	Adipose tissue	Strum et al. (2009)
miR-133a/b	PRDM-16	Increases energy expenditure; improves glucose tolerance; reduces adipogenesis	Adipose tissue	Abente et al. (2016)
miR-196a	HOX-C8	Promotes adipogenic remodeling	Adipose tissue	Abente et al. (2016)
miR-138	EID1	Regulates adipogenesis	Adipose tissue	Wang et al. (2019)
miR-210	TCF7L2	Modulates adipogenic differentiation	Adipose tissue	Ortega et al. (2010)
miR-215	CTNNBIP1, FNDC3B	Negative regulator of adipocyte differentiation	Adipose tissue	Scheideler (2016)
miR-448	KLF5	Inhibits triglyceride accumulation and adipocyte development	Adipocytes	Kinoshita et al. (2010)
miR-519d	PPARα	Promotes maturation of pre-adipocytes	Adipose tissue	Martinelli et al. (2010)
miR-142	ACSL1, ACSL4	Facilitates conversion of fatty acids to acetyl-CoA	Adipose tissue	Cruz-Gil et al. (2018)
miR-206	FASN, LXRα	Promotes de novo fatty acid synthesis	Adipose tissue	Wang and Tontonoz (2018)

Continued

Table 5.1 miRNA-Mediated regulation of adipogenesis, lipid metabolism, and inflammation in obesity.—*continued*

miRNA	Major target genes	Functional role	Target organ/ tissue	References
miR-370	ACC1, CPT1α, FASN	Regulates malonyl-CoA synthesis and mitochondrial FA transport	Liver, adipose tissue	Jones et al. (2017)
miR-544a	ACSL1, ACSL4	Enhances long-chain fatty acid activation	Adipose tissue	Jones et al. (2017)
miR-148a	HMGCR, PGC1α	Stimulates insulin gene transcription	Adipose tissue, liver	Carrer et al. (2012)
miR-335	STXBP1	Regulates fatty acid synthesis, triglycerides, and insulin	Pancreas, liver, adipose tissue	Esguerra et al. (2011)
miR-143	ERK5, GLUT, PPARγ2, MAPK7	Inhibits adipocyte differentiation; promotes insulin resistance	Liver, adipose tissue, pancreas	Rottiers and Näär (2012)
miR-223	FBXW-7	Suppresses TLR4; regulates macrophage-mediated inflammation	Adipose tissue	Deiuliis et al. (2016)
miR-200b-5p	OLR-1	Promotes pro-inflammatory signaling and angiogenesis	Adipose tissue	Ruiz-Roso et al. (2020)
miR-145	RS1, PPARγ2, C/EBPα	Suppresses adipogenesis; reduces triglyceride accumulation	Adipocytes	Abente et al. (2016)
miR-146b	SIRT1	Promotes adipogenesis by inhibiting SIRT1-FOXO1 signaling	Adipose tissue	Abente et al. (2016)
miR-155	CREB, C/EBPβ	Regulates brown-to-white adipocyte transition; modulates adipogenesis	Adipocytes	Abente et al. (2016)
miR-378/378*	ESRRG, GABPA	Regulates adipocyte differentiation and lipid synthesis	Liver, adipose tissue	Carrer et al. (2012)

(Thanikachalam et al., 2018). miR-31 regulates adipogenesis via C/EBPα, while miR-31-5p and miR-200b-5p activate pro-inflammatory signaling and angiogenesis by recognizing oxidized LDL through OLR-1 (Ruiz-Roso et al., 2020). miR-21 modulates adipogenesis in mesenchymal stem cells by targeting TGFBR2 (Gerin et al., 2010). The miR-33a/b family exerts pleiotropic effects on lipid and glucose metabolism by targeting ABCA1, CPT1A, HADHB, IRS2, and PRKAA1 (AMPK), thereby inhibiting insulin signaling and fatty acid oxidation in the liver, macrophages, and pancreatic β-cells (Kim et al., 2015). miR-34 regulates fatty acid activation and metabolic homeostasis via ACSL1, SIRT1, and VAMP2 (Cruz-Gil et al., 2018), while miR-103 and miR-107 impair adipocyte differentiation and promote insulin resistance through CAV1, DICER, PDK1, and WNT3A (Fernández-Hernando et al., 2013). miR-132 activates inflammatory pathways and enhances adipocyte proliferation through CREB signaling (Strum et al., 2009).

Several miRNAs regulate adipocyte lineage commitment and differentiation. miR-133a/b targets PRDM-16, increasing energy expenditure and reducing adipogenesis, while miR-196a suppresses HOX-C8 to promote adipogenic remodeling (Abente et al., 2016). miR-138, miR-210, and miR-215 regulate adipogenesis through EID1, TCF7L2, and CTNNBIP1/FNDC3B, respectively (Scheideler, 2016). miR-448 inhibits triglyceride accumulation via KLF5 [104], whereas miR-519d promotes adipocyte maturation through PPARα (Martinelli et al., 2010).

Lipid handling is further controlled by miR-142, miR-206, miR-370, and miR-544a, which collectively regulate fatty acid activation, malonyl-CoA synthesis, and mitochondrial fatty acid transport across adipose tissue and liver (Wang and Tontonoz, 2018; Cruz-Gil et al., 2018; "Jones, J. E. C., Esler, W. P., Patel, R., Lanba, A., Vera, N. B., Pfefferkorn, J. A., & Vernochet, C. (2017). Inhibition of acetylCoA carboxylase 1 (ACC1) and 2 (ACC2) reduces proliferation and de novo lipogenesis of EGFRvIII human glioblastoma cells. PLoS ONE, 12(1), e0169566.," no date). Insulin signaling is influenced by miR-148a, which stimulates insulin gene transcription (Wang et al., 2018), and by miR-335, which regulates fatty acid synthesis, triglyceride accumulation, and insulin production (Esguerra et al., 2011). Conversely, miR-143 suppresses adipocyte differentiation and promotes insulin resistance across metabolic organs (Rottiers and Näär, 2012).

Inflammatory miRNAs also contribute to adipose tissue dysfunction. miR-223 suppresses TLR4 expression and macrophage activation in adipose tissue (Deiuliis et al., 2016), while miR-145, miR-146b, and miR-155 regulate adipogenesis through epigenetic and transcriptional mechanisms involving PPARγ, C/EBPα, SIRT1, FOXO1, and CREB signaling (Abente et al., 2016). Finally, miR-378 and miR-378* regulate adipocyte differentiation and lipid synthesis via ESRRG and GABPA, reinforcing their role in systemic energy metabolism (Carrer et al., 2012).

Beyond adipogenesis, miRNAs also regulate adipocyte function. Adipose tissue acts as a major endocrine organ capable of secreting more than 600 adipokines, many of which have potential value as therapeutic biomarkers (Flehmig et al., 2014). Adipokines such as interleukin-6 (IL-6), tumor necrosis factor-α (TNF-α), resistin, adiponectin, apelin, and leptin, along with metabolic substrates like glucose and free fatty acids (FFAs), play pivotal roles in obesity-associated insulin resistance. These adipokines also influence the expression of miRNAs involved in adipogenesis. Obesity is further associated with increased macrophage infiltration into adipose tissue, leading to elevated secretion of inflammatory mediators such as TNF-α, CCL2, and IL-6 (Thanikachalam et al., 2018). Several miRNAs have been shown to regulate the expression of these inflammatory markers (Fig. 5.1).

5. miRNA and diabetes

Diabetes mellitus is a heterogeneous metabolic disorder characterized by pancreatic β-cell dysfunction and impaired insulin secretion, resulting in chronic hyperglycemia and widespread disturbances in carbohydrate, protein, and lipid metabolism (Tan et al., 2019). According to the World Health Organization (WHO), more than 400 million individuals currently live with diabetes worldwide, and this number is projected to rise to 552 million by 2030. Persistent loss of glycemic control leads to classical symptoms such as polyuria, glycosuria, weight loss, neuropathy, retinopathy, and renal and vascular complications, contributing to high morbidity and mortality (Ngari et al., 2020).

Diabetes has now reached epidemic proportions, particularly in low- and middle-income countries undergoing rapid socioeconomic transitions. Based on etiology and clinical features, diabetes is classified into four major types: type 1 diabetes mellitus (T1DM), type 2 diabetes mellitus (T2DM), gestational diabetes, and other specific forms. T1DM accounts for approximately 5%–10% of cases and arises from autoimmune-mediated destruction of pancreatic β-cells, resulting in absolute insulin deficiency. In contrast, T2DM represents 90%–99% of cases and is characterized by insulin resistance, defective insulin secretion, or both. Chronic hyperglycemia in both T1DM and T2DM drives macrovascular complications such as stroke, coronary artery disease (CAD), and peripheral artery disease, as well as microvascular complications including diabetic neuropathy, retinopathy, and nephropathy (Fowler, 2008).

Since their discovery, an expanding repertoire of microRNAs (miRNAs) has been implicated in the pathophysiology of diabetes mellitus (Table 5.2). miRNAs regulate diverse biological processes, including insulin resistance, pancreatic β-cell development and survival, glucose and lipid metabolism, inflammation, oxidative stress, and diabetes-associated complications (Cuperus et al., 2011). Dysregulation of miRNA expression disrupts metabolic homeostasis and contributes to disease onset and progression, positioning miRNAs as promising biomarkers and therapeutic targets (Al-Goblan et al., 2014). Importantly, miRNA-mediated regulation is highly tissue-specific and context-dependent, reflecting the complex metabolic dysregulation observed in diabetes.

5.1 Pancreatic β-cell function, miRNAs, and epigenetic control

Diabetes is closely associated with alterations in pancreatic hormone synthesis and secretion. Early evidence supporting miRNA involvement in endocrine regulation emerged from cloning studies of small RNAs in the insulin-secreting MIN6 β-cell line (Poy et al., 2004). Subsequent studies demonstrated that numerous miRNAs regulate pancreatic α- and β-cell differentiation, insulin biosynthesis, glucose-stimulated insulin secretion (GSIS), and β-cell survival (Table 5.3) (Tang et al., 2008).

Several miRNAs directly modulate insulin secretion and β-cell identity. miR-3a enhances insulin secretion by targeting SIRT1 in pancreatic β-cells (Thanikachalam et al., 2018), whereas miR-7 negatively regulates β-cell mass and insulin synthesis by targeting PAX6, p70S6K, and eIF4E (Calderari et al., 2017). The let-7 family targets HMGA2, INSR, RICTOR, RFX6, TSC1, IR2, and IGFIR, resulting in reduced adipogenesis and altered glucose metabolism across pancreatic β-cells, skeletal muscle, liver, and adipose tissue (Thanikachalam et al., 2018). miR-9, miR-24, miR-26, miR-30, miR-148, miR-182, and miR-200/141 further fine-tune insulin gene transcription and secretion by targeting key transcriptional regulators such as NeuroD1, SOX6, RFX6, and BHLHE family members (Thanikachalam et al., 2018; Calderari et al., 2017).

Table 5.2 Role of miRNAs in diabetes mellitus, insulin resistance, and metabolic memory.

Functional category	Key miRNAs	Major target genes/ pathways	Biological effects	Primary tissues	References
General metabolic regulation	Multiple miRNAs	Insulin signaling, glucose & lipid metabolism, inflammatory and oxidative stress pathways	Regulate insulin resistance, β-cell survival, metabolism, and diabetic complications	Pancreas, liver, muscle, adipose tissue	(Cuperus et al., 2011; Al-Goblan et al., 2014)
β-cell insulin secretion & identity	miR-3a	SIRT1	Enhances insulin secretion	Pancreatic β-cells	Thanikachalam et al. (2018)
	miR-7	PAX6, p70S6K, eIF4E	Reduces β-cell mass and insulin synthesis	Pancreatic islets	Calderari et al. (2017)
	Let-7 family	HMGA2, INSR, RICTOR, RFX6, TSC1, IR2, IGFIR	Reduces adipogenesis; alters glucose metabolism and insulin sensitivity	β-cells, muscle, liver, adipose tissue	Thanikachalam et al. (2018)
	miR-9, miR-24, miR-26, miR-30, miR-148, miR-182, miR-200/141	NeuroD1, SOX6, RFX6, BHLHE family	Fine-tune insulin gene transcription and secretion	Pancreatic β-cells	(Thanikachalam et al., 2018; Calderari et al., 2017)
miRNA biogenesis & β-cell function	Dicer-dependent miRNAs	miRNA maturation machinery	Loss impairs insulin synthesis, GSIS, and induces diabetes	Pancreatic β-cells	Mandelbaum et al. (2012)
	Argonaute (Ago)-associated miRNAs	miRNA–RISC complexes	Ago ablation enhances insulin production	Pancreatic β-cells	Tattikota et al. (2013)
Insulin resistance – skeletal muscle	miR-15a, miR-16	AKT3, PTCH1, PI3KR1, IRS1	Modulate insulin signaling and metabolic gene expression	Skeletal muscle	Tiwari et al. (2018)
	miR-135	IRS2	Decreases insulin-stimulated glucose uptake	Skeletal muscle	Calderari et al. (2017)
	miR-106b	Mitochondrial & inflammatory signaling	Promotes insulin resistance	Skeletal muscle	Tiwari et al. (2018)

Hepatic insulin resistance & lipid metabolism	miR-33	AMPKα, SIRT6, ABCA1, HADHB	Impairs insulin signaling, lipid oxidation, cholesterol efflux	Liver	(Thanikachalam et al., 2018; Calderari et al., 2017)
	miR-122	AMPKα1, HMGCR, G6PC	Regulates lipid and glucose homeostasis	Liver	Thanikachalam et al. (2018)
	miR-195, miR-301a, miR-320, miR-499	INSR, PTEN, PI3K–Akt pathway	Promote hepatic insulin resistance	Liver, adipocytes	Feng et al. (2016)
Oxidative stress & inflammation	miR-25, miR-423-5p, miR-483	NOX4, MAPK signaling	Increase ROS production and inflammatory signaling	Pancreatic β-cells	(Włodarski et al., 2020; Calderari et al., 2017)
	miR-211, miR-217, miR-221, miR-233, miR-543	SIRT1, Keap-1	Suppress Nrf2 signaling; increase oxidative stress	Pancreatic β-cells	Włodarski et al. (2020)
Diabetic complications	miR-21	PTEN, SMAD7	Vascular dysfunction, fibrosis	Serum, adipose tissue	Thanikachalam et al. (2018)
	miR-192	SIP1	Renal fibrosis and diabetic nephropathy	Kidney	Thanikachalam et al. (2018)
	miR-155	Immune regulatory pathways	Reduced expression associated with T2DM progression	PBMCs	Thanikachalam et al. (2018)
Metabolic memory & epigenetic regulation	Multiple miRNAs	DNMTs, HATs, HDACs, histone methyltransferases	Sustain long-term gene expression changes after hyperglycemia	Pancreas, liver, muscle, adipose tissue	(Cuperus et al., 2011; Al-Goblan et al., 2014)

Table 5.3 miRNAs Involved in diabetic complications and related metabolic disorders.

Diabetic complication	miRNA(s)	Major target genes/pathways	Functional role	Affected tissue/organ	References
Cardiovascular complications (CAD, cardiomyopathy, atherosclerosis)	miR-33a, miR-21, miR-208	WHSC2, ERG, SPRY1, CDC42, RhoA, HCN channels	Cardiac hypertrophy, reduced cardiac output, ventricular remodeling	Heart, vasculature	Iacomino and Siani (2017)
	miR-30	CTGF	Promotes cardiac fibrosis and collagen accumulation	Heart	Kantharidis et al. (2011)
	miR-126, miR-320	Spred1–ERK1/2, VEGF–IGF-1	Impaired angiogenesis, cardiac hypertrophy, long QT syndrome	Heart, endothelium	Matsuda et al. (2016)
	miR-16, miR-503, miR-24	COX-2, CCNE1/CDC25A, HMGB1	Endothelial dysfunction, inflammation, atherosclerosis	Heart, blood vessels	Kantharidis et al. (2011)
Diabetic retinopathy	miR-21, miR-146, miR-132, miR-155	Fibronectin, IRAK1, TRAF6	NF-κB activation, ICAM-1 and MCP-1 upregulation	Retinal endothelial cells	Moura et al. (2014)
	miR-29	VEGF, IRAK1, RAX, TRAF6	PKR–RAX stress signaling, early retinal injury	Retinal ganglion cells	Mastropasqua et al. (2014)
	miR-34 family	p53, VEGF pathways	Retinal epithelial dysfunction	Retinal pigment epithelium	Moura et al. (2014)
	miR-93, miR-145, miR-200, miR-455-5p	VEGF, TLR4, SOCS3	Altered angiogenesis, inflammation, migration	Retinal epithelial cells	(Kantharidis et al., 2011; Qadir et al., 2019)
Diabetic nephropathy	miR-25	PTEN, CDC42	Promotes renal fibrosis and glomerular injury	Kidney	Kantharidis et al. (2011)
	miR-93	VEGF	Microvascular injury and fibrosis	Kidney	Qadir et al. (2019)
	miR-192, miR-216a	ZEB1/2, PTEN	Mesangial expansion, ECM accumulation	Kidney	Moura et al. (2014)
	miR-377	MnSOD	Oxidative stress, fibronectin accumulation	Kidney	Wang et al. (2011)
	miR-200 family	TGF-β, ZEB1/2	EMT and renal fibrosis	Kidney	Moura et al. (2014)

Diabetic neuropathy (sensory and autonomic)	miR-27a, miR-499a	ND	Increased risk of peripheral and autonomic neuropathy	Heart, smooth muscle	(Cheng et al., 2015; Simeoli and Fierabracci, 2019)
	miR-146a	IRAK1, TRAF6	Alters neurotrophin signaling	Brain	Simeoli and Fierabracci (2019)
	miR-128a	ND	Genetic susceptibility to neuropathy	Neural tissue	Ciccacci et al. (2014)
	miR-216a, miR-217	ND	Progressive neural damage	Neural tissue	Simeoli and Fierabracci (2019)
	miR-302	PTEN	Neurotoxicity	Neural tissue	Qadir et al. (2019)
Atherosclerosis	miR-34a	ND	Plaque instability, lipid dysregulation	Plasma, vasculature	Price et al. (2014)
	miR-16, miR-503, miR-24	Inflammatory signaling pathways	Endothelial dysfunction	Blood vessels	Raitoharju et al. (2013)
NAFLD/NASH	miR-23b	TGF-β	Hepatic fibrosis	Hepatic stellate cells	(H. Chen et al., 2014)
	miR-148b	TGF-β signaling	Dysregulated fibrogenesis	Hepatic stellate cells	Koeck et al. (2014)
	miR-214	Twist, CCN2	Suppresses fibrogenic signaling	Hepatic stellate cells	(L. Chen et al., 2014)
	miR-4269, miR-4429	TGF-β	NAFLD progression	Hepatic stellate cells	Koeck et al. (2014)
	miR-103, miR-33, miR-27b, miR-34, miR-223, miR-370, miR-122	ABCA transporters, SIRT1, IRS2, SIRT6, LETF, HNF	Cholesterol and fatty acid metabolism	Liver, heart	Iacomino and Siani (2017)

Genetic ablation studies provide compelling mechanistic evidence for miRNA-dependent β-cell regulation. β-cell–specific deletion of Dicer disrupts miRNA biogenesis, leading to impaired insulin synthesis, defective GSIS, and diabetes onset (Mandelbaum et al., 2012). Conversely, targeted ablation of Argonaute proteins enhances insulin production, underscoring the regulatory complexity of miRNA-RIS + C complexes in β-cell physiology (Tattikota et al., 2013). At the cellular level, insulin secretion is initiated by membrane depolarization driven by increased ATP: ADP ratios, a process indirectly regulated by miRNAs through their effects on mitochondrial metabolism, ion channels, and vesicle trafficking (H. Chen et al., 2014).

5.2 Insulin resistance, peripheral tissues, and miRNA networks

Following nutrient intake, insulin acts on peripheral tissues, primarily the liver, skeletal muscle, and adipose tissue, to maintain glucose homeostasis. Insulin resistance is characterized by elevated blood glucose levels, reduced glucose uptake in skeletal muscle and adipose tissue, and impaired suppression of hepatic gluconeogenesis. This condition arises when peripheral tissues fail to respond adequately to physiological insulin concentrations (Peppa et al., 2010).

Multiple miRNAs regulate key components of insulin signaling pathways. miR-15a and miR-16 modulate insulin signaling and metabolic gene expression in skeletal muscle by targeting AKT3, PTCH1, PI3KR1, and IRS1 (Tiwari et al., 2018). miR-135 reduces insulin-stimulated glucose uptake via IRS2 suppression (Calderari et al., 2017), while miR-106b promotes insulin resistance through mitochondrial and inflammatory signaling pathways (Tiwari et al., 2018). Hepatic insulin resistance and lipid dysregulation are strongly influenced by miR-33, miR-122, miR-195, miR-301a, miR-320, and miR-499, which target genes involved in cholesterol transport, fatty acid oxidation, AMPK signaling, PI3K–Akt pathways, and insulin receptor function (Calderari et al., 2017; Feng et al., 2016).

5.3 miRNAs, inflammation, oxidative stress, and diabetic complications

Several miRNAs contribute to oxidative stress, inflammation, and tissue damage in diabetes. miR-25, miR-423-5p, and miR-483 regulate NOX-dependent ROS production and MAPK signaling in pancreatic β-cells (Włodarski et al., 2020; Calderari et al., 2017). miR-211, miR-217, miR-221, miR-233, and miR-543 target SIRT1 or Keap-1, leading to impaired Nrf2 signaling, increased oxidative stress, and β-cell dysfunction (Włodarski et al., 2020). miR-21 and miR-192 are implicated in vascular and renal fibrosis, contributing to diabetic nephropathy and microvascular complications (Thanikachalam et al., 2018). Reduced expression of miR-155 in T2DM patients further links immune dysregulation with disease progression (Thanikachalam et al., 2018).

6. miRNAs in other diabetic complications

Dysregulation of glucose metabolism is closely associated with long-term degenerative complications in both type 1 and type 2 diabetes mellitus. Diabetic complications are broadly categorized into macrovascular outcomes, including cardiomyopathy and atherosclerosis, and microvascular complications such as diabetic retinopathy, diabetic nephropathy, and peripheral neuropathy (Simeoli and Fierabracci, 2019). Growing evidence indicates that aberrant miRNA expression contributes significantly to the initiation and progression of these tissue-specific diabetic pathologies, linking epigenetic dysregulation to sustained organ damage (Table 5.3).

6.1 Cardiovascular complications and miRNA dysregulation

Diabetes is a major risk factor for chronic cardiovascular disorders affecting both the vasculature and myocardium, including coronary artery disease (CAD), stroke, hypertension, and atherosclerosis (Chew et al., 2013). These pathologies collectively contribute to heart failure through molecular, structural, and functional remodeling of cardiac tissue. Diabetic cardiomyopathy is characterized by impaired myocardial contractility and progressive cardiac dysfunction independent of hypertension or CAD.

Multiple miRNAs regulate pathways involved in cardiac hypertrophy, fibrosis, angiogenesis, and endothelial dysfunction. miR-33a, miR-21, and miR-208 target genes such as WHSC2, ERG, SPRY1, CDC42, RhoA, and HCN channels, contributing to reduced cardiac output and ventricular remodeling associated with CAD (Iacomino and Siani, 2017). miR-30 modulates connective tissue growth factor (CTGF), and its expression correlates with collagen accumulation and severe cardiac fibrosis (Kantharidis et al., 2011). miR-126 and miR-320 impair angiogenic signaling through Spred1–ERK1/2 and VEGF–IGF-1 pathways, contributing to long QT syndrome, cardiac hypertrophy, and reduced angiogenesis in diabetes (Matsuda et al., 2016). Endothelial dysfunction and atherosclerosis are further regulated by miR-16, miR-503, and miR-24 through COX-2, CCNE1/CDC25A, and HMGB1-mediated inflammatory signaling (Kantharidis et al., 2011).

6.2 Diabetic retinopathy and miRNA-mediated vascular dysfunction

Diabetic retinopathy is among the leading causes of blindness worldwide. Chronic hyperglycemia induces degeneration of retinal microvasculature, neuro-retinal dysfunction, and impaired insulin signaling (Mcclelland and Kantharidis, 2014). Early studies using streptozotocin-induced diabetic rat models demonstrated significant alterations in miRNA expression profiles within retinal endothelial cells, identifying miRNAs as key contributors to retinal vascular damage.

miR-21, miR-146, miR-132, and miR-155 target fibronectin, IRAK1, and TRAF6, resulting in upregulation of ICAM-1 and MCP-1 and sustained activation of NF-κB signaling in diabetic retinal endothelial cells (Moura et al., 2014). miR-29 is upregulated in retinal ganglion cells during early diabetes and regulates VEGF, IRAK1, RAX, and TRAF6, implicating PKR–RAX–mediated stress signaling in retinopathy progression (Mastropasqua et al., 2014). The miR-34 family is elevated in diabetic retinas and acts downstream of p53 and VEGF signaling in retinal pigment epithelial cells (Moura et al., 2014). Additional miRNAs, including miR-93, miR-145, miR-200, and miR-455-5p, regulate VEGF, TLR4, and SOCS3, affecting retinal epithelial cell proliferation, migration, angiogenesis, and inflammatory responses (Kantharidis et al., 2011; Qadir et al., 2019).

6.3 Diabetic nephropathy and fibrotic miRNA networks

Diabetic nephropathy is the most common cause of end-stage renal disease, affecting nearly 50% of individuals with T2DM. It is characterized by progressive glomerular injury, renal fibrosis, and eventual kidney failure, leading to high morbidity and mortality (Gohda et al., 2014). Transforming growth factor-β (TGF-β) signaling is a central driver of renal fibrosis, although multiple downstream regulatory pathways contribute to disease progression (Acikgoz et al., 2014).

Among diabetic complications, nephropathy exhibits some of the most extensive miRNA dysregulation. miR-25 promotes nephropathy by targeting PTEN and CDC42, while miR-93 correlates with microvascular injury and renal fibrosis through VEGF regulation (Kantharidis et al., 2011; Qadir et al., 2019). miR-192, miR-216a, miR-377, and the miR-200 family regulate ZEB1/2, PTEN, MnSOD, and TGF-β signaling, promoting mesangial expansion, extracellular matrix accumulation, epithelial–mesenchymal transition, and oxidative stress (Wang et al., 2011; Moura et al., 2014). These miRNA-driven pathways collectively drive progressive renal dysfunction in diabetes.

6.4 Diabetic neuropathy and neural miRNA regulation

Diabetic neuropathy represents the most prevalent and clinically challenging diabetic complication, encompassing both sensory and autonomic neuropathies. Sensory neuropathy presents as pain, paresthesia, and sensory loss, while autonomic neuropathy is associated with malignant arrhythmias, myocardial infarction, and sudden cardiac death (Deli et al., 2013).

miRNAs contribute to neuropathic outcomes by modulating inflammatory signaling, oxidative stress, and neuronal survival pathways. miR-27a and miR-499a are associated with increased incidence of cardiovascular autonomic neuropathy and diabetic peripheral neuropathy, particularly affecting cardiac and smooth muscle tissues (Cheng et al., 2015; Simeoli and Fierabracci, 2019). miR-146a regulates neurotrophin signaling through IRAK1 and TRAF6 in the brain (Simeoli and Fierabracci, 2019), while sequence variations in miR-128a and altered expression of miR-216a and miR-217 are associated with progressive neural damage in diabetes (Ciccacci et al., 2014; Simeoli and Fierabracci, 2019). miR-302 further contributes to neurotoxicity by targeting PTEN (Qadir et al., 2019).

6.5 miRNAs in atherosclerosis, NAFLD, and non-metabolic complications

Beyond classical diabetic complications, several miRNAs serve as biomarkers and regulators of non-metabolic diseases. Elevated circulating miR-34a levels have been reported in atherosclerosis, CAD, and NAFLD (Price et al., 2014). Atherosclerosis, characterized by arterial plaque formation and vascular stiffening, remains a leading cause of global mortality (Libby, 2001). miRNAs regulate lipid metabolism, inflammatory signaling, oxidative stress, and plaque stability, highlighting their therapeutic relevance (Raitoharju et al., 2013).

NAFLD encompasses a spectrum of liver disorders ranging from steatosis to cirrhosis and hepatocellular carcinoma and is characterized by hepatic lipid accumulation and inflammation (Michelotti et al., 2013). miR-23b, miR-148b, miR-214, miR-4269, and miR-4429 regulate TGF-β signaling, Twist, and CCN2 in hepatic stellate cells, influencing fibrogenesis and disease progression (H. Chen et al., 2014; Koeck et al., 2014). Cholesterol and fatty acid metabolism are further regulated by miR-103, miR-33, miR-27b, miR-34, miR-223, miR-370, and miR-122 through ABCA transporters, SIRT1, IRS2, SIRT6, LETF, and HNF pathways (Iacomino and Siani, 2017).

Collectively, these findings demonstrate that miRNAs not only reflect systemic metabolic dysfunction but also actively contribute to the persistence of diabetes-related complications across multiple organs. Through sustained alterations in gene regulation, miRNAs participate in metabolic memory, reinforcing pathological transcriptional programs even after glycemic control is achieved. This epigenetic persistence provides a mechanistic basis for long-term tissue damage in diabetes and highlights miRNAs as promising biomarkers and therapeutic targets for preventing chronic diabetic complications.

7. miRNA as disease biomarkers

miRNAs are not restricted to intracellular compartments; circulating miRNAs (c-miRNAs) have been detected in a wide range of body fluids, including serum, plasma, saliva, urine, and breast milk (Párrizas and Novials, 2016). These extracellular miRNAs were first described in humans in 2008 during studies on cancer patients (Mitchell et al., 2008). Since then, c-miRNAs have attracted significant attention due to their stability in biological fluids and their potential utility as non-invasive biomarkers for metabolic diseases. They are increasingly used for disease diagnosis, monitoring therapeutic responses, and evaluating the effects of dietary and lifestyle interventions (Arrese et al., 2015).

Extensive research has demonstrated the clinical relevance of c-miRNAs as biomarkers across diverse populations and age groups. Altered circulating miRNA profiles have been associated with type 2 diabetes mellitus (T2DM) (Willwit et al., 2017), dyslipidemia (Miao et al., 2019), metabolic syndrome (Cerda et al., 2021), cardiovascular diseases (Creemers et al., 2012), and obesity (Assmann et al., 2020). Unlike free RNA, which is rapidly degraded by RNases present in biofluids, c-miRNAs exhibit remarkable stability (Mitchell et al., 2008). This stability is attributed to their association with protective carriers such as extracellular vesicles (including exosomes, micro vesicles, and apoptotic bodies), lipoproteins such as high-density lipoproteins (HDLs) and low-density lipoproteins (LDLs), or RNA-binding proteins like Argonaute-2 (AGO2) (Li et al., 2012).

In adipose tissue, miRNA transport occurs through multiple mechanisms. The AGO2 protein complex can shuttle miRNAs within the same adipocyte to regulate target mRNAs locally (Turchinovich et al., 2011). Alternatively, miRNAs can be packaged into exosomes, microparticles, or lipoproteins and transported to distant organs, where they influence gene expression in a paracrine or endocrine manner (Bae et al., 2019). These miRNA-mRNA interactions regulate key metabolic genes involved in appetite control, adipocyte differentiation, and other adipose tissue–associated metabolic processes linked to obesity (Párrizas and Novials, 2016).

The use of circulating miRNAs as biomarkers offers several advantages, including high detection sensitivity, non-invasive sample collection, and the ability to perform multiplex analyses, which enhances diagnostic specificity and clinical applicability (Blondal et al., 2013).

Several studies have investigated alterations in miRNA expression across metabolic conditions such as insulin resistance and overweight/obesity, using diverse experimental models to identify potential biomarkers for predicting type 2 diabetes mellitus (T2DM) and cardiovascular diseases. Epigenetic profiling of circulating miRNAs (c-miRNAs) in serum or plasma has revealed obesity-specific miRNA signatures. Comparative analyses between healthy and obese individuals demonstrated significant upregulation of miR-138 and miR-376a ($P < 0.001$) and downregulation of miR-15b ($P < 0.001$) in obese subjects. Receiver operating characteristic (ROC) curve analyses showed strong diagnostic performance, with area under the curve (AUC) values of 0.9075 for miR-15b, 0.9950 for miR-138, and 0.8875 for miR-376a. Among these, miR-138 exhibited superior discriminatory power, indicating that these three miRNAs represent promising serum biomarkers for obesity (Hijmans et al., 2018).

In addition, circulating miR-130b has been identified as a potential biomarker of metabolic disorders, including metabolic syndrome (AUC 0.833, $P < 0.001$; specificity 96%, sensitivity 55%) and hypertriglyceridemia (AUC 0.758, $P < 0.01$). Mechanistically, transforming growth factor-β (TGF-β) induces the release of miR-130b from mature adipocytes. Other signaling molecules, including peroxisome proliferator-activated receptor gamma (PPARγ) ligands, cytokines, and insulin, also influence miR-130b secretion, reflecting the complex regulatory environment of adipose tissue in different biological contexts (Wang et al., 2013).

A population-based study in 120 Chinese adults aged 40–60 years identified circulating miR-223 as a biomarker of obesity. Serum miR-223 levels were significantly lower in individuals with overweight or obesity compared with those of normal weight ($P < 0.001$). Logistic regression analysis adjusted for age, sex, triglycerides, BMI, high-sensitivity C-reactive protein, and cholesterol revealed that obese individuals with miR-223 levels below 1.06 had a 2.12-fold higher risk of obesity (95% CI: 1.62–8.4, $P < 0.05$) (Wen et al., 2015). Functionally, miR-223 expressed in macrophages plays a critical role in adipocyte inflammation and metabolic regulation (Chen et al., 2012). Reduced miR-223 activity in monocytes and its dysregulation during macrophage differentiation promote pro-inflammatory activation (Cekaite et al., 2010).

Similarly, an Algerian study evaluating circulating miR-146a and miR-21 in obese and normal-weight adult men demonstrated significantly lower levels of both miRNAs in obese individuals ($P < 0.001$). This reduction was accompanied by elevated concentrations of inflammatory cytokines IL-6 and TNF-α. Inverse correlations were observed between miR-146a and IL-6/TNF-α, as well as between miR-21 and these cytokines, suggesting that miR-146a and miR-21 serve as obesity-associated biomarkers linked to systemic inflammation (Benbaibeche et al., 2022).

Further supporting the metabolic relevance of c-miRNAs, a large Swedish cohort study (Malmö Diet and Cardiovascular Cancer Cohort) involving 553 healthy individuals reported that circulating miR-483-5p levels were positively associated with insulin resistance, dyslipidemia, and obesity (Gallo et al., 2018). In a Chinese cohort, Miao et al. identified elevated circulating levels of miR-3659 and miR-151a-5p in obese adults with dyslipidemia. ROC analyses showed strong predictive value, with AUCs of 0.806 for miR-3659 and 0.769 for miR-151a-5p, indicating that miR-3659 may be a superior biomarker for dyslipidemia in obesity (Miao et al., 2019).

Intervention studies further demonstrate the dynamic nature of c-miRNAs. In a 3-month dietary and exercise intervention involving overweight and obese individuals, circulating miR-223 levels significantly increased following caloric restriction and aerobic exercise. Given its role in cholesterol metabolism and adipose tissue inflammation, miR-223 emerged as a robust biomarker of therapeutic response (Vickers et al., 2014). Similarly, a very-low-calorie diet (<800 kcal/day) study in obese women revealed significant modulation of multiple c-miRNAs associated with body weight and BMI, highlighting their responsiveness to acute weight loss (Manning et al., 2019).

Dietary bioactive compounds also influence c-miRNA expression. In a randomized crossover study in obese women, Bastos et al. demonstrated that green tea supplementation modulated oxidative stress markers and significantly altered c-miRNA profiles following consumption of a high-fat, high-saturated-fat meal. Five miRNAs with high interaction scores targeted genes involved in TGF-β, CARM1, RSK, and BMP signaling pathways, emphasizing the utility of c-miRNA profiling to uncover nutrigenomic mechanisms in obesity (Bastos et al., 2023).

Collectively, these studies indicate that circulating miRNAs reflect systemic metabolic status, respond dynamically to dietary and lifestyle interventions, and hold strong potential as non-invasive biomarkers for obesity, dyslipidemia, and metabolic disease progression.

8. Conclusions

miRNAs have fundamentally transformed our understanding of metabolic disease biology by revealing an additional regulatory layer that integrates genetic, epigenetic, and environmental signals. Evidence summarized in this chapter demonstrates that miRNAs orchestrate key metabolic pathways governing adipogenesis, insulin secretion, insulin sensitivity, inflammation, and mitochondrial function in a tissue- and context-dependent manner. Dysregulation of these miRNA networks contributes not only to the onset of obesity and diabetes but also to the persistence of disease through metabolic memory mechanisms driven by stable epigenetic alterations.

Circulating miRNAs have emerged as particularly powerful clinical tools due to their remarkable stability, accessibility, and responsiveness to metabolic status and therapeutic interventions. Their ability to reflect systemic metabolic health positions them as promising non-invasive biomarkers for early diagnosis, risk stratification, and monitoring of treatment efficacy. Moreover, advances in miRNA-targeted therapeutics, including antimiR technologies and nanocarrier-based delivery systems, have demonstrated encouraging safety and efficacy in preclinical and clinical studies. Future research integrating miRNA biology with epigenetics, systems biology, and personalized medicine is expected to accelerate the development of miRNA-based diagnostics and therapeutics, ultimately improving outcomes for patients with metabolic syndrome and diabetes.

References

Abente, E.J., Subramanian, M., Ramachandran, V., Najafi-Shoushtari, S.H., 2016. MicroRNAs in obesity-associated disorders. Arch. Biochem. Biophys. 589, 108–119. https://doi.org/10.1016/j.abb.2015.09.018.

Acikgoz, Y., Can, B., Bek, K., Acikgoz, A., Ozkaya, O., Genç, G., Sarikaya, S., 2014. The effect of simvastatin and erythropoietin on renal fibrosis in rats with unilateral ureteral obstruction. Ren. Fail. 36 (2), 252–257. https://doi.org/10.3109/0886022X.2013.836936.

Al-Goblan, A.S., Al-Alfi, M.A., Khan, M.Z., 2014. Mechanism linking diabetes mellitus and obesity. Diabetes Metab. Syndr. Obes. 7, 587–591. https://doi.org/10.2147/DMSO.S67400.

Alarcón, C.R., Lee, H., Goodarzi, H., Halberg, N., Tavazoie, S.F., 2015. N6-methyladenosine marks primary microRNAs for processing. Nature 519 (7544), 482–485. https://doi.org/10.1038/nature14281.

Ali, A.T., Hochfeld, W.E., Myburgh, R., Pepper, M.S., 2013. Adipocyte and adipogenesis. Eur. J. Cell Biol. 92 (6–7), 229–236. https://doi.org/10.1016/j.ejcb.2013.06.001.

Andersen, D.C., Jensen, C.H., Schneider, M., Nossent, A.Y., Eskildsen, T., Hansen, J.L., Teisner, B., Sheikh, S.P., 2010. MicroRNA-15a fine-tunes the level of Delta-like 1 homolog (DLK1) in proliferating 3T3-L1 preadipocytes. Exp. Cell Res. 316 (10), 1681–1691. https://doi.org/10.1016/j.yexcr.2010.04.002.

Aranda, J.F., Madrigal-Matute, J., Rotllan, N., Fernández-Hernando, C., 2013. MicroRNA modulation of lipid metabolism and oxidative stress in cardiometabolic diseases. Free Radic. Biol. Med. 64, 31–39. https://doi.org/10.1016/j.freeradbiomed.2013.07.014.

Arrese, M., Eguchi, A., Feldstein, A.E., 2015. Circulating microRNAs: emerging biomarkers of liver disease. Semin. Liver Dis. 35 (1), 43–54. https://doi.org/10.1055/s-0034-1397348.

Assmann, T.S., Riezu-Boj, J.I., Milagro, F.I., Martínez, J.A., 2020. Circulating adiposity-related microRNAs as predictors of the response to a low-fat diet in subjects with obesity. J. Cell Mol. Med. 24 (5), 2956–2967. https://doi.org/10.1111/jcmm.14920.

Azimzadeh, O., Sievert, W., Sarioglu, H., Merl-Pham, J., Yentrapalli, R., Bakshi, M.V., Janik, D., Ueffing, M., Atkinson, M.J., Multhoff, G., Tapio, S., 2015. Integrative proteomics and targeted transcriptomics analyses in

cardiac endothelial cells unravel mechanisms of long-term radiation-induced vascular dysfunction. J. Proteome Res. 14 (2), 1203–1219. https://doi.org/10.1021/pr501141b.
Bae, Y.U., Kim, Y., Lee, H., Kim, H., Jeon, J.S., Noh, H., Han, D.C., Ryu, S., Kwon, S.H., 2019. Bariatric surgery alters microRNA content of circulating exosomes in patients with obesity. Korea Obesity 27 (2), 264–271. https://doi.org/10.1002/oby.22379.
Bartel, D.P., 2009. MicroRNAs: target recognition and regulatory functions. Cell 136 (2), 215–233. https://doi.org/10.1016/j.cell.2009.01.002.
Bastos, R.V.S., Dorna, M.S., Chiuso-Minicucci, F., Felix, T.F., Fernandes, A.A.H., Azevedo, P.S., Franco, E.T., Polegato, B.F., Rogero, M.M., Mota, G.A.F., Quintanilha, B.J., Paiva, S.A.R., Zornoff, L.A.M., Reis, P.P., Minicucci, M.F., 2023. Acute green tea intake attenuates circulating microRNA expression induced by a high-fat, high-saturated meal in obese women: a randomized crossover study. JNB (J. Nutr. Biochem.) 112. https://doi.org/10.1016/j.jnutbio.2022.109203.
Benbaibeche, H., Hichami, A., Oudjit, B., Haffaf, E.M., Kacimi, G., Koceïr, E.A., Khan, N.A., 2022. Circulating mir-21 and mir-146a are associated with increased cytokines and CD36 in Algerian obese male participants. Arch. Physiol. Biochem. 128 (6), 1461–1466. https://doi.org/10.1080/13813455.2020.1775655.
Bhatt, K., Lanting, L.L., Jia, Y., Yadav, S., Reddy, M.A., Magilnick, N., Boldin, M., Natarajan, R., 2016. Anti-inflammatory role of microrna-146a in the pathogenesis of diabetic nephropathy. J. Am. Soc. Nephrol. 27 (8), 2277–2288. https://doi.org/10.1681/ASN.2015010111.
Blondal, T., Jensby Nielsen, S., Baker, A., Andreasen, D., Mouritzen, P., Wrang Teilum, M., Dahlsveen, I.K., 2013. Assessing sample and miRNA profile quality in serum and plasma or other biofluids. Methods 59 (1), S1. https://doi.org/10.1016/j.ymeth.2012.09.015.
Brandão-Lima, P.N., de Carvalho, G.B., Payolla, T.B., Sarti, F.M., Fisberg, R.M., Malcomson, F.C., Mathers, J.C., Rogero, M.M., 2023. Circulating microRNAs showed specific responses according to metabolic syndrome components and sex of adults from a population-based study. Metabolites 13 (1). https://doi.org/10.3390/metabo13010002.
Calderari, S., Diawara, M.R., Garaud, A., Gauguier, D., 2017. Biological roles of microRNAs in the control of insulin secretion and action. Physiol. Genom. 49 (1), 1–10. https://doi.org/10.1152/physiolgenomics.00079.2016.
Campolo, F., Catanzaro, G., Venneri, M.A., Ferretti, E., Besharat, Z.M., 2022. MicroRNA loaded edible nanoparticles: an emerging personalized therapeutic approach for the treatment of obesity and metabolic disorders. Theranostics 12 (6), 2631–2634. https://doi.org/10.7150/thno.71399.
Carrer, M., Liu, N., Grueter, C.E., Williams, A.H., Frisard, M.I., Hulver, M.W., Bassel-Duby, R., Olson, E.N., 2012. Control of mitochondrial metabolism and systemic energy homeostasis by microRNAs 378 and 378. Proc. Natl. Acad. Sci. U. S. A 109 (38), 15330–15335. https://doi.org/10.1073/pnas.1207605109.
Caus, M., Eritja, À., Bozic, M., 2021. Role of microRNAs in obesity-related kidney disease. Int. J. Mol. Sci. 22 (21), 11416. https://doi.org/10.3390/ijms222111416.
Cekaite, L., Clancy, T., Sioud, M., 2010. Increased miR-21 expression during human monocyte differentiation into DCs. Frontiers in Bioscience - Elite 2 (3), 818–828. https://doi.org/10.2741/e143.

Cerda, A., Amaral, A., de Oliveira, R., Moraes, T., Braga, A., Graciano-Saldarriaga, M.E., Fajardo, C., Hirata, R., 2021. Peripheral blood miRome identified miR-155 as a potential biomarker of metabolic syndrome and cardiometabolic risk in obese patients. Int. J. Mol. Sci. 22 (3), 1468. https://doi.org/10.3390/ijms22031468.

Chen, Q., Wang, H., Liu, Y., Song, Y., Lai, L., Han, Q., Cao, X., Wang, Q., Viola, J. P.B., 2012. Inducible MicroRNA-223 down-regulation promotes TLR-triggered IL-6 and IL-1β production in macrophages by targeting STAT3. PLoS One 7 (8), e42971. https://doi.org/10.1371/journal.pone.0042971.

Chen, X., Liang, H., Zhang, J., Zen, K., Zhang, C.Y., 2012. Horizontal transfer of microRNAs: molecular mechanisms and clinical applications. Protein Cell 3 (1), 28–37. https://doi.org/10.1007/s13238-012-2003-z.

Chen, H., Lan, H.Y., Roukos, D.H., Cho, W.C., 2014. Application of microRNAs in diabetes mellitus. J. Endocrinol. 222 (1), R1. https://doi.org/10.1530/JOE-13-0544.

Chen, L., Charrier, A., Zhou, Y., Chen, R., Yu, B., Agarwal, K., Tsukamoto, H., Lee, L.J., Paulaitis, M.E., Brigstock, D.R., 2014. Epigenetic regulation of connective tissue growth factor by MicroRNA-214 delivery in exosomes from mouse or human hepatic stellate cells. Hepatology 59 (3), 1118–1129. https://doi.org/10.1002/hep.26768.

Cheng, C., Kobayashi, M., Martinez, J.A., Ng, H., Moser, J.J., Wang, X., Singh, V., Fritzler, M.J., Zochodne, D.W., 2015. Evidence for epigenetic regulation of gene expression and function in chronic experimental diabetic neuropathy. JNEN (J. Neuropathol. Exp. Neurol.) 74 (8), 804–817. https://doi.org/10.1097/NEN.0000000000000219.

Chew, B.H., Shariff Ghazali, S., Ismail, M., Haniff, J., Bujang, M.A., 2013. Age ≥60years was an independent risk factor for diabetes-related complications despite good control of cardiovascular risk factors in patients with type 2 diabetes mellitus. Exp. Gerontol. 48 (5), 485–491. https://doi.org/10.1016/j.exger.2013.02.017.

Ciccacci, C., Morganti, R., Di Fusco, D., D'Amato, C., Cacciotti, L., Greco, C., Rufini, S., Novelli, G., Sangiuolo, F., Marfia, G.A., Borgiani, P., Spallone, V., 2014. Common polymorphisms in MIR146a, MIR128a and MIR27a genes contribute to neuropathy susceptibility in type 2 diabetes. Acta Diabetol. 51 (4), 663–671. https://doi.org/10.1007/s00592-014-0582-2.

Creemers, E.E., Tijsen, A.J., Pinto, Y.M., 2012. Circulating MicroRNAs: novel biomarkers and extracellular communicators in cardiovascular disease? Circ. Res. 110 (3), 483–495. https://doi.org/10.1161/CIRCRESAHA.111.247452.

Croce, C.M., Calin, G.A., 2005. miRNAs, cancer, and stem cell division. Cell 122 (1), 6–7. https://doi.org/10.1016/j.cell.2005.06.036.

Cruz-Gil, S., Sanchez-Martinez, R., De Cedron, M.G., Martin-Hernandez, R., Vargas, T., Molina, S., Herranz, J., Davalos, A., Reglero, G., De Molina, A.R., 2018. Targeting the lipid metabolic axis ACSL/SCD in colorectal cancer progression by therapeutic miRNAs: MiR-19b-1 role. JLR (J. Lipid Res.) 59 (1), 14–24. https://doi.org/10.1194/jlr.M076752.

Cummings, D.E., Schwartz, M.W., 2003. Genetics and pathophysiology of human obesity. Annu. Rev. Med. 54, 453–471. https://doi.org/10.1146/annurev.med.54.101601.152403.

Cuperus, J.T., Fahlgren, N., Carrington, J.C., 2011. Evolution and functional diversification of MIRNA genes. Plant Cell 23 (2), 431–442. https://doi.org/10.1105/tpc.110.082784.

Deiuliis, J.A., 2016. MicroRNAs as regulators of metabolic disease: pathophysiologic significance and emerging role as biomarkers and therapeutics. Int. J. Obes. 40 (1), 88–101. https://doi.org/10.1038/ijo.2015.170.

Deiuliis, J.A., Syed, R., Duggineni, D., Rutsky, J., Rengasamy, P., Zhang, J., Huang, K., Needleman, B., Mikami, D., Perry, K., Hazey, J., Rajagopalan, S., Xu, H., 2016. Visceral adipose MicroRNA 223 is upregulated in human and murine obesity and modulates the inflammatory phenotype of macrophages. PLoS One 11 (11), e0165962. https://doi.org/10.1371/journal.pone.0165962.

Deli, G., Bosnyak, E., Pusch, G., Komoly, S., Feher, G., 2013. Diabetic neuropathies: diagnosis and management. Neuroendocrinology 98 (4), 267–280. https://doi.org/10.1159/000358728.

Dogru, T., Ercin, C.N., Erdem, G., Sonmez, A., Tapan, S., Tasci, I., 2008. Increased hepatic and circulating interleukin-6 levels in human nonalcoholic steatohepatitis. Am. J. Gastroenterol. 103 (12), 3217–3218. https://doi.org/10.1111/j.1572-0241.2008.02161_17.x.

Dumortier, O., Hinault, C., Van Obberghen, E., 2013. MicroRNAs and metabolism crosstalk in energy homeostasis. Cell Metab. 18 (3), 312–324. https://doi.org/10.1016/j.cmet.2013.06.004.

Esguerra, J.L.S., Bolmeson, C., Cilio, C.M., Eliasson, L., 2011. Differential glucose-regulation of microRNAs in pancreatic islets of non-obese type 2 diabetes model goto-kakizaki rat. PLoS One 6 (4). https://doi.org/10.1371/journal.pone.0018613Sweden.

Feng, J., Xing, W., Xie, L., 2016. Regulatory roles of MicroRNAs in diabetes. Int. J. Mol. Sci. 17 (10), 1729. https://doi.org/10.3390/ijms17101729.

Fernández-Hernando, C., Ramírez, C.M., Goedeke, L., Suárez, Y., 2013. MicroRNAs in metabolic disease. Arterioscler. Thromb. Vasc. Biol. 33 (2), 178–185. https://doi.org/10.1161/ATVBAHA.112.300144.

Flehmig, G., Scholz, M., Klöting, N., Fasshauer, M., Tönjes, A., Stumvoll, M., Youn, B.S., Blüher, M., 2014. Identification of adipokine clusters related to parameters of fat mass, insulin sensitivity and inflammation. PLoS One 9 (6). https://doi.org/10.1371/journal.pone.0099785.

Fowler, M.J., 2008. Microvascular and macrovascular complications of diabetes. Clin. Diabetes 26 (2), 77–82. https://doi.org/10.2337/diaclin.26.2.77.

Friedman, R.C., Farh, K.K.H., Burge, C.B., Bartel, D.P., 2009. Most mammalian mRNAs are conserved targets of microRNAs. Genome Res. 19 (1), 92–105. https://doi.org/10.1101/gr.082701.108.

Frost, R.J.A., Olson, E.N., 2011. Control of glucose homeostasis and insulin sensitivity by the Let-7 family of microRNAs. Proc. Natl. Acad. Sci. U. S. A 108 (52), 21075–21080. https://doi.org/10.1073/pnas.1118922109.

Gallo, W., Esguerra, J.L.S., Eliasson, L., Melander, O., Herder, C., 2018. miR-483-5p associates with obesity and insulin resistance and independently associates with new onset diabetes mellitus and cardiovascular disease. PLoS One 13 (11), e0206974. https://doi.org/10.1371/journal.pone.0206974.

Gerin, I., Bommer, G.T., McCoin, C.S., Sousa, K.M., Krishnan, V., MacDougald, O.A., 2010. Roles for miRNA-378/378* in adipocyte gene expression and lipogenesis. Am. J. Physiol. Endocrinol. Metabol. 299 (2), E198. https://doi.org/10.1152/ajpendo.00179.2010.

Gohda, T., Mima, A., Moon, J.Y., Kanasaki, K., 2014. Combat diabetic nephropathy: from pathogenesis to treatment. J. Diabetes Res. 2014. https://doi.org/10.1155/2014/207140.

Ha, M., Kim, V.N., 2014. Regulation of microRNA biogenesis. Nat. Rev. Mol. Cell Biol. 15 (8), 509–524. https://doi.org/10.1038/nrm3838.

Heneghan, H.M., Miller, N., Kerin, M.J., 2010. Role of microRNAs in obesity and the metabolic syndrome. Obes. Rev. 11 (5), 354–361. https://doi.org/10.1111/j.1467-789x.2009.00659.x.

Hijmans, J.G., Diehl, K.J., Bammert, T.D., Kavlich, P.J., Lincenberg, G.M., Greiner, J.J., Stauffer, B.L., DeSouza, C.A., 2018. Influence of overweight and obesity on circulating inflammation-related microRNA. MicroRNA 7 (2), 148–154. https://doi.org/10.2174/2211536607666180402120806.

Hilton, C., Neville, M.J., Karpe, F., 2013. MicroRNAs in adipose tissue: their role in adipogenesis and obesity. Int. J. Obes. 37 (3), 325–332. https://doi.org/10.1038/ijo.2012.59.

Hulsmans, M., Dieuwke, De K., Paul, H., 2011. MicroRNAs regulating oxidative stress and inflammation in relation to obesity and atherosclerosis. FASEB J. 25 (8), 2515–2527. https://doi.org/10.1096/fj.11-181149.

Humphries, B., Wang, Z., Yang, C., 2019. MicroRNA regulation of epigenetic modifiers in breast cancer. Cancers 11 (7), 897. https://doi.org/10.3390/cancers11070897.

Hutny, M., Hofman, J., Zachurzok, A., Matusik, P., 2022. MicroRNAs as the promising markers of comorbidities in childhood obesity—a systematic review. Pediatric Obesity 17 (6). https://doi.org/10.1111/ijpo.12880.

Iacomino, G., Siani, A., 2017. Role of microRNAs in obesity and obesity-related diseases. Gene Nutr. 12 (1). https://doi.org/10.1186/s12263-017-0577-z.

Jones, J.E.C., Esler, W.P., Patel, R., Lanba, A., Vera, N.B., Pfefferkorn, J.A., Vernochet, C., 2017. Inhibition of acetylCoA carboxylase 1 (ACC1) and 2 (ACC2) reduces proliferation and de novo lipogenesis of EGFRvIII human glioblastoma cells. PLoS One 12 (1), e0169566.

Jung, U.J., Choi, M.S., 2014. Obesity and its metabolic complications: the role of adipokines and the relationship between obesity, inflammation, insulin resistance, dyslipidemia and nonalcoholic fatty liver disease. Int. J. Mol. Sci. 15 (4), 6184–6223. https://doi.org/10.3390/ijms15046184.

Kantharidis, P., Wang, B., Carew, R.M., Lan, H.Y., 2011. Diabetes complications: the microRNA perspective. Diabetes 60 (7), 1832–1837. https://doi.org/10.2337/db11-0082Australia.

Keller, A., Meese, E., 2016. Can circulating miRNAs live up to the promise of being minimal invasive biomarkers in clinical settings? Wiley Interdiscip. Rev.: RNA 7 (2), 148–156. https://doi.org/10.1002/wrna.1320.

Kim, J., Yoon, H., Horie, T., Burchett, J.M., Restivo, J.L., Rotllan, N., Ramírez, C. M., Verghese, P.B., Ihara, M., Hoe, H.S., Esau, C., Fernández-Hernando, C., Holtzman, D.M., Cirrito, J.R., Ono, K., Kim, J., 2015. Microrna-33 regulates apoe lipidation and amyloid-β metabolism in the brain. J. Neurosci. 35 (44), 14717–14726. https://doi.org/10.1523/JNEUROSCI.2053-15.2015.

Kinoshita, M., Koh, O., Horie, T., Nagao, K., Nishi, H., Kuwabara, Y., Takanabe-Mori, R., Hasegawa, K., Kita, T., Kimura, T., 2010. Regulation of adipocyte differentiation by activation of serotonin (5-HT) receptors 5-HT2AR and 5-HT2CR and involvement of MicroRNA-448-mediated repression of KLF5. Mol. Endocrinol. 24 (10), 1978–1987. https://doi.org/10.1210/me.2010-0054.

Klöting, N., Berthold, S., Kovacs, P., Schön, M.R., Fasshauer, M., Ruschke, K., Stumvoll, M., Blüher, M., 2009. MicroRNA expression in human omental and subcutaneous adipose tissue. PLoS One 4 (3). https://doi.org/10.1371/journal.pone.0004699Germany.

Koeck, E.S., Iordanskaia, T., Sevilla, S., Ferrante, S.C., Hubal, M.J., Freishtat, R.J., Nadler, E.P., 2014. Adipocyte exosomes induce transforming growth factor beta pathway dysregulation in hepatocytes: a novel paradigm for obesity-related liver disease. J. Surg. Res. 192 (2), 268–275. https://doi.org/10.1016/j.jss.2014.06.050.

Kurozumi, A., Goto, Y., Okato, A., Seki, N., 2017. DNA methylation and dysregulation of miRNA in cancer: feedback loop between dysregulated miRNAs and epigenetic pathways in cancer. Cancer Drug Discov. Dev. 0, 281–296. https://doi.org/10.1007/978-3-319-59786-7_10.

Lee, E.K., Lee, M.J., Abdelmohsen, K., Kim, W., Kim, M.M., Srikantan, S., Martindale, J.L., Hutchison, E.R., Kim, H.H., Marasa, B.S., Selimyan, R., Egan, J.M., Smith, S.R., Fried, S.K., Gorospe, M., 2011. miR-130 suppresses adipogenesis by inhibiting peroxisome proliferator-activated receptor γ expression. Mol. Cell Biol. 31 (4), 626–638. https://doi.org/10.1128/MCB.00894-10.

Li, W.Q., Chen, C., Xu, M.D., Guo, J., Li, Y.M., Xia, Q.M., Liu, H.M., He, J., Yu, H. Y., Zhu, L., 2011. The rno-miR-34 family is upregulated and targets ACSL1 in dimethylnitrosamine-induced hepatic fibrosis in rats. FEBS J. 278 (9), 1522–1532. https://doi.org/10.1111/j.1742-4658.2011.08075.x.

Li, L., Zhu, D., Huang, L., Zhang, J., Bian, Z., Chen, X., Liu, Y., Zhang, C.Y., Zen, K., 2012. Argonaute 2 complexes selectively protect the circulating MicroRNAs in cell-secreted microvesicles. PLoS One 7 (10). https://doi.org/10.1371/journal.pone.0046957China.

Libby, P., 2001. Current concepts of the pathogenesis of the acute coronary syndromes. Circulation 104 (3), 365–372. https://doi.org/10.1161/01.cir.104.3.365.

Lin, Q., Gao, Z., Alarcon, R.M., Ye, J., Yun, Z., 2009. A role of miR-27 in the regulation of adipogenesis. FEBS J. 276 (8), 2348–2358. https://doi.org/10.1111/j.1742-4658.2009.06967.x.

Mandelbaum, A.D., Melkman-Zehavi, T., Oren, R., Kredo-Russo, S., Nir, T., Dor, Y., Hornstein, E., 2012. Dysregulation of Dicer1 in beta cells impairs islet architecture and glucose metabolism. Exp. Diabetes Res. 2012. https://doi.org/10.1155/2012/470302.

Manning, P., Munasinghe, P.E., Papannarao, J.B., Gray, A.R., Sutherland, W., Katare, R., 2019. Acute weight loss restores dysregulated circulating microRNAs in individuals who are obese. J. Clin. Endocrinol. Metabol. 104 (4), 1239–1248. https://doi.org/10.1210/jc.2018-01751.

Marques-Rocha, J.L., Samblas, M., Milagro, F.I., Bressan, J., Martínez, J.A., Marti, A., 2015. Noncoding RNAs, cytokines, and inflammation-related diseases. FASEB (Fed. Am. Soc. Exp. Biol.) J. 29 (9), 3595–3611. https://doi.org/10.1096/fj.14-260323.

Martinelli, R., Nardelli, C., Pilone, V., Buonomo, T., Liguori, R., Castanò, I., Buono, P., Masone, S., Persico, G., Forestieri, P., Pastore, L., Sacchetti, L., 2010. miR-519d overexpression is associated with human obesity. Obesity 18 (11), 2170–2176. https://doi.org/10.1038/oby.2009.474.

Masoudi, F., Reza Sharifi, M., Pourfarzam, M., 2022. Investigation of the relationship between miR-33a, miR-122, erythrocyte membrane fatty acids profile, and serum lipids with components of metabolic syndrome in type 2 diabetic patients. Res. Pharm. Sci. 17 (3), 242–251. https://doi.org/10.4103/1735-5362.343078.

Mastropasqua, R., Toto, L., Cipollone, F., Santovito, D., Carpineto, P., Mastropasqua, L., 2014. Role of microRNAs in the modulation of diabetic retinopathy. Prog. Retin. Eye Res. 43, 92–107. https://doi.org/10.1016/j.preteyeres.2014.07.003.

Matsuda, A., Yan, I.K., Foye, C., Parasramka, M., Patel, T., 2016. MicroRNAs as paracrine signaling mediators in cancers and metabolic diseases. Best Pract. Res. Clin. Endocrinol. Metabol. 30 (5), 577–590. https://doi.org/10.1016/j.beem.2016.07.005.

Matsuzaki, J., Ochiya, T., 2017. Circulating microRNAs and extracellular vesicles as potential cancer biomarkers: a systematic review. Int. J. Clin. Oncol. 22 (3), 413–420. https://doi.org/10.1007/s10147-017-1104-3.

Mcclelland, A.D., Kantharidis, P., 2014. MicroRNA in the development of diabetic complications. Clin. Sci. 126 (2), 95–110. https://doi.org/10.1042/CS20130079Australia.

McGregor, R.A., Choi, M.S., 2011. microRNAs in the regulation of adipogenesis and obesity. Curr. Mol. Med. 11 (4), 304–316. https://doi.org/10.2174/156652411795677990.

Menon, A., Abd-Aziz, N., Khalid, K., Laa Poh, C., Naidu, R., 2022. miRNA: a promising therapeutic target in cancer. Int. J. Mol. Sci. 23 (19), 11502. https://doi.org/10.3390/ijms231911502.

Miao, L., Yin, R.-X., Pan, S.-L., Yang, S., Yang, D.-Z., Lin, W.-X., 2019. Circulating miR-3659 may be a potential biomarker of dyslipidemia in patients with obesity. J. Transl. Med. 17 (1). https://doi.org/10.1186/s12967-019-1776-8.

Michelotti, G.A., Machado, M.V., Diehl, A.M., 2013. NAFLD, NASH and liver cancer. Nat. Rev. Gastroenterol. Hepatol. 10 (11), 656–665. https://doi.org/10.1038/nrgastro.2013.183.

Mir, F.A., Mall, R., Iskandarani, A., Ullah, E., Samra, T.A., Cyprian, F., Parray, A., Alkasem, M., Abdalhakam, I., Farooq, F., Abou-Samra, A.B., 2022. Characteristic MicroRNAs linked to dysregulated metabolic pathways in qatari adult subjects with obesity and metabolic syndrome. Front. Endocrinol. 13. https://doi.org/10.3389/fendo.2022.937089.

Mitchell, P.S., Parkin, R.K., Kroh, E.M., Fritz, B.R., Wyman, S.K., Pogosova-Agadjanyan, E.L., Peterson, A., Noteboom, J., O'Briant, K.C., Allen, A., Lin, D.W., Urban, N., Drescher, C.W., Knudsen, B.S., Stirewalt, D.L., Gentleman, R., Vessella, R.L., Nelson, P.S., Martin, D.B., Tewari, M., 2008. Circulating microRNAs as stable blood-based markers for cancer detection. Proc. Natl. Acad. Sci. U. S. A 105 (30), 10513–10518. https://doi.org/10.1073/pnas.0804549105.

Moura, J., Børsheim, E., Carvalho, E., 2014. The role of MicroRNAs in diabetic complications—special emphasis on wound healing. Genes 5 (4), 926–956. https://doi.org/10.3390/genes5040926.

Mugambi Ngari, D., Munzi Mbisi, A., Wanjiru Njogu, T., 2020. Social cultural and economic factors affecting the practice of secondary prevention among patients with type 2 diabetes mellitus at consolata nkubu and meru level five hospital in meru county. Open J. Clin. Diagn. 10 (01), 1–17. https://doi.org/10.4236/ojcd.2020.101001.

Naveed, A., ur-Rahman, S., Abdullah, S., Naveed, M.A., 2017. A concise review of MicroRNA exploring the insights of MicroRNA regulations in bacterial, viral and metabolic diseases. Mol. Biotechnol. 59 (11–12), 518–529. https://doi.org/10.1007/s12033-017-0034-7.

O'Brien, J., Hayder, H., Zayed, Y., Peng, C., 2018. Overview of MicroRNA biogenesis, mechanisms of actions, and circulation. Front. Endocrinol. 9. https://doi.org/10.3389/fendo.2018.00402.

Ortega, F.J., Moreno-Navarrete, J.M., Pardo, G., Sabater, M., Hummel, M., Ferrer, A., Rodriguez-Hermosa, J.I., Ruiz, B., Ricart, W., Peral, B., Fernández-Real, J.M., 2010. MiRNA expression profile of human subcutaneous adipose and during adipocyte differentiation. PLoS One 5 (2). https://doi.org/10.1371/journal.pone.0009022Spain.

Otmani, K., Rouas, R., Berehab, M., Lewalle, P., 2024. The regulatory mechanisms of oncomiRs in cancer. Biomed. Pharmacother. 171, 116165. https://doi.org/10.1016/j.biopha.2024.116165.

Ouyang, S., Tang, R., Liu, Z., Ma, F., Li, Y., Wu, J., 2017. Characterization and predicted role of microRNA expression profiles associated with early childhood obesity. Mol. Med. Rep. 16 (4), 3799–3806. https://doi.org/10.3892/mmr.2017.7118.

Palmer, J.D., Soule, B.P., Simone, B.A., Zaorsky, N.G., Jin, L., Simone, N.L., 2014. MicroRNA expression altered by diet: can food be medicinal? Ageing Res. Rev. 17, 16–24. https://doi.org/10.1016/j.arr.2014.04.005.

Párrizas, M., Novials, A., 2016. Circulating microRNAs as biomarkers for metabolic disease. Best Pract. Res. Clin. Endocrinol. Metabol. 30 (5), 591–601. https://doi.org/10.1016/j.beem.2016.08.001.

Paul, S., Bravo Vázquez, L.A., Uribe, S.P., Manzanero Cárdenas, L.A., Ruíz Aguilar, M.F., Chakraborty, S., Sharma, A., 2021. Roles of microRNAs in carbohydrate and lipid metabolism disorders and their therapeutic potential. Biochimie 187, 83–93. https://doi.org/10.1016/j.biochi.2021.05.015.

Peng, Y., Yu, S., Li, H., Xiang, H., Peng, J., Jiang, S., 2014. MicroRNAs: emerging roles in adipogenesis and obesity. Cell. Signal. 26 (9), 1888–1896. https://doi.org/10.1016/j.cellsig.2014.05.006.

Peppa, M., Koliaki, C., Nikolopoulos, P., Raptis, S.A., 2010. Skeletal muscle insulin resistance in endocrine disease. J. Biomed. Biotechnol. 2010. https://doi.org/10.1155/2010/527850.

Poy, M.N., Eliasson, L., Krutzfeldt, J., Kuwajima, S., Ma, X., MacDonald, P.E., Pfeffer, S., Tuschl, T., Rajewsky, N., Rorsman, P., Stoffel, M., 2004. A pancreatic islet-specific microRNA regulates insulin secretion. Nature 432 (7014), 226–230. https://doi.org/10.1038/nature03076.

Price, N.L., Ramírez, C.M., Fernández-Hernando, C., 2014. Relevance of microRNA in metabolic diseases. Crit. Rev. Clin. Lab Sci. 51 (6), 305–320. https://doi.org/10.3109/10408363.2014.937522.

Qadir, M.M.F., Klein, D., Álvarez-Cubela, S., Domínguez-Bendala, J., Pastori, R. L., 2019. The role of microRNAs in diabetes-related oxidative stress. Int. J. Mol. Sci. 20 (21). https://doi.org/10.3390/ijms20215423.

Rahman, M.A., Islam, M.M., Ripon, M.A.R., Islam, M.M., Hossain, M.S., 2024. Regulatory roles of MicroRNAs in the pathogenesis of metabolic syndrome. Mol. Biotechnol. 66 (7), 1599–1620. https://doi.org/10.1007/s12033-023-00805-z.

Raitoharju, E., Oksala, N., Lehtimäki, T., 2013. MicroRNAs in the atherosclerotic plaque. Clin. Chem. 59 (12), 1708–1721. https://doi.org/10.1373/clinchem.2013.204917.

Reddy, M.A., Jin, W., Villeneuve, L., Wang, M., Lanting, L., Todorov, I., Kato, M., Natarajan, R., 2012. Pro-inflammatory role of MicroRNA-200 in vascular smooth muscle cells from diabetic mice. Arterioscler. Thromb. Vasc. Biol. 32 (3), 721–729. https://doi.org/10.1161/ATVBAHA.111.241109.

Rezk, N.A., Sabbah, N.A., Saad, M.S.S., 2016. Role of microRNA 126 in screening, diagnosis, and prognosis of diabetic patients in Egypt. IUBMB Life 68 (6), 452–458. https://doi.org/10.1002/iub.1502.

Rottiers, V., Näär, A.M., 2012. MicroRNAs in metabolism and metabolic disorders. Nat. Rev. Mol. Cell Biol. 13 (4), 239–251. https://doi.org/10.1038/nrm3313.

Ruiz-Roso, M.B., Gil-Zamorano, J., López de las Hazas, M.C., Tomé-Carneiro, J., Crespo, M.C., Latasa, M.J., Briand, O., Sánchez-López, D., Ortiz, A.I., Visioli, F., Martínez, J.A., Dávalos, A., 2020. Intestinal lipid metabolism genes regulated by miRNAs. Front. Genet. 11. https://doi.org/10.3389/fgene.2020.00707.

Scheideler, M., 2016. MicroRNAs in adipocyte formation and obesity. Best Pract. Res. Clin. Endocrinol. Metabol. 30 (5), 653–664. https://doi.org/10.1016/j.beem.2016.11.009.

Sekar, D., Venugopal, B., Sekar, P., Ramalingam, K., 2016. Role of microRNA 21 in diabetes and associated/related diseases. Gene 582 (1), 14–18. https://doi.org/10.1016/j.gene.2016.01.039.

Simeoli, R., Fierabracci, A., 2019. Insights into the role of MicroRNAs in the onset and development of diabetic neuropathy. Int. J. Mol. Sci. 20 (18), 4627. https://doi.org/10.3390/ijms20184627.

Slattery, M.L., Herrick, J.S., Mullany, L.E., Stevens, J.R., Wolff, R.K., 2017. Diet and lifestyle factors associated with miRNA expression in colorectal tissue. Pharmacogenomics Personalized Med. 10, 1–16. https://doi.org/10.2147/PGPM.S117796.

Sliwinska, A., Kasinska, M.A., Drzewoski, J., 2017. MicroRNAs & metabolic disorders - where are we heading? Arch. Med. Sci. 13 (4), 885–896. https://doi.org/10.5114/aoms.2017.65229.

Stavast, C.J., Erkeland, S.J., 2019. The non-canonical aspects of MicroRNAs: many roads to gene regulation. Cells 8 (11). https://doi.org/10.3390/cells8111465.

Strum, J.C., Johnson, J.H., Ward, J., Xie, H., Feild, J., Hester, A., Alford, A., Waters, K.M., 2009. MicroRNA 132 regulates nutritional stress-induced chemokine production through repression of SirT1. Mol. Endocrinol. 23 (11), 1876–1884. https://doi.org/10.1210/me.2009-0117.

Tan, S.Y., Mei Wong, J.L., Sim, Y.J., Wong, S.S., Mohamed Elhassan, S.A., Tan, S. H., Ling Lim, G.P., Rong Tay, N.W., Annan, N.C., Bhattamisra, S.K., Candasamy, M., 2019. Type 1 and 2 diabetes mellitus: a review on current treatment approach and gene therapy as potential intervention. Diabetes Metabol. Syndr.: Clin. Res. Rev. 13 (1), 364–372. https://doi.org/10.1016/j.dsx.2018.10.008.

Tang, X., Tang, G., Özcan, S., 2008. Role of microRNAs in diabetes. Biochim. Biophys. Acta, Gene Regul. Mech. 1779 (11), 697–701. https://doi.org/10.1016/j.bbagrm.2008.06.010.

Tang, J., Yao, D., Yan, H., Chen, X., Wang, L., Zhan, H., 2019. The role of MicroRNAs in the pathogenesis of diabetic nephropathy. International Journal of Endocrinology 2019, 1–8. https://doi.org/10.1155/2019/8719060.

Tattikota, S.G., Sury, M.D., Rathjen, T., Wessels, H.H., Pandey, A.K., You, X., Becker, C., Chen, W., Selbach, M., Poy, M.N., 2013. Argonaute2 regulates the pancreatic β-cell secretome. Mol. Cell. Proteomics 12 (5), 1214–1225. https://doi.org/10.1074/mcp.M112.024786Germany.

Thanikachalam, P.V., Ramamurthy, S., Wong, Z.W., Koo, B.J., Wong, J.Y., Abdullah, M.F., Chin, Y.H., Chia, C.H., Tan, J.Y., Neo, W.T., Tan, B.S., Khan, W.F., Kesharwani, P., 2018. Current attempts to implement microRNA-based diagnostics and therapy in cardiovascular and metabolic disease: a promising future. Drug Discov. Today 23 (3), 460–480. https://doi.org/10.1016/j.drudis.2017.10.020.

Tiwari, J., Gupta, G., De Jesus Andreoli Pinto, T., Sharma, R., Pabreja, K., Matta, Y., Arora, N., Mishra, A., Sharma, R., Dua, K., 2018. Role of microRNAs (miRNAs) in the pathophysiology of Diabetes mellitus.

Panminerva Med. 60 (1), 25–28. https://doi.org/10.23736/S0031-0808.17.03382-1.
Turchinovich, A., Weiz, L., Langheinz, A., Burwinkel, B., 2011. Characterization of extracellular circulating microRNA. Nucleic Acids Res. 39 (16), 7223–7233. https://doi.org/10.1093/nar/gkr254.
Unger, R.H., 2003. Minireview: weapons of lean body mass destruction: the role of ectopic lipids in the metabolic syndrome. Endocrinology 144 (12), 5159–5165. https://doi.org/10.1210/en.2003-0870.
Vickers, K.C., Landstreet, S.R., Levin, M.G., Shoucri, B.M., Toth, C.L., Taylor, R. C., Palmisano, B.T., Tabet, F., Cui, H.L., Rye, K.A., Sethupathy, P., Remaley, A.T., 2014. MicroRNA-223 coordinates cholesterol homeostasis. Proc. Natl. Acad. Sci. U. S. A 111 (40), 14518–14523. https://doi.org/10.1073/pnas.1215767111.
Wang, B., Tontonoz, P., 2018. Liver X receptors in lipid signalling and membrane homeostasis. Nat. Rev. Endocrinol. 14 (8), 452–463. https://doi.org/10.1038/s41574-018-0037-x.
Wang, B., Koh, P., Winbanks, C., Coughlan, M.T., McClelland, A., Watson, A., Jandeleit-Dahm, K., Burns, W.C., Thomas, M.C., Cooper, M.E., Kantharidis, P., 2011. MiR-200a prevents renal fibrogenesis through repression of TGF-β2 expression. Diabetes 60 (1), 280–287. https://doi.org/10.2337/db10-0892Australia.
Wang, Y.C., Li, Y., Wang, X.Y., Zhang, D., Zhang, H., Wu, Q., He, Y.Q., Wang, J. Y., Zhang, L., Xia, H., Yan, J., Li, X., Ying, H., 2013. Circulating miR-130b mediates metabolic crosstalk between fat and muscle in overweight/obesity. Diabetologia 56 (10), 2275–2285. https://doi.org/10.1007/s00125-013-2996-8.
Wang, M., Li, L., Liu, R., Song, Y., Zhang, X., Niu, W., Kumar, A.K., Guo, Z., Hu, Z., 2018. Obesity-induced overexpression of miRNA-24 regulates cholesterol uptake and lipid metabolism by targeting SR-B1. Gene 668, 196–203. https://doi.org/10.1016/j.gene.2018.05.072.
Wang, Y., Lin, L., Huang, Y., Sun, J., Wang, X., Wang, P., 2019. MicroRNA-138 suppresses adipogenic differentiation in human adipose tissue-derived mesenchymal stem cells by targeting lipoprotein lipase. Yonsei Med. J. 60 (12), 1187–1194.
Weiss, C.N., Ito, K., 2018. A macro view of MicroRNAs: the discovery of MicroRNAs and their role in hematopoiesis and hematologic disease. International Review of Cell and Molecular Biology 334, 99–175. https://doi.org/10.1016/bs.ircmb.2017.03.007.
Wen, D., Qiao, P., Wang, L., 2015. Circulating microRNA-223 as a potential biomarker for obesity. Obes. Res. Clin. Pract. 9 (4), 398–404. https://doi.org/10.1016/j.orcp.2015.01.006.
Wieckowska, A., Papouchado, B.G., Li, Z.Z., Lopez, R., Zein, N.N., Feldstein, A. E., 2008. Increased hepatic and circulating interleukin-6 levels in human nonalcoholic steatohepatitis. Am. J. Gastroenterol. 103 (6), 1372–1379. https://doi.org/10.1111/j.1572-0241.2007.01774.x.
Willeit, P., Skroblin, P., Moschen, A.R., Yin, X., Kaudewitz, D., Zampetaki, A., Barwari, T., Whitehead, M., Ramírez, C.M., Goedeke, L., Rotllan, N., Bonora, E., Hughes, A.D., Santer, P., Willeit, J., Kiechl, S., Fernández-Hernando, C., Mayr, M., 2017. Circulating microRNA-122 is associated with the risk of new-onset metabolic syndrome and type 2 diabetes. Diabetes 66 (2), 347–357. https://doi.org/10.2337/db16-0731.
Włodarski, A., Strycharz, J., Wróblewski, A., Kasznicki, J., Drzewoski, J., Śliwińska, A., 2020. The role of MicroRNAs in metabolic syndrome-related

oxidative stress. Int. J. Mol. Sci. 21 (18), 1–54. https://doi.org/10.3390/ijms21186902.

Wronska, A., 2023. The role of microRNA in the development, diagnosis, and treatment of cardiovascular disease: recent developments. J. Pharmacol. Exp. Therapeut. 384 (1), 123–132. https://doi.org/10.1124/jpet.121.001152.

Xie, H., Lim, B., Lodish, H.F., 2009. MicroRNAs induced during adipogenesis that accelerate fat cell development are downregulated in obesity. Diabetes 58 (5), 1050–1057. https://doi.org/10.2337/db08-1299.

Xu, P., Vernooy, S.Y., Guo, M., Hay, B.A., 2003. The drosophila microRNA mir-14 suppresses cell death and is required for normal fat metabolism. Curr. Biol. 13 (9), 790–795. https://doi.org/10.1016/S0960-9822(03)00250-1.

Yao, Q., Chen, Y., Xiang, Z., 2019. The roles of microRNAs in epigenetic regulation. Curr. Opin. Chem. Biol. 51, 11–17. https://doi.org/10.1016/j.cbpa.2019.01.024.

Yekta, S., Shih, I.H., Bartel, D.P., 2004. MicroRNA-directed cleavage of HOXB8 mRNA. Science 304 (5670), 594–596. https://doi.org/10.1126/science.1097434.

Zamore, P.D., Haley, B., 2005. Ribo-gnome: the big world of small RNAs. Science 309 (5740), 1519–1524. https://doi.org/10.1126/science.1111444.

Zhu, H., Ng, S.C., Segr, A.V., Shinoda, G., Shah, S.P., Einhorn, W.S., Takeuchi, A., Engreitz, J.M., Hagan, J.P., Kharas, M.G., Urbach, A., Thornton, J.E., Triboulet, R., Gregory, R.I., Altshuler, D., Daley, G.Q., 2011. The Lin28/let-7 axis regulates glucose metabolism. Cell 147 (1), 81–94. https://doi.org/10.1016/j.cell.2011.08.033.

6

Epigenetics and metabolic memory

1. Introduction

Diabetes mellitus, a chronic metabolic disorder characterized by persistent hyperglycemia, has long been recognized for its insidious capacity to inflict long-term damage on multiple organ systems. Despite advancements in glycemic control and pharmacotherapy, diabetic complications often continue to progress even after normalization of blood glucose levels, a phenomenon termed metabolic memory (Ceriello et al., 2009). Recent research has uncovered that this persistent pathological imprint is driven not solely by genetic predisposition or metabolic factors, but also by stable and heritable changes in gene expression mediated through epigenetic modifications (Keating and El-Osta, 2015).

Among these modifications, DNA methylation has emerged as a pivotal mechanism in shaping the transcriptional landscape of diabetic tissues. Through the enzymatic addition of methyl groups to cytosine residues within CpG dinucleotides, DNA methylation can stably silence gene expression without altering the underlying genetic code. This process, catalyzed by DNA methyltransferases (DNMTs), has been shown to suppress critical genes involved in antioxidant defense, insulin signaling, and glucose metabolism, thereby amplifying oxidative stress and inflammation, two central drivers of diabetic complications (Pirola et al., 2010; Villeneuve et al., 2010).

Beyond DNA methylation, the diabetic epigenome is dynamically remodeled through histone modifications, which regulate chromatin accessibility and transcriptional activity. These post-translational changes, including acetylation and methylation of histone tails, are influenced by hyperglycemia, oxidative stress, and inflammatory signals (Chen et al., 2020). The balance between activating and repressive histone marks determines whether genes that protect against oxidative injury or support metabolic flexibility are expressed or silenced (Tanwar et al., 2021).

Metabolic Memory. https://doi.org/10.1016/B978-0-443-44591-0.00012-6

Additionally, non-coding RNAs (ncRNAs), especially microRNAs and long non-coding RNAs, contribute to the establishment and maintenance of this aberrant epigenetic state. By modulating the stability and translation of target mRNAs or interacting with chromatin-modifying complexes, ncRNAs participate in reinforcing maladaptive gene expression patterns, sustaining cellular dysfunction in key metabolic tissues (Matai and Slack, 2023; DeFronzo et al., 2015).

Crucially, the epigenetic landscape is not only shaped by intrinsic disease mechanisms but is also highly responsive to environmental and lifestyle factors. Diet, physical activity, stress, sleep, and exposure to environmental toxins can all influence DNA methylation, histone modifications, and ncRNA expression (Ling and Rönn, 2014). These factors act as external cues that either exacerbate or mitigate the epigenetic reprogramming associated with metabolic memory, offering both a deeper understanding of disease progression and potential avenues for intervention (Smith et al., 2025).

This chapter explores the intricate role of epigenetic regulation in diabetes, with a particular focus on how DNA methylation, histone modifications, and non-coding RNAs contribute to the development and persistence of metabolic memory (Fig. 6.1). Furthermore, it highlights how environmental inputs modulate these mechanisms, setting the stage for innovative epigenetic therapies aimed at reversing chronic diabetic complications and improving long-term patient outcomes.

2. DNA methylation

DNA methylation is a key epigenetic mechanism that modulates gene expression without altering the underlying DNA sequence. It involves the enzymatic addition of a methyl group to the 5′ carbon of cytosine rings within CpG dinucleotides, especially those clustered in CpG islands located in gene promoter regions. This methylation often results in transcriptional repression (Bird, 2002). The process is catalyzed by DNA methyltransferases (DNMTs), where DNMT1 primarily maintains existing methylation patterns during DNA replication, while DNMT3A and DNMT3B are responsible for de novo methylation (Bestor, 2000). These enzymes help establish and propagate epigenetic memory in both physiological and pathological states, including diabetes (Villeneuve et al., 2008; Pirola et al., 2010).

In the diabetic milieu, persistent hyperglycemia initiates a cascade of molecular disturbances that result in the upregulation

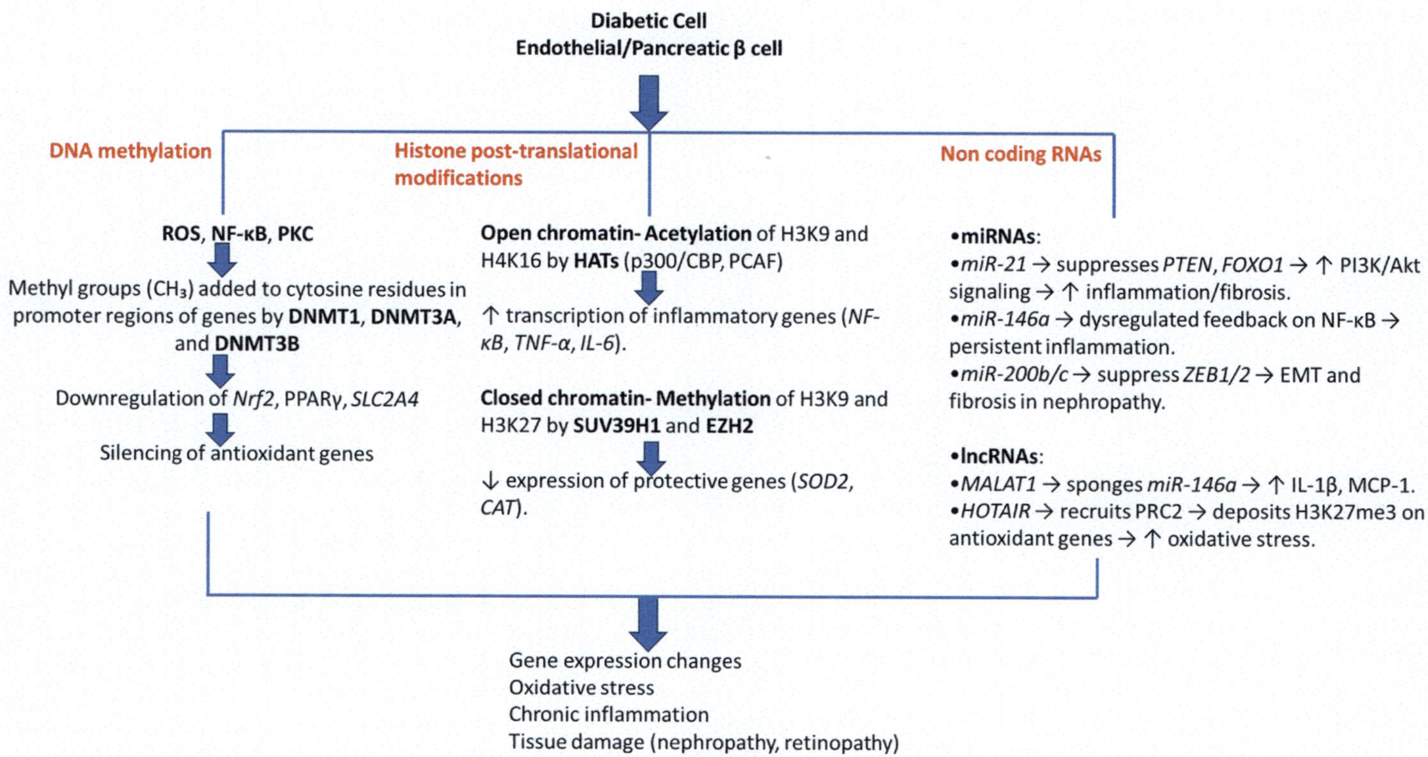

Figure 6.1 Epigenetic mechanisms underlying metabolic memory in diabetes: Hyperglycemia induces persistent epigenetic changes via DNA methylation, histone modifications, and non-coding RNAs, collectively contributing to metabolic memory. Aberrant methylation of genes like *Nrf2*, pro-inflammatory histone marks, and dysregulated miRNAs/lncRNAs perpetuate oxidative stress and inflammation even after glycemic normalization. These pathological imprinting drives long-term diabetic complications.

of DNMT expression and activity. This is mediated by increased production of reactive oxygen species (ROS), activation of protein kinase C (PKC), and stimulation of the pro-inflammatory transcription factor NF-κB (Mitro et al., 2024; Miao et al., 2014). Together, these pathways converge to enhance DNMT-mediated DNA methylation, particularly in vascular endothelial cells, renal tubular epithelial cells, and pancreatic β-cells, where the hypermethylation of protective genes exacerbates cellular dysfunction (Reddy et al., 2015).

A critical gene affected by hypermethylation is NFE2L2, which encodes Nuclear factor erythroid 2–related factor 2 (Nrf2), the master regulator of antioxidant defense. Methylation of the Nrf2 promoter reduces its transcription, leading to diminished expression of downstream antioxidant enzymes such as heme oxygenase-1 (HO-1), NAD(P)H quinone dehydrogenase 1 (NQO1), glutathione S-transferases (GSTs), and superoxide dismutases (SOD1/2) (Divyajanani et al., 2023). The downregulation of these enzymes impairs the cell's ability to neutralize ROS, contributing to persistent oxidative stress, mitochondrial dysfunction, and pro-inflammatory states, hallmarks of diabetic vascular injury (Dambal et al., 2015).

Beyond antioxidant regulation, hypermethylation also disrupts metabolic pathways crucial for maintaining insulin sensitivity and glucose homeostasis. For instance, PPARγ, a nuclear receptor vital for lipid metabolism and adipocyte differentiation, becomes epigenetically repressed in adipose tissue and skeletal muscle of diabetic individuals, contributing to insulin resistance (Hajri et al., 2021). Similarly, SLC2A4, the gene encoding glucose transporter type 4 (GLUT4), shows hypermethylation in insulin-sensitive tissues, impairing insulin-stimulated glucose uptake and exacerbating hyperglycemia (Ling et al., 2008).

These aberrant methylation changes persist even after restoration of normoglycemia (Ceriello et al., 2009). This persistence is maintained through a pathological feedback loop wherein reduced Nrf2 activity leads to increased mitochondrial ROS production, which in turn stimulates DNMT expression and perpetuates DNA hypermethylation (El-Osta et al., 2008). This cycle reinforces the silencing of protective genes and maintains a chronic inflammatory and oxidative state, facilitating the progression of long-term diabetic complications.

Recent advancements in epigenomic mapping technologies have substantiated these findings. Bisulfite sequencing offers high-resolution identification of methylated CpG sites, while chromatin immunoprecipitation followed by sequencing

(ChIP-seq) helps identify the binding of repressive complexes to methylated promoter regions (Kaluscha et al., 2022). These studies, performed in both animal models and diabetic patient tissues, consistently reveal silencing of key antioxidative and metabolic genes due to hypermethylation.

Persistent global DNA hypomethylation induced by diabetic conditions has been shown to be transmitted across cell divisions in zebrafish (Olsen et al., 2012). Similarly, sustained high glucose (HG)–induced DNAme alterations persist even after restoration of normal glucose (NG) levels, particularly in genes involved in mitochondrial homeostasis and mitochondrial DNA (mtDNA) integrity, contributing to diabetic retinopathy. These changes are functionally associated with mitochondrial dysfunction, oxidative stress, and cell death. In retinal cells, these alterations include hypermethylation of the regulatory region of DNA polymerase γ (POLG), which is required for mtDNA replication (Mishra and Kowluru, 2015); hypermethylation of mtDNA displacement-loop regions that control mtDNA transcription and replication, leading to base mismatches (Mishra and Kowluru, 2019); hypomethylation of matrix metalloproteinase-9 (MMP-9), which promotes retinal capillary cell apoptosis (Kowluru et al., 2016); and hypermethylation of genes encoding mitochondrial fusion and DNA mismatch repair proteins (Kowluru and Mohammad, 2020). These DNAme changes are further linked to sustained binding of DNMT1 to mtDNA and TET2 to MMP-9 (Mishra and Kowluru, 2016). In addition, genome-wide DNAme analyses revealed persistent methylation changes in foot fibroblasts from diabetic patients, with or without foot ulcers, even after prolonged culture under NG conditions (Park et al., 2014). Diabetes also alters DNAme at key genes associated with diabetic kidney disease (DKD) in renal proximal tubular cells (Bansal et al., 2020) and endothelial cells (ECs) in models of renal and vascular hyperglycemic memory (Paneni et al., 2012).

Given the pivotal role of DNA methylation in metabolic memory, therapeutic strategies aimed at reversing these epigenetic changes are gaining momentum. DNA methyltransferase inhibitors, such as 5-aza-2′-deoxycytidine (decitabine), have shown potential in reactivating silenced genes and restoring cellular function (Villeneuve et al., 2008). In parallel, pharmacological activators of Nrf2, such as bardoxolone methyl, sulforaphane, and curcumin, are being explored to enhance antioxidant capacity and mitigate oxidative stress (Zhou et al., 2016). Combination therapies integrating epigenetic modulators and antioxidants offer a promising avenue to disrupt metabolic memory and delay the onset of day, retinopathy, and cardiovascular disease.

3. Histone modifications

Histone modifications are critical epigenetic regulators that alter chromatin structure and control gene accessibility, thereby modulating transcriptional activity. These post translational modifications, including acetylation, methylation, phosphorylation, and ubiquitination, occur on the amino-terminal tails of histone proteins, particularly histones H3 and H4. The nature and location of these modifications determine whether chromatin adopts an open (euchromatin) or closed (heterochromatin) conformation, thereby influencing gene activation or repression (Kouzarides, 2007).

In the context of diabetes, chronic hyperglycemia induces dynamic changes in histone modification patterns, particularly promoting histone acetylation at promoters of pro-inflammatory and pro-oxidant genes. Histone acetyltransferases (HATs) such as p300/CBP and PCAF (p300/CBP-associated factor) catalyze the addition of acetyl groups to lysine residues like H3K9 and H4K16. These modifications lead to chromatin decondensation and increased accessibility of transcription factors to DNA, resulting in enhanced transcription of inflammatory genes such as NF-κB, TNF-α, and IL-6 (Brasacchio et al., 2009; Miao et al., 2014). This pro-inflammatory milieu contributes to endothelial dysfunction, leukocyte adhesion, and increased vascular permeability, key features of diabetic complications (Reddy et al., 2015).

On the other hand, repressive histone methylation marks are often found at antioxidant and metabolic regulatory gene loci in hyperglycemic conditions. Methylation at histone three lysine 9 (H3K9me3) and lysine 27 (H3K27me3), mediated by histone methyltransferases such as SUV39H1 and EZH2, contributes to transcriptional silencing. Genes encoding key antioxidant enzymes, including SOD2 and CAT, are frequently marked by these repressive modifications, leading to diminished antioxidant defenses (Keating et al., 2012; Miao et al., 2014). This silencing exacerbates mitochondrial ROS accumulation and oxidative damage, particularly in endothelial and renal cells, promoting tissue fibrosis, capillary rarefaction, and the onset of nephropathy and retinopathy (Wang et al., 2022).

Furthermore, histone deacetylases (HDACs), particularly HDAC3 and HDAC9, are found to be upregulated in diabetic tissues. These enzymes remove acetyl groups from histones, often working in complex with co-repressors to maintain transcriptional repression of protective genes, including those involved in insulin signaling and glucose uptake (Zhang et al., 2017). Inhibiting HDACs with agents like Vorinostat or trichostatin A has been shown in preclinical models to restore expression of silenced genes and reduce inflammatory and fibrotic responses (Chen et al., 2020).

Together, the interplay of activating and repressive histone marks in diabetes supports a maladaptive epigenetic landscape that promotes sustained oxidative stress, inflammation, and metabolic dysfunction, hallmarks of metabolic memory. This histone-based epigenetic programming not only sustains cellular injury long after glycemic normalization but also offers a promising target for therapeutic intervention. Emerging histone-modifying enzyme inhibitors and lifestyle interventions (e.g., exercise, intermittent fasting) capable of modulating histone marks are currently under investigation to reverse this pathological imprinting and improve long-term outcomes in diabetes management (Ling and Rönn, 2014; Natarajan et al., 2012).

Evidences suggest the implications of both local as well as global post translational histone modifications in metabolic memory. Hyperglycemia alters histone acetylation by increasing HDAC activity and reducing HAT activity in the retina and retinal endothelial cells (ECs), leading to decreased histone H3 acetylation. Importantly, these changes persist even after normalization of glucose levels, implicating global histone acetylation in the metabolic memory of diabetic retinopathy (Zhong and Kowluru, 2010). In addition to acetylation, persistent post translational histone modifications induced by high glucose at inflammatory gene loci promote sustained inflammation. Early studies demonstrated reduced levels of the repressive mark H3K9me3 and decreased occupancy of its corresponding lysine methyltransferase (KMT) Suv39h1 at promoters of inflammatory genes such as *Il6*, *Ccl2*, and *Csf2* in vascular smooth muscle cells (VSMCs) from diabetic db/db mice. These epigenetic changes persisted after prolonged culture under normoglycemic conditions and were associated with increased inflammatory gene expression and sustained cellular activation (Villeneuve et al., 2008). Similar Suv39h1-mediated PTM changes were observed at *IL6* in cardiomyocytes exposed to HG, suggesting shared epigenetic mechanisms across tissues (Yu et al., 2012).

In endothelial cells, transient HG exposure induced persistent enrichment of the activating mark H3K4me1 and increased binding of the KMT Set7 at the promoter of the NF-κB p65 subunit, even after glucose normalization. These changes were also observed in vivo and resulted in sustained expression of proatherogenic and inflammatory genes, including *VCAM1* and *CCL2* (El-Osta et al., 2008). Follow-up studies showed reduced H3K9me2 and H3K9me3 levels and increased recruitment of the demethylase LSD1 at the same promoter, further reinforcing inflammatory memory (Cooper et al., 2018). Set7-mediated H3K4me1 enrichment was subsequently identified as a key regulator of hyperglycemic memory in ECs (Okabe et al., 2012). In ECs from type 1 diabetic mice, persistent upregulation of *Serpine1* and enrichment of H3K4me3 at its promoter were observed even under normoglycemic conditions, with similar findings in normal ECs following HG exposure and glucose normalization (Takizawa et al., 2013). Notably, *SERPINE1* expression was shown to be regulated by the chromatin-associated long noncoding RNA LINC00607 located at a super-enhancer, highlighting epigenetic crosstalk between chromatin modifications and lncRNAs in vascular dysfunction and metabolic memory (Calandrelli et al., 2020).

Persistent histone PTMs also contribute to oxidative stress in diabetic complications. Poor glycemic control increased SUV420h2-mediated H4K20me3 and reduced H3K4me1 and H3K4me2 at the *Sod2* promoter in retinal tissue, leading to sustained suppression of this antioxidant gene even after restoration of euglycemia (Zhong and Kowluru, 2013). In diabetic retinas and retinal ECs, histone PTMs further impaired the activity of the redox-sensitive transcription factor Nrf2, weakening cellular antioxidant defenses (Mishra et al., 2014).

Histone modifications also regulate multiple signaling pathways relevant to diabetic complications. Thioredoxin-interacting protein (TXNIP), a pro-oxidant regulator, promoted sustained expression of cyclooxygenase-2 in retinal ECs after glucose normalization through increased promoter H3K9 acetylation and reduced H3K9me3 (Perrone et al., 2009). In renal mesangial cells and murine kidneys, HG induced persistent TXNIP upregulation via increased activating histone marks (H3K9ac, H3K4me1, and H3K4me3) and decreased repressive H3K27me3 at its promoter (De Marinis et al., 2016). Elevated TXNIP levels exacerbated oxidative stress, mitochondrial dysfunction, inflammation, fibrosis, apoptosis, and insulin resistance across multiple tissues, including the retina (Singh, 2013), kidney (Shah et al., 2015), nerves (Zhang et al., 2021), and vasculature (Myers et al., 2016). In podocytes from diabetic mice, HG induced sustained enrichment of H3K9/14ac and H3K4me1 at the *SHP-1* promoter, resulting in persistent gene activation, insulin resistance, podocyte dysfunction, and progressive nephropathy even after glucose normalization (Lizotte et al., 2016).

4. Non-coding RNAs

Non-coding RNAs (ncRNAs), particularly microRNAs (miRNAs) and long non-coding RNAs (lncRNAs), are pivotal regulators of gene expression at the post transcriptional and epigenetic levels (Table 6.1). In the context of diabetes, these

Table 6.1 Role of non-coding RNAs in metabolic memory and diabetic complications.

ncRNA type	Example	Mechanism of action	Pathological effect in diabetes	References
miRNA	**miR-21**	Targets *PTEN* and *FOXO1*, suppressing negative regulators of the PI3K/Akt pathway	Promotes inflammation, fibrosis, and insulin resistance	(Kato et al., 2009; Zhong and Kowluru, 2013)
miRNA	**miR-146a**	Negative regulator of NF-κB; dysregulated in chronic hyperglycemia	Sustains chronic inflammation via IL-6 and TNF-α dysregulation	(Bhatt et al., 2016; Feng et al., 2017)
miRNA	**miR-200b/c**	Targets *ZEB1*, *ZEB2*; mediates epithelial-to-mesenchymal transition (EMT)	Promotes renal fibrosis in diabetic nephropathy	(Kato et al., 2007; Mongroo and Rustgi, 2014)
lncRNA	**MALAT1**	Sponges miR-146a, regulates IL-1β and MCP-1 expression	Enhances inflammation in diabetic kidney and endothelium	(Puthanveetil et al., 2015; Yang et al., 2016)
lncRNA	**HOTAIR**	Recruits PRC2 to deposit H3K27me3; sponges miR-34a	Silences oxidative stress response genes, promotes vascular senescence	Li et al. (2018)
miRNAs/ lncRNAs (general)	—	Sustained expression of pro-inflammatory and stress-related genes	Contributes to metabolic memory and complications (nephropathy, retinopathy, etc.)	(Reddy et al., 2015)
Therapeutic targeting	—	Use of miRNA mimics, antisense oligonucleotides, lncRNA inhibitors	Potential reversal of metabolic memory and diabetic complications	(Natarajan et al., 2012; Li et al., 2018)

ncRNAs contribute to the phenomenon of metabolic memory by sustaining abnormal gene expression patterns long after normalization of blood glucose levels (Chen et al., 2020; Sinha et al., 2015). MicroRNAs (miRNAs) are short (~22 nucleotides) RNA molecules that bind to the 3′ untranslated region (UTR) of target messenger RNAs (mRNAs), leading to their degradation or translational repression.

Several miRNAs are consistently dysregulated in diabetic tissues. miR-21 is upregulated in endothelial cells and kidney tissues in diabetic models. It targets PTEN and FOXO1, both of which are negative regulators of the PI3K/Akt pathway. Downregulation of these genes promotes inflammation, fibrosis, and insulin resistance (Kato et al., 2009; Zhong et al., 2011). miR-146a, which normally functions as a negative feedback regulator of the NF-κB pathway during acute inflammation, is paradoxically sustained in chronic hyperglycemia. Persistent expression of miR-146a in diabetic tissues disrupts the balanced regulation of inflammatory cytokines such as IL-6 and TNF-α, leading to maladaptive chronic inflammation (Bhatt et al., 2016; Feng et al., 2017).

The miR-200 family, including miR-200b and miR-200c, contributes to epithelial-to-mesenchymal transition (EMT) and fibrosis, particularly in diabetic nephropathy, by suppressing targets such as ZEB1 and ZEB2—transcriptional repressors involved in cell polarity and extracellular matrix homeostasis (Kato et al., 2007; Mongroo and Rustgi, 2014).

Long non-coding RNAs (lncRNAs) are transcripts longer than 200 nucleotides that regulate gene expression by serving as molecular scaffolds, decoys, or guides for chromatin-modifying complexes. MALAT1 (Metastasis Associated Lung Adenocarcinoma Transcript 1) is significantly upregulated in endothelial cells and diabetic kidneys. MALAT1 binds and sequesters miR-146aReduceIL-1β and MCP-1 (Puthanveetil et al., 2015; Yang et al., 2016). HOTAIR (HOX Transcript Antisense RNA) recruits the PRC2 complex, which deposits the repressive histone mark H3K27me3 on target gene promoters, silencing genes involved in oxidative stress response and endothelial homeostasis. HOTAIR also acts as a molecular sponge for miR-34a, a regulator of vascular senescence (Li et al., 2018).

These persistent alterations in ncRNA expression form a critical part of the epigenetic memory induced by hyperglycemia. By maintaining pro-inflammatory and oxidative stress-related gene expression, these ncRNAs contribute to the development and progression of diabetic complications such as nephropathy, retinopathy, cardiomyopathy, and atherosclerosis (Reddy et al., 2015). Emerging studies suggest that targeting specific ncRNAs using antisense oligonucleotides, miRNA mimics, or lncRNA inhibitors may represent a novel therapeutic strategy for reversing metabolic memory and mitigating chronic diabetic complications (Li et al., 2018; Natarajan et al., 2012).

Evidences suggest that in human aortic endothelial cells, exposure to high glucose followed by normalization to normal glucose resulted in sustained expression of miR-125b and miR-146a-5p, persistent activation of NF-κB signaling, and continued endothelial dysfunction (Zhong et al., 2015). Similarly, genome-wide profiling of diabetic mouse hearts identified 268 miRNAs that remained dysregulated after restoration of glycemic control, suggesting a role for miRNA-mediated metabolic memory in diabetic cardiomyopathy (Costantino et al., 2016). In ECs subjected to HG-to-NG transition, NF-κB–induced miR-27a-3p signaling remained persistently activated, leading to suppression of NRF2, reduced nitric oxide (NO) bioavailability, increased reactive oxygen species (ROS), and elevated TGF-β levels. These changes promoted endothelial-to-mesenchymal transition, perivascular fibrosis, and cardiac dysfunction (Yao et al., 2022). In retinal tissues, HG exposure enhanced NF-κB p65 recruitment to the miR-23b-1 promoter, increasing miR-23b-3p expression. This miRNA targets SIRT1, resulting in enhanced NF-κB acetylation and sustained inflammatory signaling, suggesting that the miR-23b-3p/SIRT1/NF-κB feedback loop contributes to the initiation and maintenance of metabolic memory in diabetic retinopathy (Zhao et al., 2016).

LncRNAs regulate gene expression through epigenetic mechanisms and are increasingly recognized as contributors to diabetic complications; however, their role in metabolic memory remains relatively underexplored. Lnc-Ang362, an angiotensin II–induced lncRNA that regulates vascular smooth muscle cell (VSMC) proliferation (Leung et al., 2013), serves as the host transcript for miR-221 and miR-222, which promote VSMC growth and cardiomyocyte hypertrophy. These miRNAs were persistently upregulated in diabetic hearts, suggesting a potential contribution to metabolic memory (Costantino et al., 2016). Another lncRNA, lnc-MGC, which hosts approximately 40 miRNAs within the miR-379 cluster, was markedly upregulated in renal glomeruli of diabetic mice and in mesangial cells treated with HG or TGF-β. Inhibition of lnc-MGC reduced glomerular matrix accumulation, fibrosis, and hypertrophy associated with early diabetic kidney disease (DKD) (Kato et al., 2016). Expression of lnc-MGC and its associated miRNAs was driven by the endoplasmic reticulum (ER) stress–responsive transcription factor CHOP, creating a feed-forward loop that further amplified ER stress through miRNAs such as miR-379. These self-sustaining regulatory circuits may promote long-lasting molecular changes in diabetic nephropathy and contribute to metabolic memory. Nevertheless, further studies are required to firmly establish causal links between specific lncRNAs and metabolic memory mechanisms.

5. Crosstalk among epigenetic marks in the establishment of metabolic memory

Metabolic memory arises from the coordinated action of multiple epigenetic mechanisms, including DNA methylation, histone post-translational modifications, chromatin accessibility, and non-coding RNAs. These marks often act together to produce long-lasting changes in gene expression.

In diabetic mice, analysis of the angiotensinogen promoter in kidney proximal tubules showed a stepwise pattern of epigenetic changes. These changes began with increased H3K9 acetylation, followed by H3K4 trimethylation, and later DNA demethylation, resulting in enhanced gene expression. Importantly, altered DNAme and gene expression persisted even after blood glucose normalization, indicating cooperative epigenetic mechanisms underlying metabolic memory in diabetic kidney disease (DKD) (Marumo et al., 2015).

The redox gene *p66Shc* is another example of epigenetic persistence. Under diabetic conditions, *p66Shc* upregulation led to sustained ROS production, reduced nitric oxide, inflammation, and apoptosis across multiple tissues, including peripheral blood mononuclear cells, endothelial cells (ECs), kidney, heart, and blood vessels, contributing to both micro- and macrovascular complications (Francia et al., 2009). Persistent *p66Shc* expression was observed in human ECs exposed to high glucose and in diabetic mice even after restoration of normoglycemia (Paneni et al., 2012). This sustained expression was linked to promoter DNA hypomethylation and histone H3 hyperacetylation, further supporting epigenetic cooperation in metabolic memory (Paneni et al., 2012). Histone hyperacetylation was also influenced by altered SIRT1 activity (Zhou et al., 2011). Similar epigenetic changes were identified in diabetic mouse hearts, associated with reduced Dnmt3b and SIRT1 expression, along with involvement of miR-218 and miR-34a, highlighting interactions among

DNAme, histone modifications, and miRNAs in metabolic memory (Costantino et al., 2018).

In human ECs, transient high glucose exposure increased active histone marks and reduced DNA methylation at promoters of hyperglycemia-responsive genes, potentially contributing to endothelial dysfunction memory, although the persistence of these changes after normoglycemia was not assessed (Pirola et al., 2011). miRNAs can also influence metabolic memory by targeting histone-modifying enzymes. For example, in vascular smooth muscle cells from diabetic *db/db* mice, sustained upregulation of miR-125b promoted inflammatory gene expression by reducing repressive H3K9me3 marks through downregulation of its target histone methyltransferase, Suv39h1, even after culture under nondiabetic conditions (Villeneuve et al., 2010).

Further evidence comes from kidney proximal tubule epithelial cells derived from individuals with type 2 diabetes (T2D). When cultured for several passages under nondiabetic conditions, these cells retained promoter hyper-DNAme, reduced chromatin accessibility, and decreased H3K27 acetylation at key transport-related genes, including *CLDN10, CLDN14, CLDN16, SLC16A2,* and *SLC16A5.* These epigenetic alterations were associated with impaired tubular function. Additionally, T2D-derived tubular cells showed increased sensitivity to the profibrotic factor TGF-β, illustrating crosstalk between epigenetic marks and chromatin remodeling in metabolic memory of DKD (Bansal et al., 2020).

6. How environmental factors influence gene expression and metabolism

Environmental factors significantly shape epigenetic landscapes, influencing gene expression and metabolic outcomes. Diet, physical activity, stress, and exposure to toxins modulate epigenetic marks, thereby affecting metabolic health and disease susceptibility (Fig. 6.2).

6.1 Diet and nutrition

Nutritional inputs have a profound impact on epigenetic mechanisms such as DNA methylation and histone modifications, thereby influencing gene expression and long-term metabolic health (Milagro et al., 2013). Diet acts as both a substrate and regulator of epigenetic enzyme activity, linking environmental exposures to genomic outcomes.

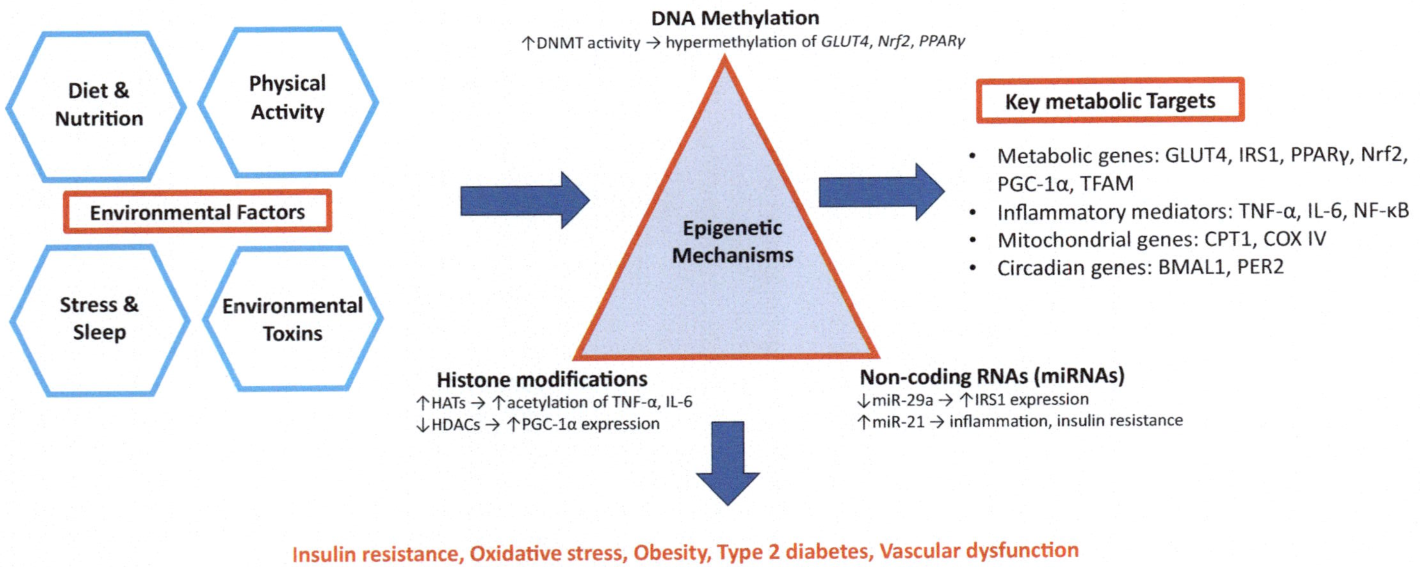

Figure 6.2 Environmental epigenetic modifiers in metabolic health and disease. Environmental and lifestyle factors modulate gene expression through epigenetic mechanisms such as DNA methylation, histone modifications, and miRNA regulation. These modifications affect metabolic gene networks and contribute to the development or prevention of chronic diseases such as diabetes and obesity. Understanding these dynamic interactions enables precision medicine strategies targeting metabolic memory and long-term disease risk.

Pro-inflammatory Diets and Epigenetic Dysregulation: Diets high in refined sugars, saturated fats, and processed foods can induce persistent epigenetic alterations that favor metabolic inflammation and insulin resistance (Stols-Gonçalves et al., 2019). These dietary patterns enhance histone acetylation at promoter regions of pro-inflammatory genes, such as TNF-α, IL-6, and NF-κB, through the activation of histone acetyltransferases (HATs) like p300/CBP and PCAF (Fernandez et al., 2009). Concurrently, high-glucose environments increase the activity of DNA methyltransferases (DNMTs), leading to aberrant methylation of key metabolic regulators. For instance, hypermethylation of the Nrf2 promoter diminishes antioxidant gene expression, worsening oxidative stress and contributing to vascular and cellular damage in diabetic tissues (Wang et al., 2022).

Role of Methyl Donor Nutrients in DNA Methylation: Nutrients that donate methyl groups are critical for maintaining appropriate DNA methylation patterns. These include Folate (vitamin B9), Vitamin B12, Choline, Betaine and Methionine.

These nutrients enter the one-carbon metabolism pathway, supporting the generation of S-adenosylmethionine (SAM), the universal methyl donor used by DNMTs (Anderson et al., 2012). Adequate intake of these micronutrients ensures normal silencing of deleterious genes and supports genome stability. For example, increased folate intake has been associated with demethylation of the PPARγ promoter, thereby enhancing insulin sensitivity and lipid metabolism (de Paula et al., 2022).

Protective Roles of Polyphenols and Omega-3 Fatty Acids: Bioactive food components such as polyphenols and omega-3 fatty acids also exert protective epigenetic effects. Polyphenols like resveratrol (found in grapes) and curcumin (from turmeric) have been shown to inhibit HATs, reducing histone acetylation at inflammatory loci, while simultaneously activating SIRT1, a histone deacetylase (HDAC) associated with anti inflammatory and longevity pathways (Donohoe and Bultman, 2012; Borra et al., 2005). These compounds also activate the Nrf2 pathway, enhancing transcription of antioxidant response element (ARE)-regulated genes such as HO-1, NQO1, and SOD, bolstering endogenous antioxidant defences (Kong et al., 2001; Ngo and Duennwald, 2022). Omega-3 fatty acids, particularly EPA and DHA, have been found to modulate histone methylation and reduce the expression of genes involved in cytokine production and lipid-induced inflammation (Sertorio et al., 2021). They may also alter miRNA profiles associated with adipogenesis and insulin signaling (Al-Mansoori et al., 2022).

6.2 Physical activity

Regular physical activity induces a spectrum of beneficial epigenetic modifications that enhance metabolic flexibility, mitochondrial biogenesis, and insulin sensitivity, particularly in skeletal muscle and adipose tissue (Barrès and Zierath, 2016; Denham et al., 2016). These changes contribute to improved glucose homeostasis and reduced risk of metabolic diseases such as type 2 diabetes and cardiovascular disease (Hawley et al., 2014).

Histone Modifications and Mitochondrial Biogenesis: Exercise increases histone acetylation, particularly H3K9ac and H4K16ac, at promoter regions of genes involved in oxidative phosphorylation and fatty acid oxidation, facilitating chromatin relaxation and gene transcription (McGee and Hargreaves, 2011). This epigenetic activation is mediated by upregulation of histone acetyltransferases (HATs) such as p300/CBP and suppression of histone deacetylases (HDACs) like HDAC5, promoting transcriptional activity in metabolic pathways (Cantó and Auwerx, 2009).

One of the central mediators of these changes is PGC-1α (Peroxisome proliferator-activated receptor gamma coactivator 1-alpha)—a master regulator of mitochondrial biogenesis. Exercise-induced phosphorylation and acetylation of PGC-1α enhances its activity, leading to increased expression of mitochondrial genes such as CPT1, TFAM, and components of the electron transport chain (e.g., NDUFB8, COX IV) (Triolo et al., 2022). This results in improved mitochondrial density and efficiency, supporting greater energy production and endurance.

Modulation of MicroRNAs and Metabolic Inflammation: Physical activity also alters the expression of specific microRNAs (miRNAs) that regulate insulin signaling, inflammation, and glucose transport (Silva et al., 2017). For instance, miR-29a and miR-223 are downregulated post-exercise, which relieves their inhibitory effects on insulin receptor substrate (IRS1) and GLUT4, enhancing insulin sensitivity (Karolina et al., 2011). miR-126, a key regulator of vascular integrity, is upregulated, promoting endothelial function and angiogenesis (de Gonzalo-Calvo et al., 2015). miR-21 and miR-146a, which are often elevated in chronic inflammatory states, are normalized with consistent aerobic training, thereby dampening NF-κB-driven inflammation (Radom-Aizik et al., 2012).

Impact on DNA Methylation: Exercise has also been shown to dynamically influence DNA methylation patterns in skeletal muscle. Acute bouts of exercise can cause hypomethylation of promoters for metabolic genes such as PPARγ, GLUT4 (SLC2A4), and TFAM, increasing their transcription (Nitert et al., 2012). This hypomethylation is transient but may become more sustained with chronic training, contributing to long-term metabolic adaptations (Laker et al., 2017).

6.3 Psychosocial stress and sleep

Chronic psychological stress and insufficient sleep exert profound effects on metabolic health, largely through epigenetic reprogramming of key genes involved in glucose and lipid metabolism (Anjaria et al., 2023). These lifestyle stressors contribute to the development and progression of insulin resistance, obesity, and type 2 diabetes (Zannas et al., 2016).

Role of Stress Hormones and Epigenetic Enzymes: Under chronic stress, elevated secretion of glucocorticoids, particularly cortisol, alters the activity of DNA methyltransferases (DNMTs) and histone deacetylases (HDACs) (Zannas and West, 2014). Cortisol binds to the glucocorticoid receptor (GR), which translocates to the nucleus and interacts with co-regulatory complexes that include DNMTs and HDACs. This interaction leads to hypermethylation of promoter regions of insulin-sensitizing genes, such as GLUT4 (SLC2A4) and IRS1 (insulin receptor substrate 1), thereby reducing their transcription and impairing insulin signaling (Sasaki et al., 2013). Simultaneously, HDACs remove acetyl groups from histones, causing chromatin condensation and suppression of anti inflammatory and metabolic genes like PPARγ and adiponectin, further exacerbating insulin resistance and adipose tissue dysfunction (Sharma and Fulton, 2013).

Effects of Sleep Deprivation on Epigenetic Marks: Sleep deprivation similarly disrupts circadian gene expression and metabolic homeostasis through altered epigenetic regulation (Saad et al., 2021). Studies have shown that reduced sleep leads to hypoacetylation of histones at the promoters of clock genes (e.g., BMAL1, PER2) and metabolic regulators, disrupting circadian rhythms and insulin sensitivity (Cai et al., 2024). Moreover, DNA methylation changes in genes such as LEP (leptin) and CRY1 impair appetite control, energy balance, and glucose metabolism (Carroll et al., 2017).

Long-Term Metabolic Consequences: These epigenetic alterations are not merely transient. Chronic exposure to stress and sleep deprivation can lead to persistent changes in gene expression, hallmarks of metabolic memory, even after cortisol levels or sleep patterns normalize (Ling and Rönn, 2014). This persistent dysregulation contributes to systemic inflammation, hepatic steatosis, impaired mitochondrial function, and increased risk for metabolic syndrome and cardiovascular disease (Diao et al., 2025).

Therapeutic Insights: Targeting the epigenetic pathways affected by stress and poor sleep holds therapeutic promise. HDAC inhibitors (e.g., valproic acid) and DNMT inhibitors (e.g., 5-aza-2′-deoxycytidine) have shown potential in reversing stress-induced metabolic dysregulation in preclinical models (Guo et al., 2025). Behavioral interventions such as cognitive-behavioral therapy (CBT) for stress, mindfulness practices, and improved sleep hygiene can also modulate stress-related hormonal outputs, potentially reversing maladaptive epigenetic patterns (Kalisch et al., 2015).

6.4 Environmental toxins

Exposure to environmental pollutants, including endocrine-disrupting chemicals (EDCs) such as bisphenol A (BPA), phthalates, polychlorinated biphenyls (PCBs), and heavy metals like arsenic, cadmium, and lead, has been strongly associated with epigenetic modifications that impair insulin signaling and promote metabolic dysregulation (Table 6.2) (La Merrill et al., 2020; Rancière et al., 2015). These compounds exert their effects through multiple pathways, most notably by inducing oxidative stress, endoplasmic reticulum (ER) stress, and mitochondrial dysfunction (Heindel and Vandenberg, 2015). For instance, BPA has been shown to increase DNA methylation at the insulin-like growth factor 2 (IGF2) gene and suppress the expression of glucose transporter type 4 (GLUT4) via altered histone acetylation, contributing to insulin resistance in adipose and muscle tissues (Ma et al., 2013; Bromer et al., 2010).

Heavy metals such as arsenic can activate DNA methyltransferases (DNMTs) and histone deacetylases (HDACs), leading to hypermethylation of the PPARγ promoter—a key gene involved in lipid metabolism and insulin sensitivity (Reichard and Puga, 2010). Additionally, cadmium exposure has been linked to the downregulation of miR-29 and upregulation of miR-21, which further disrupts insulin signaling pathways and promotes β-cell dysfunction (Fang et al., 2017).

These toxins also disrupt hormonal balance, particularly the hypothalamic-pituitary-adrenal (HPA) axis, increasing cortisol production that contributes to chronic inflammation, gluconeogenesis, and insulin resistance (Tellez-Plaza et al., 2018). Moreover, exposure during critical windows of development (e.g., in

Table 6.2 Epigenetic effects of environmental pollutants on metabolic health.

Pollutant type	Examples	Epigenetic modifications	Mechanisms of action	Target genes/ pathways	Metabolic consequences	References
Endocrine-disrupting chemicals (EDCs)	Bisphenol A (BPA), phthalates, polychlorinated biphenyls (PCBs)	- DNA hypermethylation (e.g., *IGF2*)- altered histone acetylation- changes in non-coding RNAs	- Activates DNMTs and HDACs- disrupts glucocorticoid signaling- alters chromatin accessibility	- *GLUT4* (SLC2A4)- *IGF2*- *PPARγ*- inflammatory cytokines (*IL-6, TNF-α*)	- Insulin resistance- glucose intolerance- enhanced adipogenesis- oxidative stress	(La Merrill et al., 2020; Rancière et al., 2015; Ma et al., 2013)
Heavy metals	Arsenic, cadmium, lead	- DNA hypermethylation- histone deacetylation- miRNA dysregulation (↑miR-21, ↓miR-29)	- Induces oxidative stress and ER stress- alters HPA axis signaling- upregulates DNMTs and HDACs	- *PPARγ*- *IRS1*, *GLUT4*- *Nrf2*- mitochondrial genes (e.g., *COX IV, TFAM*)	- Disrupted lipid metabolism- β-cell apoptosis- inflammation- mitochondrial dysfunction	(Fang et al., 2017; Reichard and Puga, 2010; Tellez-Plaza et al., 2018)
Persistent organic pollutants (POPs)	Dioxins, furans	- Promoter methylation- histone H3K9me3 enrichment	- Activates aryl hydrocarbon receptor (AhR)- disrupts circadian gene expression	- *BMAL1*, *PER2*- *CYP1A1*	- Altered glucose metabolism- hepatic steatosis- chronodisruption	(Skinner, 2014; Heindel and Vandenberg, 2015)
Airborne pollutants	Diesel exhaust, PM2.5	- Global DNA hypomethylation- HDAC activation- pro-inflammatory gene upregulation	- Induces reactive oxygen species (ROS)- activates NF-κB signaling	- *IL-6*, *NF-κB*, *SOD2*- *DNMT1*	- Systemic inflammation- vascular dysfunction- increased diabetes risk	(Küpers et al., 2019; Diao et al., 2025)

utero or early childhood) can cause transgenerational epigenetic inheritance, where altered methylation patterns and non-coding RNA expression profiles are passed to offspring, predisposing them to metabolic disorders (Skinner, 2014). Collectively, these environmental insults interact with the host genome through epigenetic mechanisms—including DNA methylation, histone modifications, and non-coding RNA regulation—to modulate gene expression patterns that contribute to metabolic memory and chronic disease progression in diabetes (Küpers et al., 2019).

Understanding these epigenetic-environment interactions provides a crucial foundation for developing personalized preventive and therapeutic interventions. Potential strategies include the use of epigenetic modifiers, detoxifying dietary components (e.g., sulforaphane, curcumin, resveratrol), and public health measures aimed at reducing environmental exposure, particularly in vulnerable populations (Balachandar et al., 2022).

7. Conclusion

The emerging field of epigenetics has significantly advanced our understanding of the molecular mechanisms underlying diabetic complications and the persistence of metabolic memory. Unlike genetic mutations, epigenetic modifications are dynamic and reversible, offering a compelling explanation for the sustained cellular dysfunction seen in diabetes, even after glycemic normalization. DNA methylation, histone modifications, and non-coding RNAs collectively orchestrate complex gene expression patterns that promote oxidative stress, inflammation, and vascular damage—key contributors to diabetic micro- and macrovascular complications.

Importantly, these epigenetic changes are not only influenced by hyperglycemia but are also shaped by environmental and lifestyle factors such as diet, exercise, stress, sleep, and exposure to toxins. This highlights the potential for early interventions and personalized lifestyle modifications to mitigate the long-term impact of diabetes through epigenetic reprogramming.

As research progresses, targeting the epigenetic machinery offers a promising therapeutic frontier. Pharmacological agents such as DNMT inhibitors, HDAC inhibitors, and Nrf2 activators, alongside ncRNA-based therapies, may offer novel avenues to reverse maladaptive epigenetic memory and prevent the progression of diabetic complications. However, clinical translation remains challenging, requiring a deeper understanding of tissue-specific epigenetic signatures and the development of safe, targeted delivery systems.

In conclusion, integrating epigenetic insights into diabetes management holds the potential to revolutionize both preventive and therapeutic strategies, moving us closer to precision medicine approaches that address not just blood glucose levels but the underlying molecular imprints of the disease.

References

Al-Mansoori, L., Al-Jaber, H., Prince, M.S., Elrayess, M.A., 2022. Role of inflammatory cytokines, growth factors and adipokines in adipogenesis and insulin resistance. Inflammation 45 (1), 31–44. https://doi.org/10.1007/s10753-021-01559-z.

Anderson, O.S., Sant, K.E., Dolinoy, D.C., 2012. Nutrition and epigenetics: an interplay of dietary methyl donors, one-carbon metabolism and DNA methylation. JNB (J. Nutr. Biochem.) 23 (8), 853–859. https://doi.org/10.1016/j.jnutbio.2012.03.003.

Anjaria, P., Asediya, V., Nayak, J., Koringa, P., 2023. The epigenetic landscape: how environmental cues shape gene expression. Epigenomics 15 (5), 267–270. https://doi.org/10.2217/epi-2023-0112.

Balachandar, V., Mahalaxmi, I., Neethu, R., Arul, N., Abhilash, V.G., 2022. New insights into epigenetics as an influencer: an associative study between maternal prenatal factors in autism spectrum disorder (ASD). Neurology Perspectives 2 (2), 78–86. https://doi.org/10.1016/j.neurop.2022.01.002.

Bansal, A., Balasubramanian, S., Dhawan, S., Leung, A., Chen, Z., Natarajan, R., 2020. Integrative omics analyses reveal epigenetic memory in diabetic renal cells regulating genes associated with kidney dysfunction. Diabetes 69 (11), 2490–2502. https://doi.org/10.2337/db20-0382.

Barrès, R., Zierath, J.R., 2016. The role of diet and exercise in the transgenerational epigenetic landscape of T2DM. Nat. Rev. Endocrinol. 12 (8), 441–451. https://doi.org/10.1038/nrendo.2016.87.

Bestor, T.H., 2000. The DNA methyltransferases of mammals. Hum. Mol. Genet. 9 (16), 2395–2402. https://doi.org/10.1093/hmg/9.16.2395.

Bhatt, K., Lanting, L.L., Jia, Y., Yadav, S., Reddy, M.A., Magilnick, N., Boldin, M., Natarajan, R., 2016. Anti-inflammatory role of microrna-146a in the pathogenesis of diabetic nephropathy. J. Am. Soc. Nephrol. 27 (8), 2277–2288. https://doi.org/10.1681/ASN.2015010111.

Bird, A., 2002. DNA methylation patterns and epigenetic memory. Gene Dev. 16 (1), 6–21. https://doi.org/10.1101/gad.947102.

Borra, M.T., Smith, B.C., Denu, J.M., 2005. Mechanism of human SIRT1 activation by resveratrol. J. Biol. Chem. 280 (17), 17187–17195. https://doi.org/10.1074/jbc.M501250200.

Brasacchio, D., Okabe, J., Tikellis, C., Balcerczyk, A., George, P., Baker, E.K., Calkin, A.C., Brownlee, M., Cooper, M.E., El-Osta, A., 2009. Hyperglycemia induces a dynamic cooperativity of histone methylase and demethylase enzymes associated with gene-activating epigenetic marks that coexist on the lysine tail. Diabetes 58 (5), 1229–1236. https://doi.org/10.2337/db08-1666Australia.

Bromer, J.G., Zhou, Y., Taylor, M.B., Doherty, L., Taylor, H.S., 2010. Bisphenol-A exposure in utero leads to epigenetic alterations in the developmental programming of uterine estrogen response. FASEB (Fed. Am. Soc. Exp. Biol.) J. 24 (7), 2273–2280. https://doi.org/10.1096/fj.09-140533.

Calandrelli, R., Xu, L., Luo, Y., Wu, W., Fan, X., Nguyen, T., Chen, C.J., Sriram, K., Tang, X., Burns, A.B., Natarajan, R., Chen, Z.B., Zhong, S., 2020. Stress-induced RNA–chromatin interactions promote endothelial dysfunction. Nat. Commun. 11 (1). https://doi.org/10.1038/s41467-020-18957-w.

Cantó, C., Auwerx, J., 2009. PGC-1α, SIRT1 and AMPK, an energy sensing network that controls energy expenditure. Curr. Opin. Lipidol. 20 (2), 98–105. https://doi.org/10.1097/mol.0b013e328328d0a4.

Carroll, J.E., Irwin, M.R., Levine, M., Seeman, T.E., Absher, D., Assimes, T., Horvath, S., 2017. Epigenetic aging and immune senescence in women with insomnia symptoms: findings from the women's health initiative study. Biol. Psychiatry 81 (2), 136–144. https://doi.org/10.1016/j.biopsych.2016.07.008.

Ceriello, A., Ihnat, M.A., Thorpe, J.E., 2009. The "Metabolic memory": is more than just tight glucose control necessary to prevent diabetic complications? J. Clin. Endocrinol. Metab. 94 (2), 410–415. https://doi.org/10.1210/jc.2008-1824.

Chen, Y., He, Y., Zhou, H., 2020. The potential role of lncRNAs in diabetes and diabetic microvascular complications. Endocr. J. 67 (7), 659–668. https://doi.org/10.1507/endocrj.ej19-0574.

Chen, Z., Miao, F., Braffett, B.H., Lachin, J.M., Zhang, L., Wu, X., Roshandel, D., Carless, M., Li, X.A., Tompkins, J.D., Kaddis, J.S., Riggs, A.D., Paterson, A.D., Braffet, B.H., Chen, Z., Miao, F., Zhang, L., Natarajan, R., Paterson, A.D., Natarajan, R., 2020. DNA methylation mediates development of HbA1c-associated complications in type 1 diabetes. Nat. Metab. 2 (8), 744–762. https://doi.org/10.1038/s42255-020-0231-8.

Cooper, M.E., El-Osta, A., Allen, T.J., Watson, A.M.D., Thomas, M.C., Jandeleit-Dahm, K.A.M., 2018. Metabolic karma-the atherogenic legacy of diabetes: the 2017 edwin bierman award lecture. Diabetes 67 (5), 785–790. https://doi.org/10.2337/dbi18-0010.

Costantino, S., Paneni, F., Lüscher, T.F., Cosentino, F., 2016. MicroRNA profiling unveils hyperglycaemic memory in the diabetic heart. Eur. Heart J. 37 (6), 572–576. https://doi.org/10.1093/eurheartj/ehv599.

Costantino, S., Paneni, F., Mitchell, K., Mohammed, S.A., Hussain, S., Gkolfos, C., Berrino, L., Volpe, M., Schwarzwald, C., Lüscher, T.F., Cosentino, F., 2018. Hyperglycaemia-induced epigenetic changes drive persistent cardiac dysfunction via the adaptor p66 Shc. Int. J. Cardiol. 268, 179–186. https://doi.org/10.1016/j.ijcard.2018.04.082.

Dambal, S., Shah, M., Mihelich, B., Nonn, L., 2015. The microRNA-183 cluster: the family that plays together stays together. Nucleic Acids Res. 43 (15), 7173–7188. https://doi.org/10.1093/nar/gkv703.

de Gonzalo-Calvo, D., Dávalos, A., Montero, A., García-González, Á., Tyshkovska, I., González-Medina, A., Soares, S.M.A., Martínez-Camblor, P., Casas-Agustench, P., Rabadán, M., Díaz-Martínez, Á.E., Úbeda, N., Iglesias-Gutiérrez, E., 2015. Circulating inflammatory miRNA signature in response to different doses of aerobic exercise. J. Appl. Physiol. 119 (2), 124–134. https://doi.org/10.1152/japplphysiol.00077.2015.

De Marinis, Y., Cai, M., Bompada, P., Atac, D., Kotova, O., Johansson, M.E., Garcia-Vaz, E., Gomez, M.F., Laakso, M., Groop, L., 2016. Epigenetic regulation of the thioredoxin-interacting protein (TXNIP) gene by hyperglycemia in kidney. Kidney Int. 89 (2), 342–353. https://doi.org/10.1016/j.kint.2015.12.018.

de Paula, B.M.F., de Souza Pinhel, M.A., Nicoletti, C.F., Nonino, C.B., Siqueira, F., Vannucchi, H., 2022. Folic acid supplementation modulates offspring genes involved in energy metabolism: in vivo study. Clinical Nutrition Open Science 44, 15–27. https://doi.org/10.1016/j.nutos.2022.02.002.

DeFronzo, R.A., Ferrannini, E., Groop, L., Henry, R.R., Herman, W.H., Holst, J.J., Hu, F.B., Kahn, C.R., Raz, I., Shulman, G.I., Simonson, D.C., Testa, M.A., Weiss, R., 2015. Type 2 diabetes mellitus. Nat. Rev. Dis. Primers 1. https://doi.org/10.1038/nrdp.2015.19.

Denham, J., Marques, F.Z., Bruns, E.L., O'Brien, B.J., Charchar, F.J., 2016. Epigenetic changes in leukocytes after 8 weeks of resistance exercise training. Eur. J. Appl. Physiol. 116 (6), 1245–1253. https://doi.org/10.1007/s00421-016-3382-2.

Diao, T., Liu, K., Zhou, L., Wang, Q., Lyu, J., Zhu, Z., Chen, F., Qin, W., Yang, H., Wang, C., Zhang, X., Wu, T., 2025. Sleep patterns and DNA methylation age acceleration in middle-aged and older Chinese adults. Clin. Epigenet. 17 (1). https://doi.org/10.1186/s13148-025-01898-w.

Divyajanani, S., Harithpriya, K., Ganesan, K., Ramkumar, K.M., 2023. Dietary polyphenols remodel DNA methylation patterns of NRF2 in chronic disease. Nutrients 15 (15), 3347. https://doi.org/10.3390/nu15153347.

Donohoe, D.R., Bultman, S.J., 2012. Metaboloepigenetics: Interrelationships between energy metabolism and epigenetic control of gene expression. J. Cell. Physiol. 227 (9), 3169–3177. https://doi.org/10.1002/jcp.24054.

El-Osta, A., Brasacchio, D., Yao, D., Pocai, A., Jones, P.L., Roeder, R.G., Cooper, M.E., Brownlee, M., 2008. Transient high glucose causes persistent epigenetic changes and altered gene expression during subsequent normoglycemia. J. Exp. Med. 205 (10), 2409–2417. https://doi.org/10.1084/jem.20081188Australia.

Fang, H., Xie, J., Zhang, M., Zhao, Z., Wan, Y., Yao, Y., 2017. MiRNA-21 promotes proliferation and invasion of triple-negative breast cancer cells through targeting PTEN. Merican Journal of Translational Research 9 (3), 953–961.

Feng, B., Chen, S., Gordon, A.D., Chakrabarti, S., 2017. miR-146a mediates inflammatory changes and fibrosis in the heart in diabetes. J. Mol. Cellular Cardiol. 105, 70–76. https://doi.org/10.1016/j.yjmcc.2017.03.002.

Fernandez, A.F., Rosales, C., Lopez-Nieva, P., Graña, O., Ballestar, E., Ropero, S., Espada, J., Melo, S.A., Lujambio, A., Fraga, M.F., Pino, I., Javierre, B., Carmona, F.J., Acquadro, F., Steenbergen, R.D.M., Snijders, P.J.F., Meijer, C. J., Pineau, P., Dejean, A., Lloveras, B., Capella, G., Quer, J., Buti, M., Esteban, J.L., Allende, H., Rodriguez-Frias, F., Castellsague, X., Minarovits, J., Ponce, J., Capello, D., Gaidano, G., Cigudosa, J.C., Gomez-Lopez, G., Pisano, D.G., Valencia, A., Piris, M.A., Bosch, F.X., Cahir-McFarland, E., Kieff, E., Esteller, M., 2009. The dynamic DNA methylomes of double-stranded DNA viruses associated with human cancer. Genome Res. 19 (3), 438–451. https://doi.org/10.1101/gr.083550.108Spain.

Francia, P., Cosentino, F., Schiavoni, M., Huang, Y., Perna, E., Camici, G.G., Lüscher, T.F., Volpe, M., 2009. p66Shc protein, oxidative stress, and cardiovascular complications of diabetes: the missing link. J. Mol. Med. 87 (9), 885–891. https://doi.org/10.1007/s00109-009-0499-3.

Guo, Y., Li, J., Liu, X., Ding, H., Zhang, W., 2025. Potential therapeutic targets for ischemic stroke in pre-clinical studies: epigenetic-modifying enzymes DNMT/TET and HAT/HDAC. Front. Pharmacol. 16. https://doi.org/10.3389/fphar.2025.1571276.

Hajri, T., Zaiou, M., Fungwe, T.V., Ouguerram, K., Besong, S., 2021. Epigenetic regulation of peroxisome proliferator-activated receptor gamma mediates high-fat diet-induced non-alcoholic fatty liver disease. Cells 10 (6), 1355.

Hawley, J.A., Hargreaves, M., Joyner, M.J., Zierath, J.R., 2014. Integrative biology of exercise. Cell 159 (4), 738–749. https://doi.org/10.1016/j.cell.2014.10.029.

Heindel, J.J., Vandenberg, L.N., 2015. Developmental origins of health and disease: a paradigm for understanding disease cause and prevention. Curr. Opin. Pediatr. 27 (2), 248–253. https://doi.org/10.1097/MOP.0000000000000191.

Kalisch, R., Müller, M.B., Tüscher, O., 2015. A conceptual framework for the neurobiological study of resilience. Behav. Brain Sci. 38. https://doi.org/10.1017/s0140525x1400082x.

Kaluscha, S., Domcke, S., Wirbelauer, C., Stadler, M.B., Durdu, S., Burger, L., Schübeler, D., 2022. Evidence that direct inhibition of transcription factor binding is the prevailing mode of gene and repeat repression by DNA methylation. Nat. Genet. 54 (12), 1895–1906. https://doi.org/10.1038/s41588-022-01241-6.

Karolina, D.S., Armugam, A., Tavintharan, S., Wong, M.T.K., Lim, S.C., Sum, C. F., Jeyaseelan, K., 2011. MicroRNA 144 impairs insulin signaling by inhibiting the expression of insulin receptor substrate 1 in type 2 diabetes mellitus. PLoS One 6 (8). https://doi.org/10.1371/journal.pone.0022839Singapore.

Kato, M., Zhang, J., Wang, M., Lanting, L., Yuan, H., Rossi, J.J., Natarajan, R., 2007. MicroRNA-192 in diabetic kidney glomeruli and its function in TGF-β-induced collagen expression via inhibition of E-box repressors. Proc. Natl. Acad. Sci. 104 (9), 3432–3437. https://doi.org/10.1073/pnas.0611192104.

Kato, M., Putta, S., Wang, M., Yuan, H., Lanting, L., Nair, I., Gunn, A., Nakagawa, Y., Shimano, H., Todorov, I., Rossi, J.J., Natarajan, R., 2009. TGF-β activates Akt kinase through a microRNA-dependent amplifying circuit targeting PTEN. Nat. Cell Biol. 11 (7), 881–889. https://doi.org/10.1038/ncb1897.

Kato, M., Wang, M., Chen, Z., Bhatt, K., Oh, H.J., Lanting, L., Deshpande, S., Jia, Y., Lai, J.Y.C., O'Connor, C.L., Wu, Y., Hodgin, J.B., Nelson, R.G., Bitzer, M., Natarajan, R., 2016. An endoplasmic reticulum stress-regulated lncRNA hosting a microRNA megacluster induces early features of diabetic nephropathy. Nat. Commun. 7. https://doi.org/10.1038/ncomms12864.

Keating, S.T., El-Osta, A., 2015. Epigenetics and metabolism. Circ. Res. 116 (4), 715–736. https://doi.org/10.1161/CIRCRESAHA.116.303936.

Kong, A.N.T., Owuor, E., Yu, R., Hebbar, V., Chen, C., Hu, R., Mandlekar, S., 2001. Induction of xenobiotic enzymes by the map kinase pathway and the antioxidant or electrophile response element (ARE/EpRE). Drug Metab. Rev. 33 (3–4), 255–271. https://doi.org/10.1081/DMR-120000652.

Kouzarides, T., 2007. Chromatin modifications and their function. Cell 128 (4), 693–705. https://doi.org/10.1016/j.cell.2007.02.005.

Kowluru, R.A., Mohammad, G., 2020. Epigenetics and mitochondrial stability in the metabolic memory phenomenon associated with continued progression of diabetic retinopathy. Sci. Rep. 10 (1). https://doi.org/10.1038/s41598-020-63527-1.

Kowluru, R.A., Shan, Y., Mishra, M., 2016. Dynamic DNA methylation of matrix metalloproteinase-9 in the development of diabetic retinopathy. Lab. Invest. 96 (10), 1040–1049. https://doi.org/10.1038/labinvest.2016.78.

Küpers, L.K., Monnereau, C., Sharp, G.C., Yousefi, P., Salas, L.A., Ghantous, A., Page, C.M., Reese, S.E., Wilcox, A.J., Czamara, D., Starling, A.P., Novoloaca, A., Lent, S., Roy, R., Hoyo, C., Breton, C.V., Allard, C., Just, A.C., Bakulski, K.M., Holloway, J.W., Everson, T.M., Xu, C.J., Huang, R.C., van der Plaat, D.A., Wielscher, M., Merid, S.K., Ullemar, V., Rezwan, F.I., Lahti, J., van Dongen, J., Langie, S.A.S., Richardson, T.G., Magnus, M.C., Nohr, E.A., Xu, Z., Duijts, L., Zhao, S., Zhang, W., Plusquin, M., DeMeo, D.L., Solomon, O., Heimovaara, J.H., Jima, D.D., Gao, L., Bustamante, M., Perron, P., Wright, R.O., Hertz-Picciotto, I., Zhang, H., Karagas, M.R., Gehring, U., Marsit, C.J., Beilin, L.J., Vonk, J.M., Jarvelin, M.R., Bergström, A., Örtqvist, A.K., Ewart, S., Villa, P.M., Moore, S.E., Willemsen, G., Standaert, A.R.L., Håberg, S.E., Sørensen, T.I.A., Taylor, J.A., Räikkönen, K., Yang, I.V., Kechris, K., Nawrot, T.S., Silver, M.J., Gong, Y.Y., Richiardi, L., Kogevinas, M., Litonjua, A.A., Eskenazi, B., Huen, K., Mbarek, H., Maguire, R.L., Dwyer, T., Vrijheid, M., Bouchard, L., Baccarelli, A.A., Croen, L.A., Karmaus, W., Anderson, D., de Vries, M., Sebert, S., Kere, J., Karlsson, R., Arshad, S.H., Hämäläinen, E., Routledge, M. N., Boomsma, D.I., Feinberg, A.P., Newschaffer, C.J., Govarts, E., Moisse, M., Fallin, M.D., Melén, E., Prentice, A.M., Kajantie, E., Almqvist, C., Oken, E., Dabelea, D., Boezen, H.M., Melton, P.E., Wright, R.J., Koppelman, G.H., Trevisi, L., Hivert, M.F., Sunyer, J., Munthe-Kaas, M.C., Murphy, S.K., Corpeleijn, E., Wiemels, J., Holland, N., Herceg, Z., Binder, E.B., Davey Smith, G., Jaddoe, V.W.V., Lie, R.T., Nystad, W., London, S.J., Lawlor, D.A., Relton, C.L., Snieder, H., Felix, J.F., 2019. Meta-analysis of epigenome-wide association studies in neonates reveals widespread differential DNA methylation associated with birthweight. Nat. Commun. 10 (1). https://doi.org/10.1038/s41467-019-09671-3.

La Merrill, M.A., Vandenberg, L.N., Smith, M.T., Goodson, W., Browne, P., Patisaul, H.B., Guyton, K.Z., Kortenkamp, A., Cogliano, V.J., Woodruff, T.J., Rieswijk, L., Sone, H., Korach, K.S., Gore, A.C., Zeise, L., Zoeller, R.T., 2020. Consensus on the key characteristics of endocrine-disrupting chemicals as a basis for hazard identification. Nat. Rev. Endocrinol. 16 (1), 45–57. https://doi.org/10.1038/s41574-019-0273-8.

Laker, R.C., Garde, C., Camera, D.M., Smiles, W.J., Zierath, J.R., Hawley, J.A., Barrès, R., 2017. Transcriptomic and epigenetic responses to short-term nutrient-exercise stress in humans. Sci. Rep. 7 (1). https://doi.org/10.1038/s41598-017-15420-7.

Leung, A., Trac, C., Jin, W., Lanting, L., Akbany, A., Sætrom, P., Schones, D.E., Natarajan, R., 2013. Novel long noncoding RNAs are regulated by angiotensin II in vascular smooth muscle cells. Circ. Res. 113 (3), 266–278. https://doi.org/10.1161/CIRCRESAHA.112.300849.

Li, M., Guo, Y., Wang, X.J., Duan, B.H., Li, L., 2018. HOTAIR participates in hepatic insulin resistance via regulating SIRT1. Eur. Rev. Med. Pharmacol. Sci. 22 (22), 7883–7890. https://doi.org/10.26355/eurrev-201811-16414.

Ling, C., Rönn, T., 2014. Epigenetic adaptation to regular exercise in humans. Drug Discov. Today 19 (7), 1015–1018. https://doi.org/10.1016/j.drudis.2014.03.006.

Ling, C., Del Guerra, S., Lupi, R., Rönn, T., Granhall, C., Luthman, H., Masiello, P., Marchetti, P., Groop, L., Del Prato, S., 2008. Epigenetic regulation of PPARGC1A in human type 2 diabetic islets and effect on insulin secretion. Diabetologia 51 (4), 615–622. https://doi.org/10.1007/s00125-007-0916-5.

Lizotte, F., Denhez, B., Guay, A., Gévry, N., Côté, A.M., Geraldes, P., 2016. Persistent insulin resistance in podocytes caused by epigenetic changes of SHP-1 in Diabetes. Diabetes 65 (12), 3705–3717. https://doi.org/10.2337/db16-0254.

Ma, Y., Xia, W., Wang, D.Q., Wan, Y.J., Xu, B., Chen, X., Li, Y.Y., Xu, S.Q., 2013. Hepatic DNA methylation modifications in early development of rats resulting from perinatal BPA exposure contribute to insulin resistance in adulthood. Diabetologia 56 (9), 2059–2067. https://doi.org/10.1007/s00125-013-2944-7.

Marumo, T., Yagi, S., Kawarazaki, W., Nishimoto, M., Ayuzawa, N., Watanabe, A., Ueda, K., Hirahashi, J., Hishikawa, K., Sakurai, H., Shiota, K., Fujita, T., 2015. Diabetes induces aberrant DNA methylation in the proximal tubules of the kidney. J. Am. Soc. Nephrol. 26 (10), 2388–2397. https://doi.org/10.1681/asn.2014070665.

Matai, L., Slack, F.J., 2023. MicroRNAs in age-related proteostasis and stress responses. Non-coding RNA 9 (2). https://doi.org/10.3390/ncrna9020026.

McGee, S.L., Hargreaves, M., 2011. Histone modifications and exercise adaptations. J. Appl. Physiol. 110 (1), 258–263. https://doi.org/10.1152/japplphysiol.00979.2010.

Miao, F., Chen, Z., Genuth, S., Paterson, A., Zhang, L., Wu, X., Li, S.M., Cleary, P., Riggs, A., Harlan, D.M., Lorenzi, G., Kolterman, O., Sun, W., Lachin, J.M., Natarajan, R., 2014. Evaluating the role of epigenetic histone modifications in the metabolic memory of type 1 diabetes. Diabetes 63 (5), 1748–1762. https://doi.org/10.2337/db13-1251.

Milagro, F.I., Mansego, M.L., De Miguel, C., Martínez, J.A., 2013. Dietary factors, epigenetic modifications and obesity outcomes: progresses and perspectives. Mol. Aspect. Med. 34 (4), 782–812. https://doi.org/10.1016/j.mam.2012.06.010.

Mishra, M., Kowluru, R.A., 2015. Epigenetic modification of mitochondrial DNA in the development of diabetic retinopathy. Investig. Ophthalmol. Vis. Sci. 56 (9), 5133–5142. https://doi.org/10.1167/iovs.15-16937.

Mishra, M., Kowluru, R.A., 2016. The role of DNA methylation in the metabolic memory phenomenon associated with the continued progression of diabetic retinopathy. Investig. Ophthalmol. Vis. Sci. 57 (13), 5748–5757. https://doi.org/10.1167/iovs.16-19759.

Mishra, M., Kowluru, R.A., 2019. DNA methylation—a potential source of mitochondria DNA base mismatch in the development of diabetic retinopathy. Mol. Neurobiol. 56 (1), 88–101. https://doi.org/10.1007/s12035-018-1086-9.

Mishra, M., Zhong, Q., Kowluru, R.A., 2014. Epigenetic modifications of Nrf2-mediated glutamate-cysteine ligase: implications for the development of diabetic retinopathy and the metabolic memory phenomenon associated with its continued progression. Free Radic. Biol. Med. 75, 129–139. https://doi.org/10.1016/j.freeradbiomed.2014.07.001.

Mitro, N., Verdeguer, F., Perissi, V., 2024. Epigenetics and metabolism. Front. Endocrinol. 15, 1373368.

Mongroo, P.S., Rustgi, A.K., 2014. The role of the miR-200 family in epithelial-mesenchymal transition. Cancer Biol. Ther. 10 (3), 219–222. https://doi.org/10.4161/cbt.10.3.12548.

Myers, R.B., Fomovsky, G.M., Lee, S., Tan, M., Wang, B.F., Patwari, P., Yoshioka, J., 2016. Deletion of thioredoxin-interacting protein improves cardiac inotropic reserve in the streptozotocin-induced diabetic heart. Am. J. Physiol. Heart Circ. Physiol. 310 (11), H1748. https://doi.org/10.1152/ajpheart.00051.2016.

Natarajan, R., Putta, S., Kato, M., 2012. MicroRNAs and diabetic complications. J. Cardiovasc. Transl. Res. 5 (4), 413–422. https://doi.org/10.1007/s12265-012-9368-5.

Ngo, V., Duennwald, M.L., 2022. Nrf2 and oxidative stress: a general overview of mechanisms and implications in human disease. Antioxidants 11 (12), 2345. https://doi.org/10.3390/antiox11122345.

Nitert, M.D., Dayeh, T., Volkov, P., Elgzyri, T., Hall, E., Nilsson, E., Yang, B.T., Lang, S., Parikh, H., Wessman, Y., Weishaupt, H., Attema, J., Abels, M., Wierup, N., Almgren, P., Jansson, P.A., Rönn, T., Hansson, O., Eriksson, K.F., Groop, L., Ling, C., 2012. Impact of an exercise intervention on DNA methylation in skeletal muscle from first-degree relatives of patients with type 2 diabetes. Diabetes 61 (12), 3322–3332. https://doi.org/10.2337/db11-1653Sweden.

Okabe, J., Orlowski, C., Balcerczyk, A., Tikellis, C., Thomas, M.C., Cooper, M.E., El-Osta, A., 2012. Distinguishing hyperglycemic changes by Set7 in vascular endothelial cells. Circ. Res. 110 (8), 1067–1076. https://doi.org/10.1161/CIRCRESAHA.112.266171.

Olsen, A.S., Sarras, M.P., Leontovich, A., Intine, R.V., 2012. Heritable transmission of diabetic metabolic memory in zebrafish correlates with DNA hypomethylation and aberrant gene expression. Diabetes 61 (2), 485–491. https://doi.org/10.2337/db11-0588.

Paneni, F., Mocharla, P., Akhmedov, A., Costantino, S., Osto, E., Volpe, M., Lüscher, T.F., Cosentino, F., 2012. Gene silencing of the mitochondrial adaptor p66Shc suppresses vascular hyperglycemic memory in diabetes. Circ. Res. 111 (3), 278–289. https://doi.org/10.1161/CIRCRESAHA.112.266593.

Park, L.K., Maione, A.G., Smith, A., Gerami-Naini, B., Iyer, L.K., Mooney, D.J., Veves, A., Garlick, J.A., 2014. Genome-wide DNA methylation analysis identifies a metabolic memory profile in patient-derived diabetic foot ulcer fibroblasts. Epigenetics 9 (10), 1339–1349. https://doi.org/10.4161/15592294.2014.967584.

Perrone, L., Devi, T.S., Hosoya, K.I., Terasaki, T., Singh, L.P., 2009. Thioredoxin interacting protein (TXNIP) induces inflammation through chromatin modification in retinal capillary endothelial cells under diabetic conditions. J. Cell. Physiol. 221 (1), 262–272. https://doi.org/10.1002/jcp.21852.

Pirola, L., Balcerczyk, A., Okabe, J., El-Osta, A., 2010. Epigenetic phenomena linked to diabetic complications. Nat. Rev. Endocrinol. 6 (12), 665–675. https://doi.org/10.1038/nrendo.2010.188.

Pirola, L., Balcerczyk, A., Tothill, R.W., Haviv, I., Kaspi, A., Lunke, S., Ziemann, M., Karagiannis, T., Tonna, S., Kowalczyk, A., Beresford-Smith, B., Macintyre, G., Kelong, M., Hongyu, Z., Zhu, J., El-Osta, A., 2011. Genome-wide analysis distinguishes hyperglycemia regulated epigenetic signatures of primary vascular cells. Genome Res. 21 (10), 1601–1615. https://doi.org/10.1101/gr.116095.110.

Puthanveetil, P., Chen, S., Feng, B., Gautam, A., Chakrabarti, S., 2015. Long non-coding RNA MALAT 1 regulates hyperglycaemia induced inflammatory process in the endothelial cells. J. Cell Mol. Med. 19 (6), 1418–1425. https://doi.org/10.1111/jcmm.12576.

Radom-Aizik, S., Zaldivar, F., Leu, S.Y., Adams, G.R., Oliver, S., Cooper, D.M., 2012. Effects of exercise on microRNA expression in young males peripheral blood mononuclear cells. Clin. Transl. Sci. 5 (1), 32–38. https://doi.org/10.1111/j.1752-8062.2011.00384.x.

Rancière, F., Lyons, J.G., Loh, V.H.Y., Botton, J., Galloway, T., Wang, T., Shaw, J. E., Magliano, D.J., 2015. Bisphenol A and the risk of cardiometabolic disorders: a systematic review with meta-analysis of the epidemiological evidence. Environ. Health 14 (1). https://doi.org/10.1186/s12940-015-0036-5.

Reddy, M.A., Zhang, E., Natarajan, R., 2015. Epigenetic mechanisms in diabetic complications and metabolic memory. Diabetologia 58 (3), 443–455. https://doi.org/10.1007/s00125-014-3462-y.

Reichard, J.F., Puga, A., 2010. Effects of arsenic exposure on DNA methylation and epigenetic gene regulation. Epigenomics 2 (1), 87–104. https://doi.org/10.2217/epi.09.45.

Saad, L., Zwiller, J., Kalsbeek, A., Anglard, P., 2021. Epigenetic regulation of circadian clocks and its involvement in drug addiction. Genes 12 (8), 1263. https://doi.org/10.3390/genes12081263.

Sasaki, A., de Vega, W.C., St-Cyr, S., Pan, P., McGowan, P.O., 2013. Perinatal high fat diet alters glucocorticoid signaling and anxiety behavior in adulthood. Neuroscience 240, 1–12. https://doi.org/10.1016/j.neuroscience.2013.02.044.

Sertorio, M.N., de Souza, E.A., Pisani, L.P., 2021. Update on the influence of fatty acids in epigenetic programming mechanisms. Nutrire 46 (2). https://doi.org/10.1186/s41110-021-00142-8.

Shah, A., Xia, L., Masson, E.A.Y., Gui, C., Momen, A., Shikatani, E.A., Husain, M., Quaggin, S., John, R., Fantus, I.G., 2015. Thioredoxin-interacting protein deficiency protects against diabetic nephropathy. J. Am. Soc. Nephrol. 26 (12), 2963–2977. https://doi.org/10.1681/ASN.2014050528.

Sharma, S., Fulton, S., 2013. Diet-induced obesity promotes depressive-like behaviour that is associated with neural adaptations in brain reward circuitry. Int. J. Obes. 37 (3), 382–389. https://doi.org/10.1038/ijo.2012.48.

Silva, G.J.J., Bye, A., el Azzouzi, H., Wisløff, U., 2017. MicroRNAs as important regulators of exercise adaptation. Prog. Cardiovasc. Dis. 60 (1), 130–151. https://doi.org/10.1016/j.pcad.2017.06.003.

Singh, L.P., 2013. Thioredoxin interacting protein (TXNIP) and pathogenesis of diabetic retinopathy. J. Clin. Exp. Ophthalmol. 04 (04). https://doi.org/10.4172/2155-9570.1000287.

Sinha, M., Ghatak, S., Roy, S., Sen, C.K., 2015. microRNA-200b as a switch for inducible adult angiogenesis. Antioxidants Redox Signal. 22 (14), 1257–1272. https://doi.org/10.1089/ars.2014.6065.

Skinner, M.K., 2014. Environmental stress and epigenetic transgenerational inheritance. BMC Med. 12 (1). https://doi.org/10.1186/s12916-014-0153-y.

Smith, J., Chatterjee, A., Rodger, E.J., 2025. Clinical epigenetics: recent advances and opportunities. Epigenetics Communications 5 (1). https://doi.org/10.1186/s43682-025-00038-y.

Stols-Gonçalves, D., Tristão, L.S., Henneman, P., Nieuwdorp, M., 2019. Epigenetic markers and microbiota/metabolite-induced epigenetic modifications in the pathogenesis of obesity, metabolic syndrome, type 2 diabetes, and non-alcoholic fatty liver disease. Curr. Diabetes Rep. 19 (6). https://doi.org/10.1007/s11892-019-1151-4.

Takizawa, F., Mizutani, S., Ogawa, Y., Sawada, N., 2013. Glucose-independent persistence of PAI-1 gene expression and H3K4 tri-methylation in type 1 diabetic mouse endothelium: Implication in metabolic memory. Biochem.

Biophys. Res. Commun. 433 (1), 66–72. https://doi.org/10.1016/j.bbrc.2013.02.064.

Tanwar, V.S., Reddy, M.A., Natarajan, R., 2021. Emerging role of long non-coding RNAs in diabetic vascular complications. Front. Endocrinol. 12. https://doi.org/10.3389/fendo.2021.665811.

Tellez-Plaza, M., Guallar, E., Navas-Acien, A., 2018. Environmental metals and cardiovascular disease. Br. Med. J. 362, k3435. https://doi.org/10.1136/bmj.k3435.

Triolo, M., Oliveira, A.N., Kumari, R., Hood, D.A., 2022. The influence of age, sex, and exercise on autophagy, mitophagy, and lysosome biogenesis in skeletal muscle. Skeletal Muscle 12 (1). https://doi.org/10.1186/s13395-022-00296-7.

Villeneuve, L.M., Reddy, M.A., Lanting, L.L., Wang, M., Meng, L., Natarajan, R., 2008. Epigenetic histone H3 lysine 9 methylation in metabolic memory and inflammatory phenotype of vascular smooth muscle cells in diabetes. Proc. Natl. Acad. Sci. U. S. A 105 (26), 9047–9052. https://doi.org/10.1073/pnas.0803623105.

Villeneuve, L.M., Kato, M., Reddy, M.A., Wang, M., Lanting, L., Natarajan, R., 2010. Enhanced levels of microRNA-125b in vascular smooth muscle cells of diabetic db/db mice lead to increased inflammatory gene expression by targeting the histone methyltransferase Suv39h1. Diabetes 59 (11), 2904–2915. https://doi.org/10.2337/db10-0208.

Wang, S., Zhang, X., Wang, Q., Wang, R., 2022. Histone modification in podocyte injury of diabetic nephropathy. J. Mol. Med. 100 (10), 1373–1386. https://doi.org/10.1007/s00109-022-02247-7.

Wang, Y., Zhu, J., Chen, J., Xu, R., Groth, T., Wan, H., Zhou, G., 2022. The signaling pathways induced by exosomes in promoting diabetic wound healing: a mini-review. Curr. Issues Mol. Biol. 44 (10), 4960–4976. https://doi.org/10.3390/cimb44100337.

Yang, S., Yao, H., Li, M., Li, H., Wang, F., Li, T., 2016. Long non-coding RNA MALAT1 mediates transforming growth factor beta1-induced epithelial-mesenchymal transition of retinal pigment epithelial cells. PLoS One 11 (3), e0152687. https://doi.org/10.1371/journal.pone.0152687.

Yao, Y., Song, Q., Hu, C., Da, X., Yu, Y., He, Z., Xu, C., Chen, Q., Wang, Q.K., 2022. Endothelial cell metabolic memory causes cardiovascular dysfunction in diabetes. Cardiovasc. Res. 118 (1), 196–211. https://doi.org/10.1093/cvr/cvab013.

Yu, X.Y., Geng, Y.J., Liang, J.L., Zhang, S., Lei, H.P., Zhong, S.L., Lin, Q.X., Shan, Z.X., Lin, S.G., Li, Y., 2012. High levels of glucose induce "metabolic memory" in cardiomyocyte via epigenetic histone H3 lysine 9 methylation. Mol. Biol. Rep. 39 (9), 8891–8898. https://doi.org/10.1007/s11033-012-1756-z.

Zannas, A.S., West, A.E., 2014. Epigenetics and the regulation of stress vulnerability and resilience. Neuroscience 264, 157–170. https://doi.org/10.1016/j.neuroscience.2013.12.003.

Zannas, A.S., Wiechmann, T., Gassen, N.C., Binder, E.B., 2016. Gene-stress-epigenetic regulation of FKBP5: clinical and translational implications. Neuropsychopharmacology 41 (1), 261–274. https://doi.org/10.1038/npp.2015.235.

Zhang, Q., Lenardo, M.J., Baltimore, D., 2017. 30 Years of NF-κB: a blossoming of relevance to human pathobiology. Cell 168 (1–2), 37–57. https://doi.org/10.1016/j.cell.2016.12.012.

Zhang, X., Song, Z., Yuan, Q., Lin, Z., Fan, L., Wang, H., Kong, D., Jun, H., 2021. TXNIP, a novel key factor to cause Schwann cell dysfunction in diabetic peripheral neuropathy, under the regulation of PI3K/Akt pathway inhibition-induced DNMT1 and DNMT3a overexpression. Cell Death Dis. 12 (7). https://doi.org/10.1038/s41419-021-03930-2.

Zhao, S., Li, T., Li, J., Lu, Q., Han, C., Wang, N., Qiu, Q., Cao, H., Xu, X., Chen, H., Zheng, Z., 2016. miR-23b-3p induces the cellular metabolic memory of high glucose in diabetic retinopathy through a SIRT1-dependent signalling pathway. Diabetologia 59 (3), 644–654. https://doi.org/10.1007/s00125-015-3832-0.

Zhong, Q., Kowluru, R.A., 2010. Role of histone acetylation in the development of diabetic retinopathy and the metabolic memory phenomenon. J. Cell. Biochem. 110 (6), 1306–1313. https://doi.org/10.1002/jcb.22644.

Zhong, Q., Kowluru, R.A., 2013. Epigenetic modification of Sod2 in the development of diabetic retinopathy and in the metabolic memory: role of histone methylation. Investig. Ophthalmol. Vis. Sci. 54 (1), 244–250. https://doi.org/10.1167/iovs.12-10854.

Zhong, X., Chung, A.C.K., Chen, H.Y., Meng, X.M., Lan, H.Y., 2011. Smad3-mediated upregulation of miR-21 promotes renal fibrosis. J. Am. Soc. Nephrol. 22 (9), 1668–1681. https://doi.org/10.1681/ASN.2010111168.

Zhong, X., Liao, Y., Chen, L., Liu, G., Feng, Y., Zeng, T., Zhang, J., 2015. The MicroRNAs in the pathogenesis of metabolic memory. Endocrinology 156 (9), 3157–3168. https://doi.org/10.1210/en.2015-1063.

Zhou, S., Chen, H.Z., Wan, Y.Z., Zhang, Q.J., Wei, Y.S., Huang, S., Liu, J.J., Lu, Y.B., Zhang, Z.Q., Yang, R.F., Zhang, R., Cai, H., Liu, D.P., Liang, C.C., 2011. Repression of P66Shc expression by SIRT1 contributes to the prevention of hyperglycemia-induced endothelial dysfunction. Circ. Res. 109 (6), 639–648. https://doi.org/10.1161/CIRCRESAHA.111.243592.

Zhou, Y., Zheng, J., Li, Y., Xu, D.P., Li, S., Chen, Y.M., Li, H.B., 2016. Natural polyphenols for prevention and treatment of cancer. Nutrients 8 (8). https://doi.org/10.3390/nu8080515.

7

Cardiovascular health and metabolic memory

1. Introduction

Cardiovascular disease (CVD) remains the foremost cause of morbidity and mortality among individuals with diabetes mellitus, posing a significant challenge to healthcare worldwide. The concept of diabetic cardiomyopathy was first proposed in 1974 by Robert I. Hamby and defined as myocardial structural and functional abnormalities in individuals with diabetes, occurring in the absence of hypertension, coronary artery disease, valvular disease, or other traditional cardiovascular risk factors (Hamby et al., 1974). Later studies showed that diabetic cardiomyopathy initially presents with diastolic dysfunction and vascular or microvascular impairment, progresses to systolic dysfunction, and ultimately leads to clinical heart failure. Advanced pathological features include cardiac hypertrophy, interstitial fibrosis, thickening of capillary basement membranes, capillary microangioma, and reduced capillary density (Lee and Kim, 2021). Accordingly, diabetic cardiomyopathy has classically been defined as myocardial abnormalities in patients with diabetes without coronary artery disease or hypertension (Aneja et al., 2008).

However, this strict definition has limitations, as similar myocardial abnormalities are also observed in patients with diabetes who have coexisting coronary artery disease with or without hypertension, although isolating the specific contribution of diabetes in such cases remains challenging (Miki et al., 2013). Because excluding other cardiovascular diseases in clinical practice is often unrealistic, recent definitions propose that diabetic cardiomyopathy should be described as cardiac abnormalities not fully explained by other cardiovascular or non-cardiovascular causes and likely attributable to diabetes (Li et al., 2020; Lee et al., 2019a, 2019b).

Although the precise mechanisms underlying diabetic cardiomyopathy are not fully understood, several contributory

Metabolic Memory. https://doi.org/10.1016/B978-0-443-44591-0.00007-2

processes have been proposed, including impaired mitochondrial respiration and pyruvate dehydrogenase activity, excessive reactive oxygen species generation, and dysfunction of cardiac contractile proteins and intracellular Ca^{2+} handling (Ren and Ceylan-Isik, 2004). Notably, diabetes appears to abolish the typical cardiovascular protection observed in women, with female patients exhibiting more severe myocardial electromechanical impairment and neuroregulatory dysfunction than age-matched men (Ren and Ceylan-Isik, 2004). The prevalence of diabetic cardiomyopathy continues to rise with the global increase in diabetes, yet no targeted therapies are currently available, highlighting the need for new treatment strategies (Bi et al., 2020).

Chronic hyperglycemia is considered a major driver of diabetic cardiomyopathy, acting through activation of multiple signaling pathways, including PKC, MAPK, NF-κB, SGLT2, O-GlcNAc, CREM signaling, and the renin-angiotensin-aldosterone system, ultimately promoting cardiac remodeling, cardiomyocyte apoptosis, and inflammation (Yang et al., 2015). Consequently, glycemic control has been regarded as a cornerstone in preventing diabetic complications (Afroz et al., 2019; Stettler et al., 2006). However, large clinical trials and meta-analyses, including ACCORD, ADVANCE, VADT, and UKPDS, have demonstrated that intensive glycemic control does not significantly reduce myocardial infarction or heart failure risk in patients with diabetes (Gilbert and Krum, 2015). These findings suggest that cardiovascular damage persists despite glucose normalization, a phenomenon known as hyperglycemic memory (Zakir et al., 2023). This paradox has driven growing interest in the concept of metabolic memory, the phenomenon whereby early exposure to hyperglycemia leaves a durable, deleterious imprint on vascular tissues, influencing cardiovascular outcomes long after glycemic normalization (Yao et al., 2022).

Originally identified in the context of microvascular complications, metabolic memory is now recognized as a fundamental mechanism underpinning diabetic macrovascular disease (Aschner and Ruiz, 2012). It encompasses a constellation of biochemical, molecular, and epigenetic alterations that sustain endothelial dysfunction, inflammation, and vascular remodeling, thereby accelerating atherogenesis and plaque instability. Importantly, emerging research highlights that metabolic memory is not solely driven by hyperglycemia; lipid abnormalities, including diabetic dyslipidaemia and cholesterol-driven epigenetic reprogramming, play a pivotal and often underappreciated role in perpetuating vascular injury (Tian et al., 2023).

This chapter explores the complex interplay between metabolic memory and cardiovascular health in diabetes. It examines the mechanistic pathways linking early metabolic insults to persistent vascular damage and clinical cardiovascular events, emphasizing the roles of oxidative stress, inflammation, endothelial dysfunction, and lipid-mediated toxicity. Understanding these processes is crucial for developing early and multifaceted therapeutic strategies aimed at preventing the long-term cardiovascular burden in diabetic populations. Through this lens, the chapter underscores the imperative for integrated glucose and lipid management to mitigate the cardiovascular risks imposed by metabolic memory.

2. Metabolic memory and cardiovascular disease: An overview

Metabolic memory refers to the phenomenon in which the adverse effects of early hyperglycemia continue to influence disease progression long after blood glucose levels have been normalized. Originally demonstrated in the context of microvascular complications such as retinopathy and nephropathy, this concept has since been extended to macrovascular diseases, including coronary artery disease and stroke, the primary causes of mortality in individuals with diabetes (Luna et al., 2016).

Seminal clinical trials have underscored the long-term cardiovascular implications of metabolic memory. In the Diabetes Control and Complications Trial (DCCT) and its follow-up, the Epidemiology of Diabetes Interventions and Complications (EDIC) study, patients with type 1 diabetes who received intensive insulin therapy (achieving a mean HbA1c of ~7%) experienced a substantial reduction in cardiovascular events, such as myocardial infarction, stroke, and cardiovascular death, many years after the trial ended, even when their glycemic levels later matched those of the conventionally treated group (Nathan, 2021). Similarly, the UK Prospective Diabetes Study (UKPDS) demonstrated that in patients with newly diagnosed type 2 diabetes, intensive glucose control not only reduced microvascular complications but also conferred a legacy benefit in terms of reduced myocardial infarction risk and all-cause mortality over long-term follow-up (Marso et al., 2010).

The enduring cardiovascular benefits observed in these studies suggest that early glycemic environment induces permanent or semi-permanent biological changes in vascular tissues. Mechanistically, chronic hyperglycemia leads to oxidative stress, mitochondrial dysfunction, and the formation of advanced glycation end-products (AGEs), which interact with their receptors (RAGE) to initiate and perpetuate inflammatory signaling pathways (Shen et al., 2020). These processes cause endothelial cell activation, smooth muscle cell proliferation, and alterations in vascular extracellular matrix, promoting atherogenesis and arterial stiffening. Moreover, hyperglycemia triggers epigenetic modifications, including DNA methylation and histone acetylation, that maintain a pro-inflammatory gene expression profile even in the absence of continuing hyperglycemia (Morey et al., 2019).

Importantly, these vascular changes are not easily reversible and contribute to a heightened cardiovascular risk profile that persists despite subsequent glycemic normalization. Endothelial dysfunction, marked by impaired nitric oxide (NO) production and increased vascular permeability, becomes a sustained state (Cyr et al., 2020). This is often accompanied by increased expression of adhesion molecules (e.g., ICAM-1, VCAM-1), which facilitate leukocyte infiltration and perpetuate atherosclerotic plaque development (Habas and Shang, 2018). In addition, metabolic memory has been linked to vascular smooth muscle cell senescence and macrophage dysfunction, further driving plaque instability and thrombogenesis (Uryga and Bennett, 2016).

Clinically, these insights highlight the critical need for early and aggressive intervention in diabetes management, not just to control blood sugar but also to prevent the long-term imprinting of deleterious vascular changes. The concept of metabolic memory thus represents a paradigm shift in our understanding of diabetic cardiovascular disease: it is not only current metabolic status that matters, but also the quality of metabolic control achieved during the early stages of the disease.

3. Advanced glycation end products in hyperglycemic memory and diabetic cardiomyopathy

Advanced glycation end products (AGEs) are formed by nonenzymatic reactions between sugars or their metabolites and proteins, nucleic acids, or lipids, followed by further chemical modifications. Accumulation of AGEs and increased RAGE expression promote diabetic cardiomyopathy, while inhibition of AGE formation improves cardiac function (Ma et al., 2009). AGEs alter extracellular matrix proteins such as collagen and laminin, disrupting basement membrane structure and reducing cardiac compliance, leading to diastolic dysfunction (Brownlee, 1992). AGEs also activate RAGE-dependent signaling, inducing inflammation, oxidative stress, autophagy, and apoptosis, which drive cardiac remodeling and dysfunction (Brownlee, 1992).

In fibroblasts, AGE–RAGE signaling increases TGF-β expression, fibroblast proliferation, and extracellular matrix synthesis, contributing to myocardial fibrosis (Oldfield et al., 2001). In macrophages, AGEs increase RAGE expression, promote M1 polarization, and enhance proinflammatory cytokine production, which further activates fibroblasts (Jin et al., 2015). AGEs reduce endothelial nitric oxide availability and impair endothelium-dependent vasodilation, while AGE inhibition restores vascular function. AGEs also induce VCAM-1 expression in endothelial cells, enhancing monocyte adhesion and promoting atherogenesis (Schmidt et al., 1995).

In cardiomyocytes, AGEs impair RyR2 regulation, increase intracellular Ca^{2+}, reduce mitochondrial membrane potential, and induce apoptosis, leading to cardiac dysfunction (Wang et al., 2019a, 2019b). Glycation of RyR2 and SERCA2a disrupts sarcoplasmic reticulum Ca^{2+} handling in diabetic hearts (Hamilton and Terentyev, 2019). AGEs activate PKC in an ROS-dependent manner, causing mitochondrial dysfunction and cardiomyocyte death (Yang et al., 2018). AGE modified LDL shows reduced clearance, contributing to dyslipidemia, endothelial dysfunction, and atherosclerosis, and enhances platelet aggregation and cholesterol esterification in monocytes, promoting thrombosis and vascular injury (Zoltowska et al., 2001).

The late stages of AGE formation are largely irreversible, and AGE-modified proteins such as collagen and fibrinogen become stiff and resistant to degradation (Onursal et al., 2021). Thus, persistent AGE accumulation after glucose normalization may partly explain hyperglycemic memory, highlighting the need for strategies to enhance AGE turnover and restore normal cellular function.

4. Persistent MicroRNA dysregulation in diabetic heart

MicroRNAs (miRNAs) play key roles in cardiovascular diseases by regulating fibrosis, hypertrophy, mitochondrial dynamics, apoptosis, lipid accumulation, and oxidative stress (Zhong et al., 2015). Several studies show that miRNAs also contribute to hyperglycemic memory (HGM). Zhong et al. identified miR-125b, miR-29a-3p, and miR-146a-5p as persistently altered in diabetic rat aortas despite insulin treatment. miR-125b regulates TNFAIP3, while miR-146a-5p targets TRAF6 and IRAK1 in human aortic endothelial cells, and these changes persist after transient hyperglycemia but can be reversed by modulating these miRNAs (Zhong et al., 2015).

Transient high glucose during adipogenesis can cause lasting miRNA changes in mature adipocytes, similar to chronic hyperglycemia (Strycharz et al., 2018). In retinal pigment epithelial cells, high glucose induces sustained upregulation of miR-204 and downregulation of SIRT1, promoting ER stress and apoptosis even after glucose normalization (Peng et al., 2020). In diabetic mouse hearts, 316 miRNAs are dysregulated, and 268 of these remain altered after restoring normoglycemia. These persistent miRNAs regulate pathways involved in apoptosis, fibrosis, hypertrophy, autophagy, oxidative stress, and heart failure (Costantino et al., 2016), indicating that glycemic control alone cannot fully reverse miRNA alterations in diabetes.

JunD, a protective transcription factor against oxidative stress, is epigenetically silenced by promoter hypermethylation and translational repression via miR-673 in diabetic hearts, highlighting combined regulation by miRNAs and epigenetic mechanisms in diabetic cardiomyopathy (Hussain et al., 2020). Our previous study showed that miR-320 is upregulated in diabetic hearts and enhances CD36 transcription by promoting the interaction of Ago2 with RNA polymerase II, leading to increased fatty acid uptake, lipid accumulation, apoptosis, and cardiac dysfunction. This mechanism represents a novel nuclear function of miR-320 in activating transcription via a RITA complex with Ago2. Notably, miR-320 remains persistently dysregulated after transient hyperglycemia, suggesting that miRNA-driven lipotoxicity contributes to hyperglycemic memory in diabetic cardiomyopathy (Tong and Sadoshima, 2019).

5. Mitochondrial oxidative stress in diabetic cardiomyopathy

Excess production of superoxide by the mitochondrial electron transport chain, which is converted into other reactive oxygen species (ROS), is a key mechanism in diabetic cardiovascular complications (Wang et al., 2021). In diabetes, glucose oxidation is reduced due to impaired glucose uptake and mitochondrial metabolism in cardiomyocytes (Wende et al., 2020). As a result, the heart relies mainly on fatty acid (FA) oxidation for energy. This increases β-oxidation of fatty acyl-CoA in mitochondria, leading to accumulation of acyl-CoA (Maack et al., 2018). Because the TCA cycle cannot fully oxidize this excess substrate, toxic intermediates and ROS are generated (Jubaidi et al., 2020).

Increased FA oxidation raises the supply of NADH and FADH2 to the electron transport chain, increasing the mitochondrial membrane potential. When this reaches a critical level, electron flow at complex III is blocked and electrons leak back to coenzyme Q, which transfers them to oxygen to form superoxide (Trumpower, 1990). Superoxide is the first ROS formed in mitochondria and is later converted to other ROS (Wallace, 1992). Mitochondria are required for hyperglycemia-induced superoxide generation, which then activates other ROS-producing pathways, including NADPH oxidases and uncoupled eNOS, amplifying oxidative damage (Giacco et al., 2010). Mitochondrial superoxide overproduction is considered a common upstream event linking aldose reductase activation, PKC signaling, hexosamine pathway flux, AGE formation, and RAGE signaling in hyperglycemia-induced injury (Giacco et al., 2010).

Mitochondrial oxidative stress can persist even after glucose normalization, contributing to hyperglycemic memory (HGM). Ihnat et al. showed that oxidative stress markers such as BAX, p47phox, and 3-nitrotyrosine remain elevated for 1 week after glucose normalization in endothelial and retinal cells, and this can be reduced by blocking reactive species (Ihnat et al., 2007). Among the Shc adaptor proteins, only p66Shc promotes mitochondrial ROS generation (Cosentino et al., 2008). Loss of p66Shc reduces intracellular oxidants and increases resistance to oxidative stress, and p66Shc knockout mice are protected from diabetes-induced vascular and cardiac injury (Rota et al., 2006). Activation of p66Shc persists in diabetic aortas and high glucose–treated endothelial cells even after normoglycemia is restored, due to a positive feedback loop between PKC and p66Shc (Paneni et al., 2012). Persistent p66Shc activation increases ROS, reduces nitric oxide (NO), and induces apoptosis, driving HGM-related cardiovascular damage. Silencing p66Shc reduces ROS, improves endothelial function, and prevents apoptosis in diabetic models (Paneni et al., 2013).

A vicious cycle between transglutaminase two activation and ROS production has also been reported in the aortic endothelium after transient hyperglycemia, which can be disrupted by transglutaminase inhibitors or the antioxidant N-acetylcysteine (Lee et al., 2019a, 2019b). NADPH oxidase is highly activated in cardiomyocytes of diabetic rats, causing ROS overproduction and apoptosis (Isabelle et al., 2007). Mitochondrial ROS in diabetic hearts is also regulated by miRNAs such as miR-92a-2-5p and let-7b-5p, which control mt-Cytb expression; restoring these miRNAs reduces mitochondrial ROS (Li et al., 2019). The let-7 family is also linked to hyperglycemic memory. ROS can regulate miRNA expression, with miR-210 Ind.uced by ROS (Kim, 2019), while miR-199a and miR-125b are suppressed by ROS via promoter hypermethylation (He et al., 2012). This suggests a self-perpetuating cycle between mitochondrial ROS and miRNAs that sustains HGM in diabetic cardiomyopathy.

Mitochondrial DNA (mtDNA) is highly vulnerable to oxidative damage because it is located close to the electron transport chain and lacks efficient DNA repair mechanisms (West and Shadel, 2017). Since mtDNA encodes essential subunits of oxidative phosphorylation complexes, persistent mtDNA damage caused by hyperglycemia-induced ROS can further increase ROS production, reinforcing long-term mitochondrial dysfunction and contributing to sustained diabetic cardiomyopathy.

6. DNA methylation in hyperglycemic memory (HGM) and diabetic cardiomyopathy

DNA methylation is a central epigenetic mechanism contributing to hyperglycemic memory (HGM) in diabetic cardiomyopathy (Cencioni et al., 2014). Hypomethylation of CpG sites within gene promoters generally enhances transcription, whereas CpG methylation mediated by DNA methyltransferases (DNMTs) promotes the recruitment of methyl-CpG binding domain proteins and histone deacetylases, resulting in transcriptional repression (Jayaraman, 2012). The dynamic balance between methylation and demethylation is tightly regulated by cellular metabolism. Ten-eleven translocation (TET) enzymes require α-ketoglutarate, a tricarboxylic acid (TCA) cycle intermediate, to catalyze DNA demethylation, while succinate competes with α-ketoglutarate and inhibits TET activity (Xiao et al., 2012). Notably, succinate levels are elevated in type 2 diabetes, linking metabolic perturbations to impaired DNA demethylation and persistent epigenetic alterations (Kim, 2019).

Clinical and experimental studies support the persistence of DNA methylation changes despite glycemic normalization. Analysis of samples from the DCCT/EDIC cohort revealed distinct DNA methylation profiles in individuals previously exposed to conventional glycemic control compared with those receiving intensive therapy, despite comparable HbA1c levels at follow-up (Chen et al., 2016). Similarly, zebrafish models capable of β-cell regeneration demonstrated persistent hyperglycemia-induced DNA hypomethylation at specific loci in tissues never directly exposed to hyperglycemia, correlating with impaired tissue regeneration (Olsen et al., 2012). These findings highlight DNA methylation as a stable epigenetic contributor to long-term vascular and tissue dysfunction in diabetes and a mechanistic basis for HGM.

7. Histone modifications in hyperglycemic memory and diabetic cardiomyopathy

Histone posttranslational modifications, including acetylation, methylation, phosphorylation, ubiquitylation, and sumoylation, are critical regulators of chromatin structure and gene expression in diabetes-related complications (Su et al., 2016). Among these, histone acetylation and methylation are predominant regulators of transcriptional activity. Acetylation of histones H2A, H2B, H3, and H4 is generally associated with transcriptional activation, whereas altered acetylation patterns in diabetes modulate the expression of genes involved in cardiac function and inflammation (Chen et al., 2015). Hyperglycemia reduces glucose-6-phosphate dehydrogenase activity, leading to increased global H3 and H4 acetylation (Wang et al., 2019a, 2019b). Moreover, metabolic intermediates such as acetyl-CoA, NAD+, and NADH directly regulate the activity of histone acetyltransferases (HATs) and histone deacetylases (HDACs), linking cellular metabolism to chromatin remodeling (Kouzarides, 2000). Suppression of Sirt3 under hyperglycemic conditions reduces Foxo3A deacetylation and Parkin expression, impairing mitophagy and contributing to cardiac dysfunction (Yu et al., 2017).

Persistent alterations in histone acetylation have been demonstrated in cardiac mesenchymal stem cells derived from patients with diabetes, which exhibit reduced H3K9Ac and H3K14Ac even under normoglycemic culture conditions, suggesting durable epigenetic imprinting (Rossini et al., 2011). Elevated fatty acid β-oxidation increases acetyl-CoA availability and promotes nonenzymatic mitochondrial protein hyperacetylation, impairing enzymatic activities and increasing oxidative stress (Narita et al., 2019). Hyperacetylation of cytoplasmic proteins such as p66Shc facilitates its mitochondrial translocation and enhances ROS production, further aggravating mitochondrial dysfunction (Kumar et al., 2017).

Histone lysine methylation represents a complex and relatively stable epigenetic modification, with site-specific and degree-dependent effects on gene expression, including H3K4, H3K9, and H4K20 methylation (Jayaraman, 2012). High glucose suppresses lysine methyltransferases such as KMT5A/SET8, resulting in reduced H4K20me1 at promoters of inflammatory and metabolic genes, thereby enhancing transcriptional activation in endothelial cells (Huang et al., 2021). SET8 and the histone demethylase LSD1 also regulate DNMT1 stability, highlighting cross-talk between histone methylation and DNA methylation machinery (Zhang et al., 2019).

Genome-wide epigenomic profiling in DCCT cohorts revealed increased promoter-associated H3K9 acetylation in subjects with prior poor glycemic control, with enrichment of genes involved in ROS production, apoptosis, and immune responses (Miao et al., 2014). Hyperglycemia induces persistent epigenetic activation of inflammatory pathways through sustained enrichment of activating histone marks (e.g., H3K4me1) and loss of repressive marks (e.g., H3K9me2/3) at promoters of NF-κB-p65, IL-6, TNF-α, COX-2, VCAM-1, and MCP-1, mediated by enzymes such as Set7 and LSD1 (Yu et al., 2012; Okabe et al., 2012). Importantly, these histone modifications persist even after normalization of glucose levels, providing a molecular basis for sustained inflammatory signaling in HGM (Okabe et al., 2012).

Notably, hyperglycemia-induced suppression of epigenetic regulators, including SIRT1 and SET8, remains irreversible upon restoration of normoglycemia, further reinforcing epigenetic memory (Chen et al., 2018). Histone methylation marks such as H3K27me3 and H4K20me3 exhibit slow turnover rates, contributing to long-term stability of chromatin states (Zee et al., 2010). Additionally, histone-modifying enzymes tend to associate with the chromatin states they generate, creating positive feedback loops that stabilize epigenetic patterns across nucleosome clusters, thereby encoding durable "epigenetic memory" (Schotta et al., 2002). Stochastic modeling of nucleosome modifications further supports the concept of bistable chromatin states capable of maintaining long-term transcriptional programs despite fluctuating metabolic environments (Dodd et al., 2007).

8. Mechanisms linking metabolic memory to heart disease

The pathophysiological mechanisms underlying the cardiovascular manifestations of metabolic memory involve a complex interplay of molecular, cellular, and tissue-level changes that persist long after glycemic normalization (Nusca et al., 2018). These alterations impact vascular structure and function, contributing to the development and progression of atherosclerosis and increasing the risk of cardiovascular events.

8.1 Endothelial dysfunction

The endothelium, a monolayer of cells lining the blood vessels, plays a critical role in maintaining vascular tone and homeostasis. In the context of sustained hyperglycemia, endothelial cells experience significant oxidative stress due to increased mitochondrial production of reactive oxygen species (ROS) (Busik et al., 2008). Hyperglycemia also enhances the formation of advanced glycation end-products (AGEs), which interact with their receptor (RAGE) on endothelial cells, further amplifying oxidative and inflammatory signaling (Yao and Brownlee, 2010).

One of the earliest manifestations of this stress is the reduction in nitric oxide (NO) bioavailability, a crucial vasodilator and antiatherogenic molecule. Diminished NO levels impair endothelium-dependent relaxation and promote vasoconstriction, which increases vascular resistance (Malekmohammad et al., 2020). Additionally, endothelial cells in a hyperglycemic environment express higher levels of adhesion molecules such as VCAM-1 and ICAM-1, facilitating the recruitment of monocytes and lymphocytes to the vessel wall, a key initiating event in the formation of atherosclerotic plaques (Gustavsson et al., 2010). Importantly, these endothelial impairments persist due to lasting epigenetic changes and the continuous activation of damaging signaling cascades, even after glucose levels are brought under control.

8.2 Chronic inflammation

One of the hallmark features of metabolic memory is a sustained pro-inflammatory state that contributes to ongoing vascular injury. Prolonged hyperglycemia activates inflammatory transcription factors such as nuclear factor-kappa B (NF-κB) and activator protein-1 (AP-1). These factors initiate the transcription of a broad array of pro-inflammatory cytokines (e.g., IL-1β, IL-6, TNF-α) and chemokines (e.g., MCP-1) that maintain immune cell infiltration into vascular tissues (Indira and Abhilash, 2013).

In patients who achieve normoglycemia later in life, the inflammatory response does not fully resolve due to epigenetic reprogramming of immune and vascular cells (Davis and Gallagher, 2019). Studies have shown persistent histone modifications and altered DNA methylation patterns in endothelial and immune cells exposed to high glucose, which lead to a form of "inflammatory memory." This state of low-grade, chronic inflammation contributes not only to atherosclerotic plaque initiation but also to its growth and destabilization, increasing the risk of adverse cardiovascular outcomes such as stroke or myocardial infarction (Matter et al., 2024).

8.3 Vascular remodeling and plaque instability

Beyond inflammation and endothelial dysfunction, metabolic memory also contributes to structural changes in blood vessels, a process known as vascular remodeling. Hyperglycemia and the resultant metabolic disturbances upregulate matrix metalloproteinases (MMPs), enzymes that degrade the extracellular matrix (ECM) and disrupt the fibrous cap of atherosclerotic plaques. Persistent MMP activity, even in the absence of ongoing hyperglycemia, renders plaques more vulnerable to rupture (Berg and Miksztowicz, 2015).

Simultaneously, fibroblasts and vascular smooth muscle cells (VSMCs) exposed to a hyperglycemic environment may undergo phenotypic switching, increasing ECM deposition and contributing to arterial stiffness (Chakraborty et al., 2021). These changes culminate in the formation of unstable, lipid-rich plaques with thin fibrous caps, highly prone to rupture and subsequent thrombus formation. This type of plaque instability is a key mechanism underlying acute coronary syndromes, including myocardial infarction and sudden cardiac death, particularly in patients with diabetes (Fahed and Jang, 2021) Fig. 7.1.

9. The role of lipids and cholesterol in metabolic memory

While hyperglycemia is a major instigator of metabolic memory, lipid dysregulation also exerts a profound and lasting impact on cardiovascular health. In diabetes, altered lipid metabolism, characterized by dyslipidemia and persistent lipotoxic stress, plays a synergistic role with glucose abnormalities in promoting vascular injury (Chinen et al., 2007). Lipid-mediated effects often persist long after glycemic normalization, further reinforcing the chronic nature of metabolic memory in the cardiovascular system (Lockridge and Hanover, 2022).

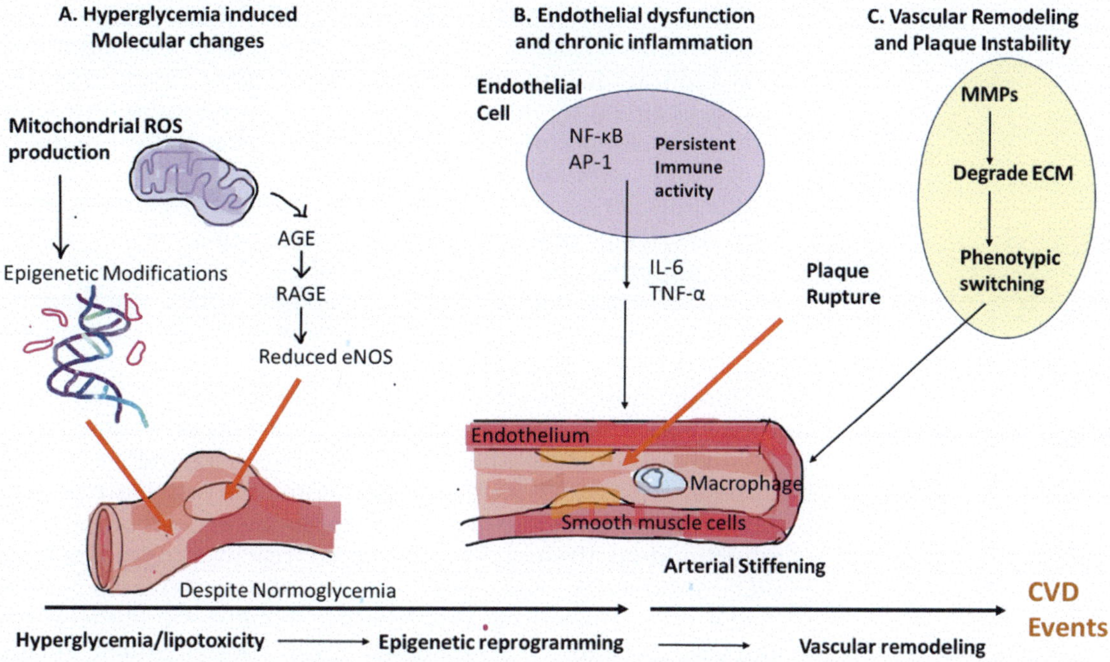

Figure 7.1 Mechanistic insights into cardiovascular complications driven by metabolic memory. The image illustrates the molecular and cellular mechanisms of cardiovascular complications in metabolic memory, highlighting endothelial dysfunction, chronic inflammation, and vascular remodeling. Key pathways include ROS generation, AGEs-RAGE interaction, cytokine release, and MMP-mediated plaque instability.

9.1 Diabetic dyslipidemia and lipotoxicity

Individuals with both type 1 and type 2 diabetes frequently exhibit a distinct pattern of lipid abnormalities collectively referred to as diabetic dyslipidemia. This condition is characterized by elevated fasting and postprandial triglyceride levels, primarily driven by increased hepatic very-low-density lipoprotein (VLDL) production and impaired clearance due to defective lipoprotein lipase (LPL) activity (Hirano, 2018). Compounding this, individuals often display an increased concentration of small, dense low-density lipoprotein (LDL) particles, which are particularly atherogenic. These smaller particles exhibit a higher affinity for arterial wall retention and are more susceptible to oxidative modification, enhancing their capacity to initiate and propagate atherosclerotic plaque development (*Feingold and Grunfeld, 2023*). Additionally, high-density lipoprotein (HDL) cholesterol levels are typically reduced, which diminishes the efficiency of reverse cholesterol transport and weakens HDL's antiinflammatory and antioxidant functions.

This triad, hypertriglyceridemia, small dense LDL, and low HDL, creates a highly atherogenic lipid profile that promotes lipid infiltration into the subendothelial space. Here, oxidized LDL is engulfed by macrophages, transforming them into foam cells, the hallmark of early atherosclerotic lesions (Mushenkova et al., 2021). Notably, research indicates that this dyslipidemic profile may persist even after achieving optimal glycemic control. The underlying contributors to this phenomenon include persistent insulin resistance, hepatic steatosis, and reduced expression of lipid-clearing enzymes and receptors, which continue to impair lipid metabolism independently of blood glucose normalization (Klisic et al., 2017).

Furthermore, elevated levels of circulating free fatty acids (FFAs) and atherogenic lipoproteins contribute to lipotoxicity, a pathological process wherein excess lipids accumulate in non-adipose tissues such as the myocardium and vascular endothelium (Sletten et al., 2018). This ectopic fat deposition leads to mitochondrial dysfunction, increased reactive oxygen species (ROS) production, and apoptosis of cardiomyocytes and endothelial cells, collectively exacerbating diabetic cardiomyopathy and vascular injury (Ferrara et al., 2019). These lipotoxic effects, much like those induced by hyperglycemia, can lead to persistent molecular and epigenetic alterations that "memorize" cellular stress and inflammation (Meulders et al., 2023). As a result, even in the absence of ongoing hyperglycemia, the damage to vascular tissues may continue unabated, contributing to the phenomenon of metabolic memory and the continued progression of atherosclerosis in diabetic individuals.

9.2 Oxidized LDL and endothelial damage

A particularly harmful consequence of diabetic dyslipidemia is the formation of oxidized low-density lipoprotein (oxLDL), a modified, highly reactive form of LDL cholesterol. OxLDL is generated when LDL particles become oxidized by reactive oxygen species (ROS) within the arterial intima, a process that transforms these otherwise inert lipoproteins into potent pro-inflammatory and cytotoxic agents (Trpkovic et al., 2015). These oxidized particles interact with specific endothelial and immune cell receptors, most notably LOX-1 (lectin-like oxidized LDL receptor-1), which mediates many of the deleterious effects of oxLDL. Upon ligand binding, LOX-1 initiates a pathological cascade that exacerbates vascular injury and accelerates atherosclerotic progression (Barreto et al., 2021).

One of the immediate consequences of LOX-1 activation is the induction of oxidative stress, largely through the stimulation of NADPH oxidase, a major enzymatic source of ROS in vascular tissues (Chan et al., 2018). This oxidative burst contributes to lipid peroxidation, DNA damage, and mitochondrial dysfunction in endothelial cells. Simultaneously, oxLDL triggers endothelial activation, characterized by the upregulation of cell adhesion molecules such as ICAM-1 (intercellular adhesion molecule-1) and VCAM-1 (vascular cell adhesion molecule-1). These molecules facilitate leukocyte adhesion and transmigration into the vessel wall, intensifying local inflammation and plaque formation (Sohrabi et al., 2020).

Moreover, chronic exposure to oxLDL leads to endothelial apoptosis and premature senescence, impairing vascular regeneration and contributing to persistent endothelial dysfunction, a critical early event in atherogenesis (Oh et al., 2017). Importantly, the effects of oxLDL are not entirely reversible upon normalization of lipid levels. This is due to the persistent activation of redox-sensitive transcription factors such as NF-κB (nuclear factor kappa-light-chain-enhancer of activated B cells) and AP-1 (activator protein 1), which sustain a pro-inflammatory gene expression profile. This enduring molecular imprint, often referred to as "oxidative memory", reflects the epigenetic and transcriptional changes induced by prior oxidative insults (Zingg et al., 2021). Over time, this memory hampers endothelial healing, maintains a pro-atherogenic microenvironment, and contributes to the progression of vascular complications in diabetes, even when traditional risk factors are adequately managed.

9.3 Cholesterol-driven epigenetic reprogramming

Emerging evidence suggests that cholesterol and its derivatives can act as epigenetic modulators, influencing gene expression patterns in a long-lasting manner. In particular, intracellular cholesterol accumulation in vascular smooth muscle cells (VSMCs), macrophages, and endothelial cells can alter histone acetylation and methylation, as well as DNA methylation profiles (Kumar et al., 2013).

One critical example involves the eNOS (endothelial nitric oxide synthase) gene. Cholesterol-mediated hypermethylation of the eNOS promoter region leads to its silencing, thereby reducing nitric oxide production and sustaining endothelial dysfunction (Kumar et al., 2013). Such changes can persist even after cholesterol-lowering interventions, highlighting the enduring impact of early cholesterol exposure on vascular biology.

Additionally, cholesterol metabolites like oxysterols may influence the activity of epigenetic enzymes such as histone deacetylases (HDACs) and DNA methyltransferases (DNMTs), promoting the expression of genes that support inflammation, fibrosis, and thrombosis (de Medina et al., 2022). These modifications reinforce pro-atherogenic cellular phenotypes, serving as another molecular layer of cardiovascular metabolic memory.

10. Interactions between glycemic and lipid memory

Metabolic memory in diabetes arises from a complex interplay between fluctuations in blood glucose levels and persistent lipid abnormalities. While hyperglycemia has long been recognized as a primary driver of vascular complications, mounting evidence demonstrates that dyslipidemia significantly reinforces and amplifies the harmful effects initiated by elevated glucose (Parhofer, 2015). This combined influence creates a synergistic relationship that accelerates vascular damage far beyond what either factor could cause alone.

One of the key mechanisms by which hyperglycemia and dyslipidemia interact is through enhanced oxidative stress (Bai et al., 2015). Elevated glucose levels increase mitochondrial production of reactive oxygen species (ROS), which damages cellular components and impairs normal vascular function. Concurrently, atherogenic lipids, particularly oxLDL, further exacerbate ROS generation (Hasheminasabgorji and Jha, 2021). This cumulative oxidative environment overwhelms endogenous antioxidant defences, perpetuating cellular injury and dysfunction within the vascular endothelium.

The synergy between glycemic and lipid abnormalities also contributes to cumulative endothelial injury (Beverly and Budoff, 2020). Hyperglycemia impairs nitric oxide (NO) bioavailability, which is crucial for vasodilation and vascular homeostasis. Simultaneously, lipid abnormalities such as elevated small dense LDL particles infiltrate the arterial intima, where they promote foam cell formation and atherosclerotic plaque development (Vekic et al., 2022). These parallel processes weaken endothelial integrity and accelerate the progression of atherosclerosis.

Moreover, the interaction sustains chronic activation of inflammatory signaling pathways. Persistent hyperglycemia primes transcription factors like NF-κB to maintain a pro-inflammatory state, while lipids stimulate additional inflammatory cascades through receptors such as LOX-1 and toll-like receptors (Bagheri et al., 2024). This ongoing inflammation recruits immune cells and perpetuates vascular remodelling and plaque instability, key contributors to cardiovascular events.

Taken together, these mechanisms illustrate how metabolic memory is not simply a result of prior hyperglycemia but is deeply influenced by the concurrent presence of lipid abnormalities. This highlights the necessity of early and comprehensive management strategies that simultaneously address both glucose and lipid control. By doing so, clinicians can better prevent the long-term cardiovascular complications that define diabetic vascular disease and improve patient outcomes.

11. Therapeutic implications

11.1 Early multifactorial intervention

The concept of metabolic memory underscores the critical importance of initiating comprehensive treatment strategies early in the course of diabetes. The landmark Steno-2 trial provided compelling evidence supporting a multifactorial intervention approach, which combines intensive glycemic control with lipid-lowering therapies, antihypertensive medications, and lifestyle modifications such as diet and exercise (Gæde et al., 2019). In this randomized controlled study involving patients with type 2 diabetes and microalbuminuria, those receiving the multifactorial treatment showed a significant reduction in cardiovascular morbidity and mortality compared to standard care (Oellgaard et al., 2018). These benefits persisted long after the trial ended, highlighting how early aggressive management can prevent or delay the establishment of metabolic memory and its associated vascular damage. This trial remains a cornerstone in reinforcing the notion that addressing multiple risk factors simultaneously is essential to mitigating long-term cardiovascular risk.

11.2 Statins and beyond

Statins have become a mainstay in cardiovascular risk reduction for people with diabetes, primarily through their potent LDL cholesterol-lowering effects (Kapur and Musunuru, 2008). Beyond lipid lowering, statins exhibit pleiotropic properties, including antiinflammatory, antioxidative, and plaque-stabilizing actions, which may directly counteract several pathological mechanisms involved in metabolic memory (Zhang et al., 2024). By reducing

Table 7.1 HDAC inhibitors in cardiovascular diseases.

Class	Inhibitor Name	Target Enzyme(s)	Mechanism of action	Effects in cardiovascular diseases	References
HDAC inhibitor	Trichostatin A (TSA)	HDAC1, HDAC2, HDAC3 (Class I and II)	Reversible inhibition of histone deacetylation → chromatin relaxation and gene reactivation	Improves endothelial function; suppresses hypertrophy and fibrosis	Guo et al. (2017), Lei et al.
HDAC inhibitor	Vorinostat (SAHA)	Class I and II HDACs	Increases acetylation of histones and non-histone proteins	Reduces vascular inflammation, oxidative stress, and cardiac remodeling	Yoon and Eom (2016)
HDAC inhibitor	Valproic Acid (VPA)	HDAC1, HDAC2	Epigenetic modulation through HDAC inhibition	Enhances angiogenesis, attenuates cardiac hypertrophy and improves myocardial infarction outcomes	Tian et al. (2019)
HDAC inhibitor	Sodium Butyrate	Class I and IIa HDACs	Histone acetylation, antiinflammatory and antioxidative effects	Protects against atherosclerosis and ischemic injury	Zhang et al. (2017)

vascular inflammation and improving endothelial function, statins help attenuate the persistent vascular injury seen in diabetic patients. Furthermore, newer lipid-modulating agents such as PCSK9 inhibitors and bempedoic acid are gaining prominence for their ability to lower LDL-C effectively, especially in statin-intolerant patients or those requiring further LDL reduction (Gunta et al., 2023). Emerging therapies targeting liver X receptor (LXR) agonists are also under investigation, given their potential to influence cholesterol metabolism and inflammatory pathways in vascular cells, offering hope for directly modulating lipid-driven components of metabolic memory (Ma et al., 2009).

11.3 Epigenetic therapies

As research into the molecular underpinnings of metabolic memory advances, epigenetic modifications have emerged as promising therapeutic targets. Persistent changes in DNA methylation and histone acetylation patterns sustain the maladaptive gene expression profiles contributing to chronic inflammation, oxidative stress, and endothelial dysfunction. Novel pharmacologic agents such as histone deacetylase (HDAC) inhibitors (Table 7.1) and DNA methyltransferase (DNMT) inhibitors are being explored for their ability to reverse these epigenetic marks and restore normal cellular function (Stenzig et al., 2018; Zhang et al., 2025). While primarily investigated in oncology, these epigenetic drugs hold potential for cardiovascular applications by reprogramming vascular cells and dampening the persistent pro-atherogenic signaling established during early hyperglycemic episodes. Future clinical trials are needed to establish the safety and efficacy of such epigenetic therapies in the context of diabetic cardiovascular disease.

12. Conclusion

Cardiovascular disease in diabetes is not only a result of current metabolic status but also of past metabolic insults encoded in the molecular memory of vascular cells. The concept of metabolic memory underscores the critical importance of early and sustained glycemic and lipid control in reducing long-term cardiovascular risk. A deeper understanding of how glucose and lipid disturbances jointly contribute to this memory will guide the development of more effective, targeted interventions to improve cardiovascular outcomes in individuals with diabetes.

References

Afroz, A., Ali, L., Karim, M.N., Alramadan, M.J., Alam, K., Magliano, D.J., Billah, B., 2019. Glycaemic control for people with type 2 diabetes mellitus in Bangladesh - an urgent need for optimization of management plan. Sci. Rep. 9 (1). https://doi.org/10.1038/s41598-019-46766-9.

Aneja, A., Tang, W.H.W., Bansilal, S., Garcia, M.J., Farkouh, M.E., 2008. Diabetic cardiomyopathy: insights into pathogenesis, Diagnostic challenges, and therapeutic options. Am. J. Med. 121 (9), 748–757. https://doi.org/10.1016/j.amjmed.2008.03.046.

Aschner, P.J., Ruiz, A.J., 2012. Metabolic memory for vascular disease in diabetes. Diabetes Technol. Therapeut. 14 (1), S68. https://doi.org/10.1089/dia.2012.0012.

Bagheri, B., Khatibiyan Feyzabadi, Z., Nouri, A., Azadfallah, A., Mahdizade Ari, M., Hemmati, M., Darban, M., Alavi Toosi, P., Banihashemian, S.Z., 2024. Atherosclerosis and toll-like Receptor4 (TLR4), lectin-like oxidized low-density lipoprotein-1 (LOX-1), and proprotein convertase subtilisin/kexin Type9 (PCSK9). Mediat. Inflamm. 2024 (1), 5830491.

Bai, J., Zheng, S., Jiang, D., Han, T., Li, Y., Zhang, Y., Liu, W., Cao, Y., Hu, Y., 2015. Oxidative stress contributes to abnormal glucose metabolism and insulin sensitivity in two hyperlipidemia models. Int. J. Clin. Exp. Pathol. 8 (10), 13193–13200.

Barreto, J., Karathanasis, S.K., Remaley, A., Sposito, A.C., 2021. Role of LOX-1 (Lectin-Like oxidized low-density lipoprotein receptor 1) as a cardiovascular risk predictor mechanistic insight and potential clinical use. Arterioscler. Thromb. Vasc. Biol. 41 (1), 153–166. https://doi.org/10.1161/ATVBAHA.120.315421.

Berg, G., Miksztowicz, V., 2015. Metalloproteinases in the pathogenesis and progression of metabolic syndrome: potential targets for improved outcomes. Metalloproteinases Med. 51. https://doi.org/10.2147/MNM.S88993.

Beverly, J.K., Budoff, M.J., February 1, 2020. Atherosclerosis: pathophysiology of insulin resistance, hyperglycemia, hyperlipidemia, and inflammation. J. Diabetes 12 (2), 102–104.

Bi, Y., Zhang, Y., Ren, J., 2020. Phosphoinositide 3-kinase therapy in diabetic cardiomyopathy: unravelling an enigma. Am. J. Physiol. Heart Circ. Physiol. 318 (5), H1029. https://doi.org/10.1152/ajpheart.00160.2020.

Brownlee, M., 1992. Glycation products and the pathogenesis of diabetic complications. Diabetes Care 15 (12), 1835–1843. https://doi.org/10.2337/diacare.15.12.1835.

Busik, J.V., Mohr, S., Grant, M.B., 2008. Hyperglycemia-Induced reactive oxygen species toxicity to endothelial cells is dependent on paracrine mediators. Diabetes 57 (7), 1952–1965. https://doi.org/10.2337/db07-1520.

Cencioni, C., Spallotta, F., Greco, S., Martelli, F., Zeiher, A.M., Gaetano, C., 2014. Epigenetic mechanisms of hyperglycemic memory. Int. J. Biochem. Cell Biol. 51 (1), 155–158. https://doi.org/10.1016/j.biocel.2014.04.014.

Chakraborty, R., Chatterjee, P., Dave, J.M., Ostriker, A.C., Greif, D.M., Rzucidlo, E.M., Martin, K.A., 2021. Targeting smooth muscle cell phenotypic switching in vascular disease. JVS-Vascular Science 2, 79–94. https://doi.org/10.1016/j.jvssci.2021.04.001.

Chan, S.H., Hung, C.H., Shih, J.Y., Chu, P.M., Cheng, Y.H., Lin, H.C., Hsieh, P.L., Tsai, K.L., 2018. Exercise intervention attenuates hyperhomocysteinemia-induced aortic endothelial oxidative injury by regulating SIRT1 through mitigating NADPH oxidase/LOX-1 signaling. Redox Biol. 14, 116–125. https://doi.org/10.1016/j.redox.2017.08.016.

Chen, Y., Du, J., Zhao, Y.T., et al., 2015. HDAC inhibition improves myocardial function. Cardiovasc. Diabetol. 14, 99.

Chen, Z., Miao, F., Paterson, A.D., et al., 2016. Persistence of DNA methylation and metabolic memory. Proc. Natl. Acad. Sci. U. S. A 113 (21), E3002–E3011.

Chen, X., Wu, Q., Jiang, H., Wang, J., Zhao, Y., Xu, Y., Zhu, M., 2018. SET8 is involved in the regulation of hyperglycemic memory in human umbilical endothelial cells. Acta Biochim. Biophys. Sin. 50 (7), 635–642. https://doi.org/10.1093/abbs/gmy051.

Chinen, I., Shimabukuro, M., Yamakawa, K., Higa, N., Matsuzaki, T., Noguchi, K., Ueda, S., Sakanashi, M., Takasu, N., 2007. Vascular lipotoxicity: endothelial dysfunction via fatty-acid-induced reactive oxygen species overproduction in obese Zucker diabetic fatty rats. Endocrinology 148 (1), 160–165. https://doi.org/10.1210/en.2006-1132Japan.

Cosentino, F., Francia, P., Camici, G.G., et al., 2008. p66Shc protein in aging and cardiovascular disease. Arterioscler. Thromb. Vasc. Biol. 28 (4), 622–628.

Costantino, S., Paneni, F., Lüscher, T.F., Cosentino, F., 2016. MicroRNA profiling unveils hyperglycaemic memory in the diabetic heart. Eur. Heart J. 37 (6), 572–576. https://doi.org/10.1093/eurheartj/ehv599.

Cyr, A.R., Huckaby, L.V., Shiva, S.S., Zuckerbraun, B.S., 2020. Nitric oxide and endothelial dysfunction. Crit. Care Clin. 36 (2), 307–321. https://doi.org/10.1016/j.ccc.2019.12.009.

Davis, F.M., Gallagher, K.A., 2019. Epigenetic mechanisms in monocytes/macrophages regulate inflammation in cardiometabolic and vascular disease. Arterioscler. Thromb. Vasc. Biol. 39 (4), 623–634. https://doi.org/10.1161/ATVBAHA.118.312135.

de Medina, P., Silvente-Poirot, S., Poirot, M., 2022. Oxysterols are potential physiological regulators of ageing. Ageing Res. Rev. 77, 101615. https://doi.org/10.1016/j.arr.2022.101615.

Dodd, I.B., Micheelsen, M.A., Sneppen, K., Thon, G., 2007. Epigenetic memory by nucleosome modification. Cell 129 (4), 813–822.

Fahed, A.C., Jang, I.K., 2021. Plaque erosion and acute coronary syndromes: phenotype, molecular characteristics and future directions. Nat. Rev. Cardiol. 18 (10), 724–734. https://doi.org/10.1038/s41569-021-00542-3.

Feingold, K.R., Grunfeld, C., June 2, 2023. Diabetes and dyslipidemia. In: InDiabetes and Cardiovascular Disease. Springer International Publishing, Cham, pp. 425–472.

Ferrara, D., Montecucco, F., Dallegri, F., Carbone, F., 2019. Impact of different ectopic fat depots on cardiovascular and metabolic diseases. J. Cell. Physiol. 234 (12), 21630–21641. https://doi.org/10.1002/jcp.28821.

Gæde, P., Oellgaard, J., Kruuse, C., Rossing, P., Parving, H.H., Pedersen, O., 2019. Beneficial impact of intensified multifactorial intervention on risk of stroke: outcome of 21 years of follow-up in the randomised Steno-2 Study. Diabetologia 62 (9), 1575–1580. https://doi.org/10.1007/s00125-019-4920-3.

Giacco, F., Brownlee, M., Schmidt, A.M., 2010. Oxidative stress and diabetic complications. Circ. Res. 107 (9), 1058–1070. https://doi.org/10.1161/circresaha.110.223545.

Gilbert, R.E., Krum, H., 2015. Heart failure in diabetes: effects of anti-hyperglycaemic drug therapy. Lancet 385 (9982), 2107–2117. https://doi.org/10.1016/S0140-6736(14)61402-1.

Gunta, S.P., O'Keefe, J.H., O'Keefe, E.L., Lavie, C.J., 2023. PCSK9 inhibitor, ezetimibe, and bempedoic acid: evidence-based therapies for statin-intolerant patients. Prog. Cardiovasc. Dis. 79, 12–18. https://doi.org/10.1016/j.pcad.2023.02.007.

Guo, Y., Li, Z., Shi, C., Li, J., Yao, M., Chen, X., 2017. Trichostatin A attenuates oxidative stress-mediated myocardial injury through the FoxO3a signaling pathway. Int. J. Mol. Med. 40 (4), 999–1008. https://doi.org/10.3892/ijmm.2017.3101.

Gustavsson, C., Agardh, C.D., Zetterqvist, A.V., Nilsson, J., Agardh, E., Gomez, M.F., 2010. Vascular cellular adhesion molecule-1 (VCAM-1) expression in mice retinal vessels is affected by both hyperglycemia and hyperlipidemia. PLoS One 5 (9), 1–12. https://doi.org/10.1371/journal.pone.0012699Sweden.

Habas, K., Shang, L., 2018. Alterations in intercellular adhesion molecule 1 (ICAM-1) and vascular cell adhesion molecule 1 (VCAM-1) in human endothelial cells. Tissue Cell 54, 139–143. https://doi.org/10.1016/j.tice.2018.09.002.

Hamby, R.I., Zoneraich, S., Sherman, L., 1974. Diabetic cardiomyopathy. JAMA, J. Am. Med. Assoc. 229 (13), 1749–1754. https://doi.org/10.1001/jama.1974.03230510023016.

Hamilton, S., Terentyev, D., 2019. Altered intracellular calcium homeostasis and arrhythmogenesis in the aged heart. Int. J. Mol. Sci. 20 (10), 2386. https://doi.org/10.3390/ijms20102386.

Hasheminasabgorji, E., Jha, J.C., 2021. Dyslipidemia, diabetes and atherosclerosis: role of inflammation and ros-redox-sensitive factors. Biomedicines 9 (11). https://doi.org/10.3390/biomedicines9111602.

He, J., Xu, Q., Jing, Y., Agani, F., Qian, X., Carpenter, R., Jiang, B.H., 2012. Reactive oxygen species regulate ERBB2 and ERBB3 expression via miR-199a/125b and DNA methylation. EMBO Rep. 13 (12), 1116.

Hirano, T., 2018. Pathophysiology of diabetic dyslipidemia. J. Atherosclerosis Thromb. 25 (9), 771–782. https://doi.org/10.5551/jat.rv17023.

Huang, T., Li, X., Wang, F., et al., 2021. CREB/KMT5A complex regulates PTP1B. Cell Death Dis. 12 (4), 333.

Hussain, S., Khan, A.W., Akhmedov, A., Suades, R., Costantino, S., Paneni, F., Caidahl, K., Mohammed, S.A., Hage, C., Gkolfos, C., Björck, H., Pernow, J., Lund, L.H., Lüscher, T.F., Cosentino, F., 2020. Hyperglycemia induces myocardial dysfunction via epigenetic regulation of JunD. Circ. Res. 127 (10), 1261–1273. https://doi.org/10.1161/CIRCRESAHA.120.317132.

Ihnat, M.A., Thorpe, J.E., Kamat, C.D., et al., 2007. ROS mediate cellular memory of high glucose. Diabetologia 50 (7), 1523–1531.

Indira, M., Abhilash, P.A., 2013. Role of NF-kappa B (NF-κB) in diabetes. Forum Immunopathol. Dis. Ther. 4 (2), 111–132. https://doi.org/10.1615/forumimmundisther.2013008396.

Isabelle, M., Vergeade, A., Moritz, F., et al., 2007. NADPH oxidase inhibition prevents cardiac dysfunction. J. Mol. Cell. Cardiol. 42 (2), 326–332.

Jayaraman, S., 2012. Epigenetic mechanisms of metabolic memory. Circ. Res. 110 (8), 1039–1041.

Jin, X., Yao, T., Zhou, Z., Zhu, J., Zhang, S., Hu, W., Shen, C., 2015. Advanced glycation end products enhance macrophage polarization into M1 phenotype via RAGE/NF-κB. BioMed Res. Int. 2015, 732450.

Jubaidi, F.F., Zainalabidin, S., Mariappan, V., Budin, S.B., 2020. Mitochondrial dysfunction in diabetic cardiomyopathy. Int. J. Mol. Sci. 21 (17), 6043.

Kapur, N.K., Musunuru, K., 2008. Clinical efficacy and safety of statins in managing cardiovascular risk. Vasc. Health Risk Manag. 4 (2), 341–353.

Kim, M., 2019. DNA methylation in type 2 diabetes. Genomics & Informatics 17 (4), e38.

Klisic, A., Kavaric, N., Jovanovic, M., Zvrko, E., Skerovic, V., Scepanovic, A., Medin, D., Ninic, A., 2017. Association between unfavorable lipid profile and glycemic control in patients with type 2 diabetes mellitus. J. Res. Med. Sci. 22 (1). https://doi.org/10.4103/jrms.jrms_284_17.

Kouzarides, T., 2000. Acetylation: a regulatory modification. EMBO J. 19 (6), 1176–1179.

Kumar, A., Kumar, S., Vikram, A., Hoffman, T.A., Naqvi, A., Lewarchik, C.M., Kim, Y.R., Irani, K., 2013. Histone and DNA methylation-mediated epigenetic downregulation of endothelial kruppel-like factor 2 by low-density lipoprotein cholesterol. Arterioscler. Thromb. Vasc. Biol. 33 (8), 1936–1942. https://doi.org/10.1161/ATVBAHA.113.301765.

Kumar, S., Kim, Y.R., Vikram, A., Naqvi, A., Li, Q., Kassan, M., Kumar, V., Bachschmid, M.M., Jacobs, J.S., Kumar, A., Irani, K., 2017. Sirtuin1-regulated lysine acetylation of p66Shc governs diabetes-induced vascular oxidative stress and endothelial dysfunction. Proc. Natl. Acad. Sci. U. S. A 114 (7), 1714–1719. https://doi.org/10.1073/pnas.1614112114.

Lee, W.S., Kim, J., 2021. Application of animal models in diabetic cardiomyopathy. Diabetes and Metabolism Journal 45 (2), 129–145. https://doi.org/10.4093/DMJ.2020.0285.

Lee, M.M.Y., McMurray, J.J.V., Lorenzo-Almorós, A., Kristensen, S.L., Sattar, N., Jhund, P.S., Petrie, M.C., 2019a. Diabetic cardiomyopathy. Heart 105 (4), 337–345.

Lee, J.Y., Lee, Y.J., Jeon, H.Y., et al., 2019b. Transglutaminase 2–ROS vicious cycle. FASEB (Fed. Am. Soc. Exp. Biol.) J. 33 (11), 12655–12667.

Lei L, Chen M, Wang C, Jiang X, Li Y, Wang W, Li S, Zhao L, Sheng R, Han J, Zhang Y. Trichostatin D as a novel KLF2 activator attenuates TNFα-induced endothelial inflammati .

Li, H., Dai, B., Fan, J., et al., 2019. miRNA-92a-2-5p and let-7b-5p in mitochondrial translation. Mol. Ther. Nucleic Acids 17, 424–435.

Li, H., Fan, J., Chen, C., Wang, D.W., 2020. Subcellular microRNAs in diabetic cardiomyopathy. Ann. Transl. Med. 8 (23). https://doi.org/10.21037/atm-20-2205, 1602–1602.

Lockridge, A., Hanover, J.A., 2022. A nexus of lipid and O-Glcnac metabolism in physiology and disease. Front. Endocrinol. 13. https://doi.org/10.3389/fendo.2022.943576.

Luna, P., Guarner, V., Farías, J.M., Hernández-Pacheco, G., Martínez, M., 2016. Importance of metabolic memory in the development of vascular complications in diabetic patients. J. Cardiothorac. Vasc. Anesth. 30 (5), 1369–1378. https://doi.org/10.1053/j.jvca.2016.02.008.

Ma, H., Li, S.Y., Xu, P., Babcock, S.A., Dolence, E.K., Brownlee, M., Li, J., Ren, J., 2009. Advanced glycation endproduct (AGE) accumulation and AGE receptor (RAGE) up-regulation contribute to the onset of diabetic cardiomyopathy. J. Cell Mol. Med. 13 (8 B), 1751–1764. https://doi.org/10.1111/j.1582-4934.2008.00547.xChina.

Maack, C., Lehrke, M., Backs, J., et al., 2018. Heart failure and diabetes: a state-of-the-art review. Eur. Heart J. 39 (48), 4243–4254.

Malekmohammad, K., Sewell, R.D.E., Rafieian-Kopaei, M., 2020. Mechanisms of medicinal plant activity on nitric oxide (NO) bioavailability as prospective treatments for atherosclerosis. Curr. Pharm. Des. 26 (22), 2591–2601. https://doi.org/10.2174/1381612826666200318152049.

Marso, S.P., Kennedy, K.F., House, J.A., McGuire, D.K., 2010. The effect of intensive glucose control on all-cause and cardiovascular mortality, myocardial infarction and stroke in persons with type 2 diabetes mellitus: a systematic review and meta-analysis. Diabetes Vasc. Dis. Res. 7 (2), 119–130. https://doi.org/10.1177/1479164109353367.

Matter, M.A., Paneni, F., Libby, P., Frantz, S., Stähli, B.E., Templin, C., Mengozzi, A., Wang, Y.J., Kündig, T.M., Räber, L., Ruschitzka, F., Matter, C.M., 2024. Inflammation in acute myocardial infarction: the good, the bad and the ugly. Eur. Heart J. 45 (2), 89–103. https://doi.org/10.1093/eurheartj/ehad486.

Meulders, B., Marei, W.F.A., Xhonneux, I., Bols, P.E.J., Leroy, J.L.M.R., 2023. Effect of lipotoxicity on mitochondrial function and epigenetic programming during bovine in vitro embryo production. Sci. Rep. 13 (1). https://doi.org/10.1038/s41598-023-49184-0.

Miao, F., Chen, Z., Genuth, S., et al., 2014. Histone modifications in metabolic memory. Diabetes 63 (5), 1748–1762.

Miki, T., Yuda, S., Kouzu, H., Miura, T., 2013. Diabetic cardiomyopathy: pathophysiology and clinical features. Heart Fail. Rev. 18 (2), 149–166. https://doi.org/10.1007/s10741-012-9313-3.

Morey, M., O'Gaora, P., Pandit, A., Hélary, C., Mukhopadhyay, P., 2019. Hyperglycemia acts in synergy with hypoxia to maintain the pro-inflammatory phenotype of macrophages. PLoS One 14 (8), e0220577. https://doi.org/10.1371/journal.pone.0220577.

Mushenkova, N.V., Bezsonov, E.E., Orekhova, V.A., Popkova, T.V., Starodubova, A.V., Orekhov, A.N., 2021. Recognition of oxidized lipids by macrophages and its role in atherosclerosis development. Federation Biomedicines 9 (8). https://doi.org/10.3390/biomedicines9080915.

Narita, T., Weinert, B.T., Choudhary, C., 2019. Functions and mechanisms of non-histone protein acetylation. Nat. Rev. Mol. Cell Biol. 20 (3), 156–174. https://doi.org/10.1038/s41580-018-0081-3.

Nathan, D.M., 2021. Realising the long-term promise of insulin therapy: the DCCT/EDIC study. Diabetologia 64 (5), 1049–1058. https://doi.org/10.1007/s00125-021-05397-4.

Nusca, A., Tuccinardi, D., Albano, M., Cavallaro, C., Ricottini, E., Manfrini, S., Pozzilli, P., Di Sciascio, G., 2018. Glycemic variability in the development of cardiovascular complications in diabetes. Diabetes Metabol. Res. Rev. 34 (8). https://doi.org/10.1002/dmrr.3047.

Oellgaard, J., Gæde, P., Rossing, P., Rørth, R., Køber, L., Parving, H.H., Pedersen, O., 2018. Reduced risk of heart failure with intensified multifactorial intervention in individuals with type 2 diabetes and microalbuminuria: 21 years of follow-up in the randomised Steno-2 study. Diabetologia 61 (8), 1724–1733. https://doi.org/10.1007/s00125-018-4642-y.

Oh, S.-T., Park, H., Yoon, H.J., Yang, S.Y., Martins, M.J., 2017. Long-term treatment of native LDL induces senescence of cultured human endothelial cells. Oxid. Med. Cell. Longev. 2017 (1). https://doi.org/10.1155/2017/6487825.

Okabe, J., Orlowski, C., Balcerczyk, A., et al., 2012. Set7 in endothelial hyperglycemic changes. Circ. Res. 110 (8), 1067–1076.

Oldfield, M.D., Bach, L.A., Forbes, J.M., Nikolic-Paterson, D., McRobert, A., Thallas, V., Atkins, R.C., Osicka, T., Jerums, G., Cooper, M.E., 2001. Advanced glycation end products cause epithelial–myofibroblast transdifferentiation via RAGE. J. Clin. Investig. 108 (12), 1853–1863.

Olsen, A.S., Sarras Jr., M.P., Leontovich, A., Intine, R.V., 2012. Heritable diabetic metabolic memory in zebrafish. Diabetes 61 (2), 485–491.

Onursal, C., Dick, E., Angelidis, I., Schiller, H.B., Staab-Weijnitz, C.A., 2021. Collagen biosynthesis, processing, and maturation in lung ageing. Front. Med. 8, 593874.

Paneni, F., Mocharla, P., Akhmedov, A., et al., 2012. Gene silencing of p66Shc suppresses hyperglycemic memory. Circ. Res. 111 (3), 278–289.

Paneni, F., Volpe, M., Lüscher, T.F., Cosentino, F., 2013. SIRT1, p66Shc, and Set7/9 in vascular memory. Diabetes 62 (6), 1800–1807.

Parhofer, K.G., 2015. Interaction between glucose and lipid metabolism: more than diabetic dyslipidemia. Diabetes & Metabolism Journal 39 (5), 353. https://doi.org/10.4093/dmj.2015.39.5.353.

Peng, Q.H., Tong, P., Gu, L.M., Li, W.J., 2020. Astragalus polysaccharide attenuates metabolic memory. Biosci. Rep. 40 (1), BSR20192121.

Ren, J., Ceylan-Isik, A.F., 2004. Diabetic cardiomyopathy: do women differ from men? Endocrine 25 (2), 73–83.

Rossini, A., Frati, C., Lagrasta, C., et al., 2011. Distinctive properties of human cardiac and bone marrow stromal cells. Cardiovasc. Res. 89 (3), 650–660.

Rota, M., LeCapitaine, N., Hosoda, T., et al., 2006. p66Shc deletion prevents diabetic cardiac aging. Circ. Res. 99 (1), 42–52.

Schmidt, A.M., Hori, O., Chen, J.X., Li, J.F., Crandall, J., Zhang, J., Cao, R., Yan, S.D., Brett, J., Stern, D., 1995. Advanced glycation endproducts interacting with their endothelial receptor induce expression of vascular cell adhesion molecule-1 (VCAM-1) in cultured human endothelial cells and in mice. A potential mechanism for the accelerated vasculopathy of diabetes. J. Clin. Investig. 96 (3), 1395–1403. https://doi.org/10.1172/JCI118175.

Schotta, Ebert, Krauss, et al., 2002. EMBO J. 21 (5), 1121–1131.

Shen, C.Y., Lu, C.H., Wu, C.H., Li, K.J., Kuo, Y.M., Hsieh, S.C., Yu, C.L., 2020. The development of maillard reaction, and advanced glycation end product (Age)-receptor for age (rage) signaling inhibitors as novel therapeutic strategies for patients with age-related diseases. Molecules 25 (23). https://doi.org/10.3390/molecules25235591.

Sletten, A.C., Peterson, L.R., Schaffer, J.E., 2018. Manifestations and mechanisms of myocardial lipotoxicity in obesity. J. Intern. Med. 284 (5), 478–491. https://doi.org/10.1111/joim.12728.

Sohrabi, Y., Lagache, S.M.M., Voges, V.C., Semo, D., Sonntag, G., Hanemann, I., Kahles, F., Waltenberger, J., Findeisen, H.M., 2020. OxLDL-mediated immunologic memory in endothelial cells. J. Mol. Cell. Cardiol. 146, 121–132. https://doi.org/10.1016/j.yjmcc.2020.07.006.

Stenzig, J., Schneeberger, Y., Löser, A., Peters, B.S., Schaefer, A., Zhao, R.R., Ng, S.L., Höppner, G., Geertz, B., Hirt, M.N., Tan, W., Wong, E., Reichenspurner, H., Foo, R.S.Y., Eschenhagen, T., 2018. Pharmacological inhibition of DNA methylation attenuates pressure overload-induced cardiac hypertrophy in rats. J. Mol. Cell. Cardiol. 120, 53–63. https://doi.org/10.1016/j.yjmcc.2018.05.012.

Stettler, C., Allemann, S., Jüni, P., Cull, C.A., Holman, R.R., Egger, M., Krähenbühl, S., Diem, P., 2006. Glycemic control and macrovascular disease in types 1 and 2 diabetes mellitus: meta-analysis of randomized trials. Am. Heart J. 152 (1), 27–38. https://doi.org/10.1016/j.ahj.2005.09.015.

Strycharz, J., Świderska, E., Wróblewski, A., Podolska, M., Czarny, P., Szemraj, J., Balcerczyk, A., Drzewoski, J., Kasznicki, J., Śliwińska, A., 2018. Hyperglycemia alters miRNA patterns during adipogenesis. Nutrients 10 (11), 1774.

Su, X., Wellen, K.E., Rabinowitz, J.D., 2016. Metabolic control of methylation and acetylation. Curr. Opin. Chem. Biol. 30, 52–60. https://doi.org/10.1016/j.cbpa.2015.10.030.

Tian, S., Lei, I., Gao, W., Liu, L., Guo, Y., Creech, J., Herron, T.J., Xian, S., Ma, P. X., Eugene Chen, Y., Li, Y., Alam, H.B., Wang, Z., 2019. HDAC inhibitor valproic acid protects heart function through Foxm1 pathway after acute myocardial infarction. EBioMedicine 39, 83–94. https://doi.org/10.1016/j.ebiom.2018.12.003.

Tian, H., Zhao, X., Zhang, Y., Xia, Z., 2023. Abnormalities of glucose and lipid metabolism in myocardial ischemia-reperfusion injury. Biomed. Pharmacother. 163, 114827. https://doi.org/10.1016/j.biopha.2023.114827.

Tong, M., Sadoshima, J., 2019. Nuclear miR-320 controls lipotoxicity. Circ. Res. 125 (12), 1121–1123. https://doi.org/10.1161/circresaha.119.316199.

Trpkovic, A., Resanovic, I., Stanimirovic, J., Radak, D., Mousa, S.A., Cenic-Milosevic, D., Jevremovic, D., Isenovic, E.R., 2015. Oxidized low-density lipoprotein as a biomarker of cardiovascular diseases. Crit. Rev. Clin. Lab Sci. 52 (2), 70–85. https://doi.org/10.3109/10408363.2014.992063.

Trumpower, B.L., 1990. The protonmotive Q cycle. Energy transduction by coupling of proton translocation to electron transfer by the cytochrome bc1 complex. J. Biol. Chem. 265 (20), 11409–11412. https://doi.org/10.1016/s0021-9258(19)38410-8.

Uryga, A.K., Bennett, M.R., 2016. Ageing induced vascular smooth muscle cell senescence in atherosclerosis. J. Physiol. (Paris) 594 (8), 2115–2124. https://doi.org/10.1113/JP270923.

Vekic, J., Zeljkovic, A., Cicero, A.F.G., Janez, A., Pantea Stoian, A., Sonmez, A., Rizzo, M., 2022. Atherosclerosis development and progression: the role of atherogenic small, dense LDL. Medicina 58 (2), 299. https://doi.org/10.3390/medicina58020299.

Wallace, D.C., 1992. Diseases of the mitochondrial DNA. Annu. Rev. Biochem. 61, 1175–1212. https://doi.org/10.1146/annurev.bi.61.070192.005523.

Wang, M., Hu, J., Yan, L., et al., 2019a. High glucose induces G6PD ubiquitination. FASEB (Fed. Am. Soc. Exp. Biol.) J. 33 (5), 6296–6310.

Wang, J., Tang, Z., Zhang, Y., Qiu, C., Zhu, L., Zhao, N., Liu, Z., 2019b. Matrine alleviates AGEs-induced cardiac dysfunction. Eur. J. Pharmacol. 842, 118–124.

Wang, D., Yin, Y., Wang, S., et al., 2021. FGF1ΔHBS prevents diabetic cardiomyopathy. Signal Transduct. Targeted Ther. 6 (1), 133.

Wende, A.R., Schell, J.C., Ha, C.M., et al., 2020. Myocardial glucose utilization and mitochondrial dysfunction. Diabetes 69 (10), 2094–2111.

West, A.P., Shadel, G.S., 2017. Mitochondrial DNA in innate immune responses and inflammatory pathology. Nat. Rev. Immunol. 17 (6), 363–375.

Xiao, M., Yang, H., Xu, W., et al., 2012. Inhibition of α-KG-dependent demethylases by fumarate and succinate. Genes Dev. 26 (12), 1326–1338.

Yang, L., Zhao, D., Ren, J., Yang, J., 2015. Endoplasmic reticulum stress and protein quality control in diabetic cardiomyopathy. Biochim. Biophys. Acta Mol. Basis Dis. 1852 (2), 209–218. https://doi.org/10.1016/j.bbadis.2014.05.006.

Yang, Y.C., Tsai, C.Y., Chen, C.L., Kuo, C.H., Hou, C.W., Cheng, S.Y., Aneja, R., Huang, C.Y., Kuo, W.W., 2018. Pkcδ activation is involved in ROS-mediated mitochondrial dysfunction and apoptosis in cardiomyocytes exposed to advanced glycation end products (AGEs). Aging and Disease 9 (4), 647–663. https://doi.org/10.14336/AD.2017.0924.

Yao, D., Brownlee, M., 2010. Hyperglycemia-induced reactive oxygen species increase expression of the receptor for advanced glycation end products (RAGE) and RAGE ligands. Diabetes 59 (1), 249–255. https://doi.org/10.2337/db09-0801.

Yao, Y., Song, Q., Hu, C., Da, X., Yu, Y., He, Z., Xu, C., Chen, Q., Wang, Q.K., 2022. Endothelial cell metabolic memory causes cardiovascular dysfunction in diabetes. Cardiovasc. Res. 118 (1), 196–211. https://doi.org/10.1093/cvr/cvab013.

Yoon, S., Eom, G.H., 2016. HDAC and HDAC inhibitor: from cancer to cardiovascular diseases. Chonnam medical journal 52 (1).

Yu, X.Y., Geng, Y.J., Liang, J.L., et al., 2012. Histone H3K9 methylation in metabolic memory. Mol. Biol. Rep. 39 (9), 8891–8898.

Yu, W., Gao, B., Li, N., et al., 2017. Sirt3 deficiency exacerbates diabetic cardiac dysfunction. Biochim. Biophys. Acta, Mol. Basis Dis. 1863 (8), 1973–1983.

Zakir, M., Ahuja, N., Surksha, M.A., Sachdev, R., Kalariya, Y., Nasir, M., Kashif, M., Shahzeen, F., Tayyab, A., Khan, M.S.moazzam, Junejo, M., Kumar, F.N.U.M., Varrassi, G., Kumar, S., Khatri, M., Mohamad, T., 2023. Cardiovascular complications of diabetes: from microvascular to macrovascular pathways. Cureus 15 (9). https://doi.org/10.7759/cureus.45835.

Zee, B.M., Levin, R.S., Xu, B., LeRoy, G., Wingreen, N.S., Garcia, B.A., 2010. In vivo residue-specific histone methylation dynamics. J. Biol. Chem. 285 (5), 3341–3350. https://doi.org/10.1074/jbc.M109.063784.

Zhang, L., Du, J., Yano, N., Wang, H., Zhao, Y.T., Dubielecka, P.M., Zhuang, S., Chin, Y.E., Qin, G., Zhao, T.C., 2017. Sodium butyrate protects -against high fat diet-induced cardiac dysfunction and metabolic disorders in type II diabetic mice. J. Cell. Biochem. 118 (8), 2395–2408. https://doi.org/10.1002/jcb.25902.

Zhang, H., Gao, Q., Tan, S., et al., 2019. SET8 prevents excessive DNA methylation. Nucleic Acids Res. 47 (17), 9053–9068.

Zhang, X., Feng, H., Han, Y., Yuan, X., Jiang, M., Wang, W., Gao, L., 2024. Plaque stabilization and regression, from mechanisms to surveillance and clinical strategies. Rev. Cardiovasc. Med. 25 (12). https://doi.org/10.31083/j.rcm2512459.

Zhang, L.Y., Wang, Y.Y., Wen, R., Zhang, T.N., Yang, N., 2025. Role of histone deacetylase and inhibitors in cardiovascular diseases. Cell Prolif. 58 (12). https://doi.org/10.1111/cpr.70077.

Zhong, X., Liao, Y., Chen, L., Liu, G., Feng, Y., Zeng, T., Zhang, J., 2015. The MicroRNAs in the pathogenesis of metabolic memory. Endocrinology 156 (9), 3157–3168. https://doi.org/10.1210/en.2015-1063.

Zingg, J.-M., Vlad, A., Ricciarelli, R., 2021. Oxidized LDLs as signaling molecules. Antioxidants 10 (8), 1184. https://doi.org/10.3390/antiox10081184.

Zoltowska, M., Ziv, E., Delvin, E., Stan, S., Bar-On, H., Kalman, R., Levy, E., 2001. Circulating lipoproteins and hepatic sterol metabolism in Psammomys obesus prone to obesity, hyperglycemia and hyperinsulinemia. Atherosclerosis 157 (1), 85–96.

8

Obesity and metabolic memory

1. Introduction

Obesity has emerged as one of the most pressing public health challenges of the 21st century, affecting more than 650 million adults worldwide and driving a surge in metabolic diseases such as type 2 diabetes, cardiovascular disorders, and non-alcoholic fatty liver disease (Mohajan and Mohajan, 2023). Traditionally, obesity management has focused on the balance between caloric intake and energy expenditure, emphasizing the role of current lifestyle behaviors in driving weight gain and metabolic disruption (Kushner, 2018). However, this approach often fails to account for the persistent metabolic barriers that many individuals face, even after adopting healthier habits or achieving weight loss.

Recent advances in metabolic science have introduced a paradigm-shifting concept: metabolic memory, the phenomenon by which the body retains a long-lasting imprint of past metabolic states, particularly those shaped by chronic overnutrition, sedentary behavior, and inflammation. This "memory" is not simply a psychological or behavioral echo of previous habits but a biologically encoded legacy that affects hormonal regulation, energy metabolism, immune function, and gene expression (Dong et al., 2024). It helps explain why so many individuals regain weight after dieting, why insulin resistance can persist despite weight normalization, and why metabolic health improvements often lag behind lifestyle changes (Hinte et al., 2024).

Epigenetic changes are important contributors to the development and progression of obesity-related metabolic comorbidities. Diet, physical activity, hormones, and environmental exposures shape the epigenome by altering cellular metabolism and the availability of metabolites required for DNA and histone modifications. Diet regulates levels of acetyl-CoA, short-chain fatty acids, NAD^+, SAM, and UDP-GlcNAc, thereby influencing histone acetylation, DNA and histone methylation, and O-GlcNAcylation, which affect genes involved in mitochondrial function, inflammation, insulin resistance, and lipid metabolism

Metabolic Memory. https://doi.org/10.1016/B978-0-443-44591-0.00003-5

(Elshorbagy et al., 2013; Felix et al., 2021). Physical activity enhances mitochondrial biogenesis and energy metabolism, modifies DNA methylation and histone marks in skeletal muscle, and induces exercise "memory" through persistent epigenetic changes, with effects varying by training status, exercise type, and diet composition (Sexton et al., 2023).

Hormones interact directly with epigenetic enzymes and regulate their expression, while epigenetic modifications also control hormone signaling, hormonal disorders such as Cushing's syndrome and polycystic ovarian syndrome are associated with altered histone marks and DNA methylation linked to metabolic dysfunction (Bjune et al., 2022; García-Eguren et al., 2022). Endocrine-disrupting chemicals (EDCs) act as obesogens by disrupting hormone action and inducing heritable epimutations, with transgenerational obesity reported after exposure to compounds such as BPA and DDT (Skinner et al., 2018). Metabolic epigenetic circadian crosstalk further explains tissue-specific effects of diet, sleep loss, and exercise on DNA methylation and histone acetylation (Greco et al., 2020), while EDC-induced epigenetic alterations are enriched in hormone-responsive and lipid-rich tissues such as adipose tissue, liver, brain, and reproductive organs (Jefferson et al., 2023). Together, these stable yet reversible epigenetic changes can encode a form of metabolic memory, allowing prior obesogenic or metabolic exposures to exert long-lasting effects on gene expression and disease risk even after normalization of lifestyle factors.

Understanding metabolic memory is essential to reframing the narrative of obesity from one of personal failure to one grounded in physiological resilience and complexity. Rather than viewing obesity solely as a product of willpower or poor choices, this perspective acknowledges that past exposures, particularly prolonged periods of metabolic stress, can shape future responses, making it more difficult for individuals to achieve or maintain metabolic health (Alum, 2025).

This chapter delves into the intricate relationship between obesity and metabolic memory. It begins by exploring how obesity alters core metabolic processes, including energy expenditure, insulin signaling, adipose tissue function, and hormonal regulation. It then examines the scientific evidence linking past diet and physical activity to current metabolic states, highlighting the epigenetic, inflammatory, and endocrine pathways through which metabolic memory operates. Finally, it presents evidence-based strategies to break the cycle of metabolic memory, ranging from prolonged lifestyle interventions and nutrigenomic approaches to microbiome modulation, behavioural therapy, and pharmacological aids.

As we move toward an era of precision medicine and digital health, recognizing and addressing metabolic memory will be crucial in designing interventions that are not only more effective but also more compassionate and personalized. This chapter offers a roadmap for doing just that, by honouring the biological weight of the past while unlocking the potential for sustainable metabolic transformation in the future.

2. Obesity and metabolism

Obesity is defined as an excessive accumulation of body fat that presents significant risks to health and is associated with a host of chronic conditions including type 2 diabetes, cardiovascular disease, and certain cancers (Scully et al., 2021). Traditionally attributed to a simple imbalance between energy intake and energy expenditure, obesity is now recognized as a multifactorial metabolic disease with complex physiological underpinnings (Fig. 8.1) (Yárnoz-Esquiroz et al., 2022). Metabolism, which includes the myriad biochemical processes that sustain life, such as energy production, storage, and utilization, plays a pivotal role in the onset and persistence of obesity (Power and Thomas, 2011).

One of the primary metabolic components affected in obesity is the Basal Metabolic Rate (BMR), which refers to the amount of energy the body requires at rest to maintain vital functions such as breathing, circulation, and cellular repair. In individuals with

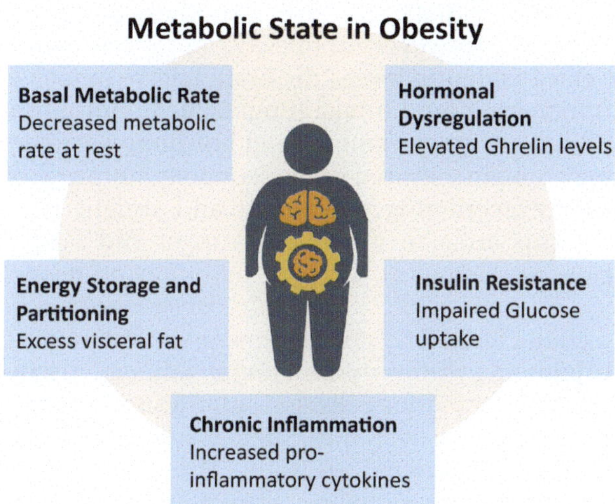

Figure 8.1 Metabolic dysfunctions underlying obesity. This figure illustrates the key physiological disturbances in obesity. These interconnected mechanisms contribute to persistent metabolic dysfunction and weight retention.

obesity, especially those undergoing weight loss, the body often adapts through a phenomenon known as adaptive thermogenesis, wherein the BMR decreases more than expected (Bastías-Pérez et al., 2020). This makes sustaining weight loss particularly challenging, as the body becomes more efficient at conserving energy, leading to a plateau in weight reduction and promoting weight regain.

Another critical metabolic feature of obesity is energy storage and partitioning. In a healthy metabolic state, energy from food is efficiently used or stored as glycogen and fat. However, in obesity, the body becomes biased toward excessive fat storage, particularly in visceral adipose tissue, fat that accumulates around internal organs. This type of fat is not merely a passive storage depot but acts as an active endocrine organ, secreting pro-inflammatory cytokines and adipokines that disrupt metabolic regulation and promote insulin resistance (Friedman et al., 2024).

Insulin resistance is one of the hallmark features of metabolic dysfunction in obesity (Tong et al., 2022). In this state, the body's tissues, particularly muscle, liver, and fat, become less responsive to insulin, a hormone critical for glucose uptake and utilization. As a result, blood glucose levels rise, prompting the pancreas to secrete even more insulin. This chronic hyperinsulinemia not only fails to correct the underlying resistance but also enhances lipogenesis (fat creation), suppresses fat breakdown, and contributes to further fat accumulation (Smith et al., 2020).

Hormonal dysregulation significantly contributes to the pathophysiology of obesity. Leptin, a hormone produced by adipocytes, typically signals satiety to the hypothalamus and regulates energy balance. However, in obesity, leptin resistance develops, despite elevated leptin levels, the brain fails to perceive satiety, leading to increased food intake (Engin, 2024). Additionally, levels of ghrelin, the hunger-stimulating hormone secreted by the stomach, may remain elevated or inadequately suppressed after meals, further exacerbating overeating and weight gain (Rossi et al., 2021). This imbalance between hunger and satiety hormones creates a physiological drive to maintain or regain weight.

Obesity is also characterized by chronic low-grade inflammation, primarily originating from dysfunctional adipose tissue (Khanna et al., 2022). Enlarged fat cells and infiltrating immune cells release pro-inflammatory cytokines, such as tumor necrosis factor-alpha (TNF-α) and interleukin-6 (IL-6). These inflammatory mediators disrupt insulin signaling, impair mitochondrial function, and exacerbate metabolic inflexibility, making it more difficult for the body to switch between fuel sources efficiently (Cortez et al., 2013). This inflammatory state is both a consequence and a driver of metabolic dysfunction, creating a vicious cycle that sustains obesity.

Understanding the dynamic and interconnected nature of these metabolic disturbances is essential. It reveals why obesity is not merely a matter of willpower or calorie counting but a deeply rooted metabolic condition. Importantly, it also provides the biological foundation upon which the concept of metabolic memory rests, wherein past metabolic insults, such as prolonged poor diet and inactivity, leave lasting molecular and physiological imprints that continue to affect metabolic health even after behavioral changes have been implemented.

3. How past diet and exercise influence current metabolism?

A growing body of research supports that the concept of metabolic memory, is particularly relevant in the context of obesity, where historical dietary patterns and physical activity levels can continue to shape metabolic outcomes long after visible weight has been lost or normalized (Dulloo and Montani, 2015). Despite a transition to healthier behaviors, individuals may face persistent metabolic challenges due to adaptations programmed by their previous lifestyle.

One of the most common manifestations of this phenomenon is post diet weight regain. Individuals who have lost weight, especially after prolonged periods of obesity, often encounter metabolic adaptation, a process by which the body lowers its resting metabolic rate (RMR) in response to reduced energy intake and body mass (Martin et al., 2022). This adaptation is not merely proportional to the amount of weight lost but often exceeds predictions, leading to a disproportionate drop in energy expenditure. Simultaneously, hunger-regulating hormones such as ghrelin increase, while satiety signals such as leptin decrease, making it physiologically more difficult to maintain the reduced weight. These hormonal shifts increase food cravings and drive energy conservation, tipping the energy balance toward weight regain (Chao et al., 2017).

Additionally, insulin resistance can persist even after substantial weight loss. In individuals with a history of chronic hyperinsulinemia, elevated insulin levels due to prolonged overnutrition, the cellular pathways involved in glucose uptake may remain dysfunctional (Schmitz et al., 2016). Although weight normalization can improve insulin sensitivity, epigenetic changes, mitochondrial dysfunction, and residual inflammation often hinder a complete reversal (Gasmi et al., 2021). This lingering insulin resistance can impair glucose handling and promote fat storage, particularly under conditions of minor dietary indiscretion.

Past dietary habits also influence fat distribution patterns, which significantly impact metabolic health. Overnutrition, especially in early life or during critical developmental windows, has been shown to predispose individuals to increased visceral adiposity, the accumulation of fat around internal organs (Morris, 2009). Unlike subcutaneous fat, visceral fat is more metabolically active and secretes higher levels of inflammatory cytokines and adipokines (Kolb, 2022). Even if total body weight returns to normal, the preferential deposition of fat in visceral stores increases the risk for metabolic syndrome, type 2 diabetes, and cardiovascular disease.

A lesser-known but critical consequence of long-term poor dietary habits is inflammatory priming of the immune system. Chronic exposure to excessive nutrients, particularly saturated fats and refined sugars, can "train" innate immune cells such as macrophages and neutrophils into a heightened inflammatory state. This phenomenon, known as trained immunity, leads to a persistently elevated inflammatory tone even in the absence of overt stimuli (Ochando et al., 2023). The resulting low-grade systemic inflammation disrupts insulin signaling, alters lipid metabolism, and contributes to ongoing metabolic dysfunction.

Therefore, the metabolic consequences of past dietary and activity patterns are not easily erased. They imprint on endocrine function, gene expression, tissue-specific metabolism, and immune system behavior, creating a resilient metabolic phenotype that resists change. Recognizing and addressing this legacy is essential in designing more effective obesity treatments that go beyond weight loss and focus on restoring metabolic integrity at a deeper, more durable level.

4. Epigenetic dysregulation in obesity

Obesity is associated with widespread alterations in DNA methylation across key metabolic tissues, reflecting the integration of environmental inputs such as diet, physical activity, and hormonal signals into long-term gene regulation. Diet-induced changes in one-carbon metabolism alter S-adenosylmethionine (SAM) availability, influencing DNA methyltransferase activity and methylation patterns (Sanderson et al., 2019). In humans, plasma SAM levels correlate positively with fat mass, truncal adiposity, insulin resistance (HOMA-IR), and overfeeding-induced weight gain (Lind et al., 2018). In adipose tissue, differential DNA methylation is linked to insulin resistance and metabolic syndrome, with consistent methylation expression changes observed in genes regulating mitochondrial function, integrin signaling, lipid metabolism, and glucose homeostasis (Arner et al., 2016; Sharma et al., 2020). Genome-wide analyses of blood DNA methylation identified loci associated with BMI and future type 2 diabetes risk, including ABCG1, which predicts incident T2D independently of adiposity (Do et al., 2023). Importantly, DNA methylation changes can persist after weight loss, contributing to "epigenetic memory" that predisposes individuals to weight regain (Hinte et al., 2024), and can also be transmitted across generations following obesogenic exposures such as endocrine-disrupting chemicals (EDCs) (Jung et al., 2022; Skinner et al., 2018).

Histone modifications dynamically respond to nutrient availability and cellular metabolism in obesity, linking metabolic state to chromatin accessibility and transcriptional control. Obesogenic diets alter acetyl-CoA and NAD^+ availability, reshaping histone acetylation through histone acetyltransferases and sirtuin deacetylases (Tam et al., 2020; Carrer et al., 2017). Exercise-induced changes in histone marks, including H3K4me1 and H3K27ac, modulate enhancer activity in skeletal muscle genes involved in oxidative metabolism and mitochondrial biogenesis (Williams et al., 2021). In mouse models, histone-modifying enzymes play causal roles in obesity-related phenotypes: KMT2D/MLL4 promotes hepatic steatosis through H3K4me1 at PPARγ2-binding sites (Kim et al., 2016), PHF2 protects against diet-induced steatohepatitis by erasing repressive H3K9me2 marks at ChREBP target genes (Bricambert et al., 2018), and EZH2 regulates lipid uptake and adipocyte hypertrophy via H3K27 methylation (Yiew et al., 2019). Persistent histone modifications in adipocytes following high-fat diet exposure underlie obesogenic "epigenetic memory," predisposing to accelerated weight regain after weight loss (Hinte et al., 2024), highlighting the long-term chromatin imprinting of prior metabolic stress.

Obesity is associated with altered expression of miRNAs that regulate insulin sensitivity, adipogenesis, mitochondrial metabolism, and inflammatory pathways. Epigenetic regulation of miRNA genes is influenced by metabolic and redox states, with reactive oxygen species (ROS) modulating miRNA expression through promoter hypermethylation or transcriptional control (Louwagie and Vu, 2024). Exercise and dietary interventions induce dynamic changes in miRNA profiles in skeletal muscle and circulation, contributing to metabolic remodelling and improved insulin sensitivity (Kovac et al., 2024; Müller et al., 2024). In animal models, obesity-associated miRNA dysregulation contributes to impaired mitochondrial function and lipid handling, while EDC exposure induces heritable epigenetic alterations affecting regulatory elements that control appetite and energy homeostasis (Tolu et al., 2025). Together, these findings suggest that miRNAs act as both mediators and biomarkers of obesogenic stress, potentially participating in feed-forward loops with DNA methylation and histone modifications to sustain metabolic dysfunction across time and, in some contexts, across generations (Odimegwu et al., 2024).

5. Strategies for breaking the cycle of metabolic memory in obesity

While metabolic memory presents a formidable obstacle in the management of obesity, it is not immutable. Advances in our understanding of metabolic plasticity have revealed that with the right combination of interventions, applied consistently and over the long term, it is possible to reprogram dysfunctional metabolic pathways and attenuate the lingering effects of past lifestyle habits. The key lies in adopting multifaceted and sustained strategies that go beyond short-term fixes to effect lasting physiological change (Fig. 8.2).

5.1 Prolonged lifestyle intervention

Metabolic memory is not formed overnight, and similarly, it cannot be erased by transient efforts. Sustained lifestyle modification, over months or even years, is essential to disrupt entrenched metabolic patterns (Wadden et al., 2020). Long-term caloric restriction, regular physical activity, and nutrient-dense dietary choices are necessary to restore hormonal balance, improve insulin sensitivity, and shift body composition favorably.

One effective approach is intermittent fasting or periodic caloric restriction, which has been shown to modulate critical metabolic processes. These interventions can stimulate autophagy, a cellular cleansing process that removes damaged organelles and improves mitochondrial efficiency (Hwangbo et al., 2020). Additionally, fasting regimens enhance insulin sensitivity and reduce chronic inflammation, both of which are central to countering metabolic dysfunction (Liang et al., 2021).

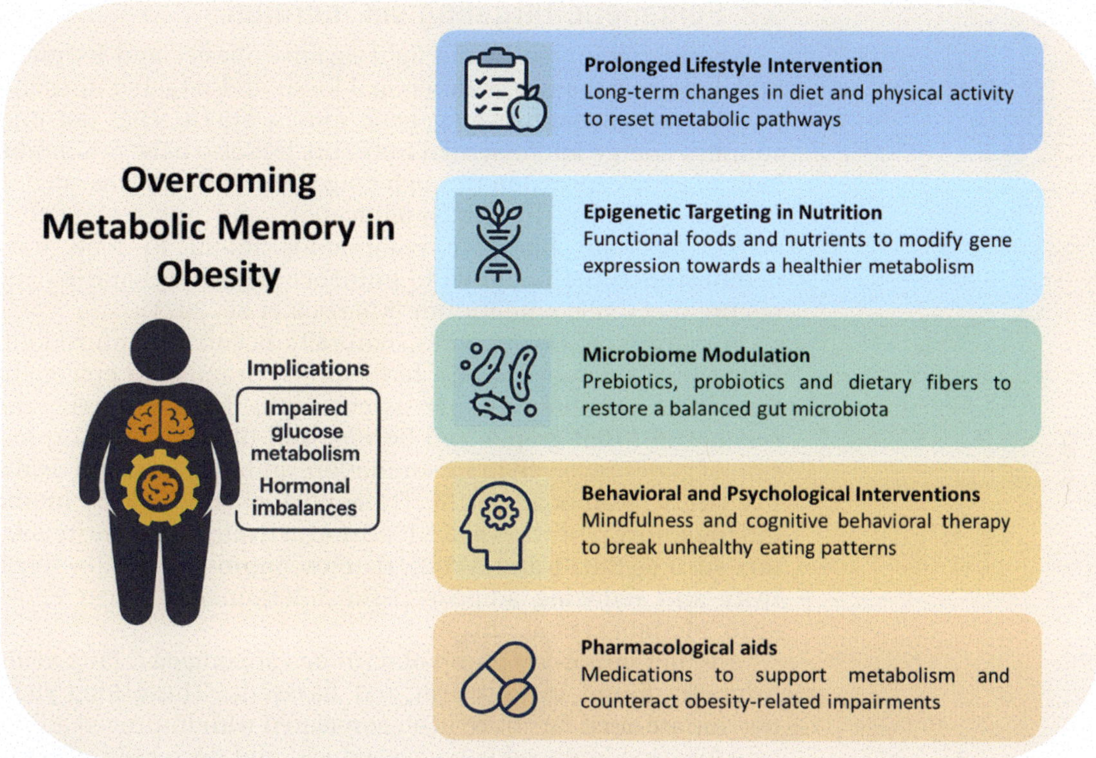

Figure 8.2 Overcoming metabolic memory in obesity: A multifaceted approach. This infographic presents five synergistic strategies, lifestyle intervention, nutritional epigenetics, microbiome modulation, behavioral therapy, and pharmacological aids, aimed at reversing metabolic memory in obesity. Each component targets a distinct yet interconnected mechanism to restore metabolic health.

Physical activity, particularly resistance training and high-intensity interval training (HIIT), plays a pivotal role in this transformation. Unlike steady-state cardio, these forms of exercise stimulate mitochondrial biogenesis, enhance muscle glucose uptake, and promote epigenetic remodeling of key metabolic genes (Crea, 2024). Resistance training also helps preserve or increase lean muscle mass, which in turn elevates basal metabolic rate (BMR), offsetting the adaptive thermogenesis commonly seen after weight loss (Mukherjee et al., 2020).

Furthermore, exercise acts as a natural antiinflammatory agent, reducing the secretion of pro-inflammatory adipokines and improving immune cell function. These benefits are not merely acute but accumulate over time, gradually reshaping the metabolic landscape.

5.2 Epigenetic targeting via nutrition

An emerging area in the fight against obesity and its metabolic legacy is the use of functional foods and targeted nutrients to reverse maladaptive epigenetic modifications. Diet not only supplies energy and essential nutrients but also acts as a modulator of gene expression through epigenetic mechanisms such as DNA methylation, histone modification, and non-coding RNA activity. Certain bioactive compounds found in food have demonstrated the potential to influence these mechanisms and restore metabolic equilibrium (Mierziak et al., 2021).

For instance, polyphenols, naturally occurring antioxidants found in plant-based foods, have shown promise in epigenetic regulation. Compounds such as curcumin (from turmeric) and resveratrol (from grapes and berries) can modulate the expression of genes involved in inflammation, adipogenesis, and oxidative stress (Tian et al., 2016). These phytochemicals may inhibit inflammatory pathways like NF-κB and activate metabolic regulators such as SIRT1 and AMPK, thereby improving insulin sensitivity and reducing adipose tissue inflammation (Tian et al., 2016; Mojtabavi et al., 2023).

Another important group of nutrients are omega-3 fatty acids, primarily found in fatty fish and flaxseeds. These long-chain polyunsaturated fats have been associated with improved adipocyte function, reduced hepatic steatosis, and decreased systemic inflammation (Lee et al., 2020). Omega-3s may also influence DNA methylation patterns in genes involved in lipid metabolism, contributing to a more metabolically favorable gene expression profile (Frankhouser et al., 2022).

Incorporating such nutrigenomic strategies into daily dietary patterns holds promise in reversing or mitigating the epigenetic imprints of obesity, thus breaking the cycle of metabolic memory and enabling more successful weight management outcomes.

5.3 Microbiome modulation

The gut microbiome, a dynamic community of trillions of microorganisms residing in the gastrointestinal tract, has emerged as a crucial player in energy homeostasis, immune regulation, and metabolic signaling. Past dietary habits, particularly those high in saturated fats and refined sugars, can induce long-lasting shifts in the composition and function of the gut microbiota, reinforcing obesity-related inflammation and insulin resistance (Deledda et al., 2021). Consequently, restoring a healthy microbial balance is a strategic avenue for reversing metabolic memory.

One key approach involves the use of prebiotics and probiotics. Prebiotics, non-digestible fibers that serve as food for beneficial bacteria, can stimulate the growth of antiinflammatory bacterial strains, improve gut barrier integrity, and promote metabolic flexibility (Liu et al., 2022; Camilleri, 2021). Probiotics, on the other hand, introduce beneficial live microorganisms that can suppress harmful bacterial populations, enhance short-chain fatty acid (SCFA) production, and modulate host immune responses (Liu et al., 2022; Camilleri, 2021).

A fiber-rich diet supports microbial diversity and increases the production of SCFAs such as butyrate, propionate, and acetate, which serve as signaling molecules influencing energy metabolism, inflammation, and satiety regulation (Zhao et al., 2019). These SCFAs also interact with G-protein-coupled receptors and influence the secretion of gut hormones like GLP-1 and PYY, thereby enhancing insulin sensitivity and appetite control (Alhabeeb et al., 2021).

By actively reshaping the gut microbiome through dietary interventions and supplementation, individuals may be able to counteract the microbial imprint left by years of poor dietary choices and restore a more balanced metabolic environment.

5.4 Behavioral and psychological interventions

Behavioral patterns formed during periods of weight gain and poor lifestyle choices can become deeply ingrained, contributing to the persistence of metabolic memory. Thus, breaking the cycle of obesity is not only a biological challenge but also a psychological one. Interventions targeting cognitive, emotional, and behavioral components are essential to achieving long-term success (Steptoe and Frank, 2023).

Mindful eating has emerged as an effective strategy to recalibrate the brain's reward and appetite systems. By cultivating conscious awareness of hunger and satiety cues, individuals learn to differentiate between physiological hunger and emotional or environmental triggers for eating (Warren et al., 2017). This practice helps reduce binge eating, emotional eating, and mindless snacking, common behaviors associated with weight regain and poor metabolic outcomes.

Additionally, Cognitive Behavioral Therapy (CBT) offers structured psychological support to address the cognitive distortions and maladaptive habits surrounding food, body image, and self-regulation. CBT assists individuals in identifying negative thought patterns, such as all-or-nothing thinking or self-defeating beliefs, and replacing them with healthier, goal-oriented behaviors

(Cha et al., 2025). These interventions are particularly effective in managing relapse prevention, enhancing motivation, and fostering sustainable behavioral change, all of which are critical to reversing the behavioral conditioning that underlies metabolic memory.

5.5 Pharmacological aids

For individuals with persistent metabolic impairments despite lifestyle interventions, pharmacological agents may provide necessary support to override metabolic inertia. These medications can modulate pathways related to appetite regulation, insulin signaling, and energy expenditure, key nodes that are often altered in those with a history of obesity.

GLP-1 receptor agonists (Table 8.1) have shown profound efficacy in reducing appetite, promoting weight loss, and improving glycemic control (Camilleri and Lupianez-Merly, 2024). They mimic the action of glucagon-like peptide-1, enhancing insulin secretion and slowing gastric emptying, which supports better postprandial glucose regulation and satiety. SGLT2 inhibitors, primarily used in the management of type 2 diabetes, promote urinary glucose excretion, thereby lowering blood glucose levels and facilitating modest weight reduction. These agents also provide cardiorenal protective benefits, making them valuable in obese patients with metabolic syndrome or type 2 diabetes (Vallon and Thomson, 2017).

Metformin, one of the most commonly prescribed antidiabetics drugs, improves hepatic insulin sensitivity, suppresses hepatic glucose production, and modulates the gut microbiota (Lee et al., 2018). It also appears to influence epigenetic markers and may reduce inflammation, offering additional benefits in breaking the cycle of metabolic memory (Li et al., 2022). In select cases, the integration of pharmacotherapy with lifestyle and behavioral interventions can provide a multidimensional approach to obesity treatment, especially for those who face persistent metabolic resistance or comorbidities (Lv et al., 2022).

6. Future perspectives

As our understanding of metabolic memory deepens, the future of obesity treatment is moving toward precision medicine—a model that recognizes individual variation in genetics, environment, and lifestyle. Advances in genomic, epigenomic, transcriptomic, and metabolomic profiling offer unprecedented opportunities to identify biomarkers that reflect an individual's

Table 8.1 GLP-1 receptor agonists and related therapies (Wang et al., 2023).

Drug	Type	Dosing frequency	Typical dose	Indications	Key effects
Beinaglutide (BN)	Short-acting	3x/day	0.1–0.2 mg	T2DM, obesity, NASH	↓ BMI, glucose, inflammation, ↑ insulin sensitivity
Exenatide (EX)	Short-acting	2x/day	0.2 μg/kg	T2DM, obesity, PCOS	↓ glucose, appetite, ↑ insulin, nausea common
Lixisenatide (LIXI)	Long-acting (daily)	1x/day	Variable	T2DM	↓ HbA1c, cholesterol, well-tolerated
Liraglutide (LIR)	Long-acting (daily)	1x/day	1.2–3 mg	T2DM, obesity	↓ appetite, glucose, body weight (up to 9.2 kg)
Semaglutide (SMG)	Long-acting (weekly)	1x/week	1–2.4 mg	T2DM, obesity	↓ weight (up to 15.3 kg), mild GI effects
Dulaglutide (DUL)	Long-acting (weekly)	1x/week	0.75–4.5 mg	T2DM	↓ weight (~2.9 kg), potential for pancreatitis
Exenatide-LAR	Long-acting (weekly)	1x/week	2 mg	T2DM, obesity	Sustained release, ~3.7 kg weight loss
PEG loxenatide (PEX-168)	Long-acting (weekly)	1x/week	0.03–0.33 mg/kg	T2DM, obesity	↓ weight (up to 3.3 kg), mild GI effects
Tirzepatide	Dual GIPR/GLP-1R	1x/week	5–15 mg	T2DM, obesity	↓ weight (5.4–11.7 kg), more effective than GLP-1 alone
Peptide 20	Triple GIPR/GLP-1R/GCGR	Experimental	N/A	Obesity	↑ energy expenditure, ↓ weight (animal studies)

metabolic history and risk of persistent dysregulation. These molecular insights can guide personalized therapeutic strategies, ensuring that interventions are biologically congruent with each person's metabolic trajectory and responsiveness.

In addition, digital health technologies are revolutionizing how we monitor and manage metabolism in real-time. Tools such as continuous glucose monitors (CGMs), wearable fitness trackers, and AI-powered diet and activity apps can dynamically track metabolic responses to food, exercise, stress, and sleep. This enables just-in-time adjustments to diet, medication, or behavior and enhances patient engagement and adherence. Furthermore, machine learning algorithms can analyze these data streams to detect early signs of metabolic drift and suggest preemptive interventions, creating a feedback-informed, adaptive care model.

As these technologies become more accessible, they hold the potential to democratize precision obesity care, shifting the paradigm from generalized guidelines to data-driven, individualized treatment plans that can better address the complexities of metabolic memory.

7. Conclusion

Metabolic memory presents a formidable but not insurmountable challenge in the treatment of obesity. It underscores the fact that health outcomes are shaped not only by current behaviors but also by the accumulated effects of past dietary patterns, physical activity levels, and metabolic insults. This recognition compels a shift in both patient and clinician expectations—away from short-term fixes and toward long-term, holistic, and personalized interventions.

Although reversing metabolic memory requires sustained effort, research and clinical evidence affirm that with persistent lifestyle modification, strategic nutritional and behavioral therapies, and appropriate pharmacological or microbiome-targeted interventions, the negative legacy of past metabolic dysfunction can be overcome. The integration of precision medicine and digital health tools promises to further refine our approach, making metabolic rehabilitation more effective and accessible.

Ultimately, transforming obesity care means acknowledging the weight of the past while embracing the possibilities of the future. By combining insights from cutting-edge science with patient-centered care, we can break the cycle of metabolic memory and pave the way toward lasting metabolic health.

References

Alhabeeb, H., AlFaiz, A., Kutbi, E., AlShahrani, D., Alsuhail, A., AlRajhi, S., Alotaibi, N., Alotaibi, K., AlAmri, S., Saleh, A., AlJohani, N., 2021. Gut hormones in health and obesity: The upcoming role of short chain fatty acids. Nutrients 13 (2), 481. https://doi.org/10.3390/nu13020481.

Alum, E.U., 2025. Metabolic memory in obesity: Can early-life interventions reverse lifelong risks? Obes. Med. 55, 100610. https://doi.org/10.1016/j.obmed.2025.100610.

Arner, P., Sahlqvist, A.S., Sinha, I., Xu, H., Yao, X., Waterworth, D., Rajpal, D., Loomis, A.K., Freudenberg, J.M., Johnson, T., Thorell, A., Näslund, E., Ryden, M., Dahlman, I., 2016. The epigenetic signature of systemic insulin resistance in obese women. Diabetologia 59 (11), 2393–2405. https://doi.org/10.1007/s00125-016-4074-5.

Bastías-Pérez, M., Zagmutt, S., Soler-Vázquez, M.C., Serra, D., Mera, P., Herrero, L., 2020. Impact of adaptive thermogenesis in mice on the treatment of obesity. Cells 9 (2), 316. https://doi.org/10.3390/cells9020316.

Bjune, J.I., Strømland, P.P., Jersin, R.Å., Mellgren, G., Dankel, S.N., 2022. Metabolic and epigenetic regulation by estrogen in adipocytes. Front. Endocrinol. 13. https://doi.org/10.3389/fendo.2022.828780. https://www.frontiersin.org/journals/endocrinology#.

Bricambert, J., Alves-Guerra, M.C., Esteves, P., Prip-Buus, C., Bertrand-Michel, J., Guillou, H., Chang, C.J., Vander Wal, M.N., Canonne-Hergaux, F., Mathurin, P., Raverdy, V., Pattou, F., Girard, J., Postic, C., Dentin, R., 2018. The histone demethylase Phf2 acts as a molecular checkpoint to prevent NAFLD progression during obesity. Nat. Commun. 9 (1). https://doi.org/10.1038/s41467-018-04361-y. http://www.nature.com/ncomms/index.html.

Camilleri, M., 2021. Human intestinal barrier: Effects of stressors, diet, prebiotics, and probiotics. Clin. Transl. Gastroenterol. 12 (1), e00308. https://doi.org/10.14309/ctg.0000000000000308.

Camilleri, M., Lupianez-Merly, C., 2024. Effects of GLP-1 and other gut hormone receptors on the gastrointestinal tract and implications in clinical practice. Am. J. Gastroenterol. 119 (6), 1028–1037. https://doi.org/10.14309/ajg.0000000000002519.

Carrer, A., Parris, J.L.D., Trefely, S., Henry, R.A., Montgomery, D.C., Torres, A., Viola, J.M., Kuo, Y.M., Blair, I.A., Meier, J.L., Andrews, A.J., Snyder, N.W., Wellen, K.E., 2017. Impact of a high-fat diet on tissue Acyl-CoA and histone acetylation levels. J. Biol. Chem. 292 (8), 3312–3322. https://doi.org/10.1074/jbc.M116.750620.

Cha, J.Y., Kim, S.Y., Lim, Y.W., Choi, K.H., Shin, I.S., 2025. Comparative effectiveness of cognitive behavioral therapy and behavioral therapy in obesity: A systematic review and network meta-analysis. J. Clin. Psychol. Med. Settings 32 (1), 96–110. https://doi.org/10.1007/s10880-023-10000-6.

Chao, A.M., Jastreboff, A.M., White, M.A., Grilo, C.M., Sinha, R., 2017. Stress, cortisol, and other appetite-related hormones: Prospective prediction of 6-month changes in food cravings and weight. Obesity 25 (4), 713–720. https://doi.org/10.1002/oby.21790. http://onlinelibrary.wiley.com/journal/10.1002/(ISSN)1930-739X.

Cortez, M., Carmo, L.S., Rogero, M.M., Borelli, P., Fock, R.A., 2013. A high-fat diet increases IL-1, IL-6, and TNF-α production by increasing NF-κb and attenuating PPAR-γ expression in bone marrow mesenchymal stem cells. Inflammation 36 (2), 379–386. https://doi.org/10.1007/s10753-012-9557-z.

Crea, E., 2024. Effects of repeated high-intensity interval training interventions on oxidative metabolism adaptations in human skeletal muscle.

Deledda, A., Annunziata, G., Carlo Tenore, G., Palmas, V., Manzin, A., Velluzzi, F., 2021. Diet-derived antioxidants and their role in inflammation, obesity and gut microbiota modulation. Antioxidants 10 (5), 708. https://doi.org/10.3390/antiox10050708.

Do, W.L., Sun, D., Meeks, K., Dugué, P.A., Demerath, E., Guan, W., Li, S., Chen, W., Milne, R., Adeyemo, A., Agyemang, C., Nassir, R., Manson, J.A.E., Shadyab, A.H., Hou, L., Horvath, S., Assimes, T.L., Bhatti, P., Jordahl, K.M., Baccarelli, A.A., Smith, A.K., Staimez, L.R., Stein, A.D., Whitsel, E.A., Narayan, K.M.V., Conneely, K.N., 2023. Epigenome-wide meta-analysis of BMI in nine cohorts: Examining the utility of epigenetically predicted BMI.

Am. J. Hum. Genet. 110 (2), 273–283. https://doi.org/10.1016/j.ajhg.2022.12.014.

Dong, H., Sun, Y., Nie, L., Cui, A., Zhao, P., Leung, W.K., Wang, Q., 2024. Metabolic memory: Mechanisms and diseases. Signal Transduct. Targeted Ther. 9 (1). https://doi.org/10.1038/s41392-024-01755-x. https://www.nature.com/sigtrans.

Dulloo, A.G., Montani, J.-P., 2015. Pathways from dieting to weight regain, to obesity and to the metabolic syndrome: An overview. Obes. Rev. 16 (S1), 1–6. https://doi.org/10.1111/obr.12250.

Elshorbagy, A.K., Nijpels, G., Valdivia-Garcia, M., Stehouwer, C.D.A., Ocke, M., Refsum, H., Dekker, J.M., 2013. S-adenosylmethionine is associated with fat mass and truncal adiposity in older adults. J. Nutr. 143 (12), 1982–1988. https://doi.org/10.3945/jn.113.179192.

Engin, A., 2024. The mechanism of leptin resistance in obesity and therapeutic perspective. Obes. Lipotoxicity 1460, 463–487. https://doi.org/10.1007/978-3-031-63657-8_16.

Felix, J.B., Cox, A.R., Hartig, S.M., 2021. Acetyl-CoA and metabolite fluxes regulate white adipose tissue expansion. Trends Endocrinol. Metabol. 32 (5), 320–332. https://doi.org/10.1016/j.tem.2021.02.008.

Frankhouser, D.E., Steck, S., Sovic, M.G., Belury, M.A., Wang, Q., Clinton, S.K., Bundschuh, R., Yan, P.S., Yee, L.D., 2022. Dietary omega-3 fatty acid intake impacts peripheral blood DNA methylation -anti-inflammatory effects and individual variability in a pilot study. JNB (J. Nutr. Biochem.) 99. https://doi.org/10.1016/j.jnutbio.2021.108839. www.elsevier.com/locate/jnutbio.

Friedman, M.I., Sørensen, T.I.A., Taubes, G., Lund, J., Ludwig, D.S., 2024. Trapped fat: obesity pathogenesis as an intrinsic disorder in metabolic fuel partitioning. Obes. Rev. 25 (10). https://doi.org/10.1111/obr.13795. http://onlinelibrary.wiley.com/journal/10.1111/(ISSN)1467-789X.

García-Eguren, G., González-Ramírez, M., Vizán, P., Giró, O., Vega-Beyhart, A., Boswell, L., Mora, M., Halperin, I., Carmona, F., Gracia, M., Casals, G., Squarcia, M., Enseñat, J., Vidal, O., Di Croce, L., Hanzu, F.A., 2022. Glucocorticoid-induced fingerprints on visceral adipose tissue transcriptome and epigenome. J. Clin. Endocrinol. Metabol. 107 (1), 150–166. https://doi.org/10.1210/clinem/dgab662.

Gasmi, A., Noor, S., Menzel, A., Dosa, A., Pivina, L., Bjørklund, G., 2021. Obesity and insulin resistance: associations with chronic inflammation, genetic and epigenetic factors. Curr. Med. Chem. 28 (4), 800–826. https://doi.org/10.2174/0929867327666200824112056.

Greco, C.M., Cervantes, M., Fustin, J.M., Ito, K., Ceglia, N., Samad, M., Shi, J., Koronowski, K.B., Forne, I., Ranjit, S., Gaucher, J., Kinouchi, K., Kojima, R., Gratton, E., Li, W., Baldi, P., Imhof, A., Okamura, H., Sassone-Corsi, P., 2020. S-adenosyl-l-homocysteine hydrolase links methionine metabolism to the circadian clock and chromatin remodeling. Sci. Adv. 6 (51). https://doi.org/10.1126/sciadv.abc5629. https://advances.sciencemag.org/content/advances/6/51/eabc5629.full.pdf.

Hinte, L.C., Castellano-Castillo, D., Ghosh, A., Melrose, K., Gasser, E., Noé, F., Massier, L., Dong, H., Sun, W., Hoffmann, A., Wolfrum, C., Rydén, M., Mejhert, N., Blüher, M., von Meyenn, F., 2024. Adipose tissue retains an epigenetic memory of obesity after weight loss. Nature 636 (8042), 457–465. https://doi.org/10.1038/s41586-024-08165-7.

Hwangbo, D.S., Lee, H.Y., Abozaid, L.S., Min, K.J., 2020. Mechanisms of lifespan regulation by calorie restriction and intermittent fasting in model organisms. Nutrients 12 (4). https://doi.org/10.3390/nu12041194. https://www.mdpi.com/2072-6643/12/4/1194/pdf.

Jefferson, T.B., Wang, T., Jefferson, W.N., Li, Y., Hamilton, K.J., Wade, P.A., Williams, C.J., Korach, K.S., 2023. Multiple tissue-specific epigenetic alterations regulate persistent gene expression changes following developmental DES exposure in mouse reproductive tissues. Epigenetics 18 (1). https://doi.org/10.1080/15592294.2022.2139986. http://www.tandfonline.com/toc/kepi20/current.

Jung, Y.H., Wang, H.L.V., Ruiz, D., Bixler, B.J., Linsenbaum, H., Xiang, J.F., Forestier, S., Shafik, A.M., Jin, P., Corces, V.G., 2022. Recruitment of CTCF to an Fto enhancer is responsible for transgenerational inheritance of BPA-induced obesity. Proc. Natl. Acad. Sci. U. S. A 119 (50). https://doi.org/10.1073/pnas.2214988119. https://www.pnas.org/doi/10.1073/pnas.2214988119.

Khanna, D., Khanna, S., Khanna, P., Kahar, P., Patel, B.M., 2022. Obesity: A chronic low-grade inflammation and its markers. Cureus 14 (2). https://doi.org/10.7759/cureus.22711.

Kim, D.H., Kim, J., Kwon, J.S., Sandhu, J., Tontonoz, P., Lee, S.K., Lee, S., Lee, J. W., 2016. Critical roles of the histone methyltransferase MLL4/KMT2D in murine hepatic steatosis directed by ABL1 and PPARγ2. Cell Rep. 17 (6), 1671–1682. https://doi.org/10.1016/j.celrep.2016.10.023.

Kolb, H., 2022. Obese visceral fat tissue inflammation: from protective to detrimental? BMC Med. 20 (1). https://doi.org/10.1186/s12916-022-02672-y.

Kovac, L., Gancheva, S., Jähnert, M., Sehgal, R., Mastrototaro, L., Schlensak, M., Granderath, F.A., Rittig, K., Roden, M., Schürmann, A., Kahl, S., Ouni, M., 2024. Different effects of bariatric surgery on epigenetic plasticity in skeletal muscle of individuals with and without type 2 diabetes. Diabetes Metabol. 50 (5), 101561. https://doi.org/10.1016/j.diabet.2024.101561.

Kushner, R.F., 2018. Weight loss strategies for treatment of obesity: Lifestyle management and pharmacotherapy. Prog. Cardiovasc. Dis. 61 (2), 246–252. https://doi.org/10.1016/j.pcad.2018.06.001.

Lee, C.H., Fu, Y., Yang, S.J., Chi, C.C., 2020. Effects of Omega-3 polyunsaturated fatty acid supplementation on non-alcoholic fatty liver: A systematic review and meta-analysis. Nutrients 12 (9), 1–20. https://doi.org/10.3390/nu12092769.

Lee, H., Lee, Y., Kim, J., An, J., Lee, S., Kong, H., Song, Y., Lee, C.K., Kim, K., 2018. Modulation of the gut microbiota by metformin improves metabolic profiles in aged obese mice. Gut Microbes 9 (2), 155–165. https://doi.org/10.1080/19490976.2017.1405209.

Li, M., Bao, L., Zhu, P., Wang, S., 2022. Effect of metformin on the epigenetic age of peripheral blood in patients with diabetes mellitus. Front. Genet. 13. https://doi.org/10.3389/fgene.2022.955835.

Liang, B.J., Liao, S.R., Huang, W.X., Huang, C., Liu, H.S., Shen, W.Z., 2021. Intermittent fasting therapy promotes insulin sensitivity by inhibiting nlrp3 inflammasome in rat model. Ann. Palliat. Med. 10 (5), 5299–5309. https://doi.org/10.21037/apm-20-2410.

Lind, M.V., Lauritzen, L., Vestergaard, H., Hansen, T., Pedersen, O., Kristensen, M., Ross, A.B., 2018. One-carbon metabolism markers are associated with cardiometabolic risk factors. Nutr. Metabol. Cardiovasc. Dis. 28 (4), 402–410. https://doi.org/10.1016/j.numecd.2018.01.005.

Liu, Y., Wang, J., Wu, C., 2022. Modulation of gut microbiota and immune system by probiotics, pre-biotics, and post-biotics. Front. Nutr. 8. https://doi.org/10.3389/fnut.2021.634897.

Louwagie, A., Vu, L.P., 2024. Emerging interactions between RNA methylation and chromatin architecture. Curr. Opin. Genet. Dev. 89, 102270. https://doi.org/10.1016/j.gde.2024.102270.

Lv, N., Kringle, E.A., Ma, J., 2022. Integrated behavioral interventions for adults with comorbid obesity and depression: A systematic review. Curr. Diabetes Rep. 22 (4), 157–168. https://doi.org/10.1007/s11892-022-01458-z.

Martin, A., Fox, D., Murphy, C.A., Hofmann, H., Koehler, K., 2022. Tissue losses and metabolic adaptations both contribute to the reduction in resting metabolic rate following weight loss. Int. J. Obes. 46 (6), 1168–1175. https://doi.org/10.1038/s41366-022-01090-7.

Mierziak, J., Kostyn, K., Boba, A., Czemplik, M., Kulma, A., Wojtasik, W., 2021. Influence of the bioactive diet components on the gene expression regulation. Nutrients 13 (11), 3673. https://doi.org/10.3390/nu13113673.

Mohajan, D., Mohajan, H.K., 2023. Obesity and its related diseases: A new escalating alarming in global health. J. Innov. Med. Res. 2 (3), 12–23. https://doi.org/10.56397/jimr/2023.03.04.

Mojtabavi, S., Amin, S., Aboulfazli, S., Ali, K., Najafi, M., Jafari-Sabet, M., Ziar, A., Ebrahimi, N., Habibeh Mirmajidi, S., Ataee, R., 2023. Evaluation of curcumin effect on Il6, Sirt1, TNFα and NFkB expression of liver tissues in diabetic mice with STZ. J. Diabetes Metab. Disord. 22 (1), 205–215. https://doi.org/10.1007/s40200-022-01090-4.

Morris, M.J., 2009. Early life influences on obesity risk: Maternal overnutrition and programming of obesity. Expert Rev. Endocrinol. Metabol. 4 (6), 625–637. https://doi.org/10.1586/eem.09.45Australia. http://www.expert-reviews.com/doi/pdf/10.1586/eem.09.45.

Mukherjee, S.D., Koch, L.G., Britton, S.L., Novak, C.M., 2020. Aerobic capacity modulates adaptive thermogenesis: Contribution of non-resting energy expenditure. Physiol. Behav. 225, 113048. https://doi.org/10.1016/j.physbeh.2020.113048.

Müller, L., Hoffmann, A., Bernhart, S.H., Ghosh, A., Zhong, J., Hagemann, T., Sun, W., Dong, H., Noé, F., Wolfrum, C., Dietrich, A., Stumvoll, M., Massier, L., Blüher, M., Kovacs, P., Chakaroun, R., Keller, M., 2024. Blood methylation pattern reflects epigenetic remodelling in adipose tissue after bariatric surgery. EBioMedicine 106, 105242. https://doi.org/10.1016/j.ebiom.2024.105242.

Ochando, J., Mulder, W.J.M., Madsen, J.C., Netea, M.G., Duivenvoorden, R., 2023. Trained immunity — basic concepts and contributions to immunopathology. Nat. Rev. Nephrol. 19 (1), 23–37. https://doi.org/10.1038/s41581-022-00633-5.

Odimegwu, C.L., Uwaezuoke, S.N., Chikani, U.N., Mbanefo, N.R., Adiele, K.D., Nwolisa, C.E., Eneh, C.I., Ndiokwelu, C.O., Okpala, S.C., Ogbuka, F.N., Odo, K.E., Ohuche, I.O., Obiora-Izuka, C.E., 2024. Targeting the epigenetic marks in type 2 diabetes mellitus: Will epigenetic therapy Be a valuable adjunct to pharmacotherapy? Diabetes Metab. Syndr. Obes. 17, 3557–3576. https://doi.org/10.2147/DMSO.S479077.

Power, C., Thomas, C., 2011. Changes in BMI, duration of overweight and obesity, and glucose metabolism: 45 Years of follow-up of a birth cohort. Diabetes Care 34 (9), 1986–1991. https://doi.org/10.2337/dc10-1482.

Rossi, E., Cassioli, E., Gironi, V., Idrizaj, E., Garella, R., Squecco, R., Baccari, M. C., Maggi, M., Vignozzi, L., Comeglio, P., Ricca, V., Castellini, G., 2021. Ghrelin as a possible biomarker and maintaining factor in patients with eating disorders reporting childhood traumatic experiences. Eur. Eat. Disord. Rev. 29 (4), 588–599. https://doi.org/10.1002/erv.2831.

Sanderson, S.M., Gao, X., Dai, Z., Locasale, J.W., 2019. Methionine metabolism in health and cancer: A nexus of diet and precision medicine. Nat. Rev. Cancer 19 (11), 625–637. https://doi.org/10.1038/s41568-019-0187-8.

Schmitz, J., Evers, N., Awazawa, M., Nicholls, H.T., Brönneke, H.S., Dietrich, A., Mauer, J., Blüher, M., Brüning, J.C., 2016. Obesogenic memory can confer long-term increases in adipose tissue but not liver inflammation and insulin resistance after weight loss. Mol. Metabol. 5 (5), 328–339. https://doi.org/10.1016/j.molmet.2015.12.001.

Scully, T., Ettela, A., LeRoith, D., Gallagher, E.J., 2021. Obesity, type 2 diabetes, and cancer risk. Front. Oncol. 10. https://doi.org/10.3389/fonc.2020.615375. http://www.frontiersin.org/Oncology/about.

Sexton, C.L., Godwin, J.S., McIntosh, M.C., Ruple, B.A., Osburn, S.C., Hollingsworth, B.R., Kontos, N.J., Agostinelli, P.J., Kavazis, A.N., Ziegenfuss, T.N., Lopez, H.L., Smith, R., Young, K.C., Dwaraka, V.B., Frugé, A.D., Mobley, C.B., Sharples, A.P., Roberts, M.D., 2023. Skeletal muscle DNA methylation and mRNA responses to a bout of higher versus lower load resistance exercise in previously trained men. Cells 12 (2). https://doi.org/10.3390/cells12020263. https://www.mdpi.com/journal/cells.

Sharma, N.K., Comeau, M.E., Montoya, D., Pellegrini, M., Howard, T.D., Langefeld, C.D., Das, S.K., 2020. Integrative analysis of glucometabolic traits, adipose tissue dna methylation, and gene expression identifies epigenetic regulatory mechanisms of insulin resistance and obesity in African Americans. Diabetes 69 (12), 2779–2793. https://doi.org/10.2337/db20-0117.

Skinner, M.K., Ben Maamar, M., Sadler-Riggleman, I., Beck, D., Nilsson, E., McBirney, M., Klukovich, R., Xie, Y., Tang, C., Yan, W., 2018. Alterations in sperm DNA methylation, non-coding RNA and histone retention associate with DDT-induced epigenetic transgenerational inheritance of disease. Epigenetics Chromatin 11 (1). https://doi.org/10.1186/s13072-018-0178-0.

Smith, G.I., Shankaran, M., Yoshino, M., Schweitzer, G.G., Chondronikola, M., Beals, J.W., Okunade, A.L., Patterson, B.W., Nyangau, E., Field, T., Sirlin, C. B., Talukdar, S., Hellerstein, M.K., Klein, S., 2020. Insulin resistance drives hepatic de novo lipogenesis in nonalcoholic fatty liver disease. J. Clin. Investig. 130 (3), 1453–1460. https://doi.org/10.1172/JCI134165.

Steptoe, A., Frank, P., 2023. Obesity and psychological distress. Philos. Trans. R. Soc. B 378 (1888). https://doi.org/10.1098/rstb.2022.0225.

Tam, B.T., Murphy, J., Khor, N., Morais, J.A., Santosa, S., Regulation, A.-C.A., 2020. OXPHOS integrity and leptin levels are different in females with childhood vs adulthood onset of obesity. Endocrinology 161 (11). https://doi.org/10.1210/endocr/bqaa142.

Tian, Y., Ma, J., Wang, W., Zhang, L., Jia, X., Wang, K., Li, D., 2016. Resveratrol supplement inhibited the NF-κB inflammation pathway through activating AMPKα-SIRT1 pathway in mice with fatty liver. Mol. Cell. Biochem. 422 (1–2), 75–84. https://doi.org/10.1007/s11010-016-2807-x.

Tolu, S.S., Viny, A.D., Amengual, J.E., Pro, B., Bates, S.E., 2025. Getting the right combination to break the epigenetic code. Nat. Rev. Clin. Oncol. 22 (2), 117–133. https://doi.org/10.1038/s41571-024-00972-1.

Tong, Y., Xu, S., Huang, L., Chen, C., 2022. Obesity and insulin resistance: Pathophysiology and treatment. Drug Discov. Today 27 (3), 822–830. https://doi.org/10.1016/j.drudis.2021.11.001.

Vallon, V., Thomson, S.C., 2017. Targeting renal glucose reabsorption to treat hyperglycaemia: the pleiotropic effects of SGLT2 inhibition. Diabetologia 60 (2), 215–225. https://doi.org/10.1007/s00125-016-4157-3.

Wadden, T.A., Tronieri, J.S., Butryn, M.L., 2020. Lifestyle modification approaches for the treatment of obesity in adults. Am. Psychol. 75 (2), 235–251. https://doi.org/10.1037/amp0000517.

Wang, J.Y., Wang, Q.W., Yang, X.Y., Yang, W., Li, D.R., Jin, J.Y., Zhang, X.F., 2023. GLP– 1 receptor agonists for the treatment of obesity: role as a promising approach. Front. Endocrinol. 14, 1085799.

Warren, J.M., Smith, N., Ashwell, M., 2017. A structured literature review on the role of mindfulness, mindful eating and intuitive eating in changing eating behaviours: effectiveness and associated potential mechanisms. Nutr. Res. Rev. 30 (2), 272–283. https://doi.org/10.1017/S0954422417000154.

Williams, K., Carrasquilla, G.D., Ingerslev, L.R., Hochreuter, M.Y., Hansson, S., Pillon, N.J., Donkin, I., Versteyhe, S., Zierath, J.R., Kilpeläinen, T.O., Barrès, R., 2021. Epigenetic rewiring of skeletal muscle enhancers after exercise training supports a role in whole-body function and human health. Mol. Metabol. 53. https://doi.org/10.1016/j.molmet.2021.101290. http://www.elsevier.com/wps/find/journaldescription.cws_home/728618/description.

Yárnoz-Esquiroz, P., Olazarán, L., Aguas-Ayesa, M., Perdomo, C.M., García-Goñi, M., Silva, C., Fernández-Formoso, J.A., Escalada, J., Montecucco, F., Portincasa, P., Frühbeck, G., 2022. Obesities': position statement on a complex disease entity with multifaceted drivers. Eur. J. Clin. Invest. 52 (7). https://doi.org/10.1111/eci.13811. http://onlinelibrary.wiley.com/journal/10.1111/(ISSN)1365-2362.

Yiew, N.K.H., Greenway, C., Zarzour, A., Ahmadieh, S., Goo, B., Kim, D., Benson, T.W., Ogbi, M., Tang, Y.L., Chen, W., Stepp, D., Patel, V., Hilton, R., Lu, X.Y., Hui, D.Y., Kim, H.W., Weintraub, N.L., 2019. Enhancer of zeste homolog 2 (EZH2) regulates adipocyte lipid metabolism independent of adipogenic differentiation: Role of apolipoprotein e. J. Biol. Chem. 294 (21), 8577–8591. https://doi.org/10.1074/jbc.RA118.006871.

Zhao, J., Bai, Y., Tao, S., Zhang, G., Wang, J., Liu, L., Zhang, S., 2019. Fiber-rich foods affected gut bacterial community and short-chain fatty acids production in pig model. J. Funct.Foods 57, 266–274. https://doi.org/10.1016/j.jff.2019.04.009.

9

Intergenerational transmission of metabolic memory

1. Introduction

Recent advances have expanded the concept of metabolic memory beyond individual lifespans, pointing to a phenomenon of intergenerational metabolic memory, where transient metabolic states in one generation influence the metabolic health of future generations (Godfrey et al., 2010). This transmission is not driven by changes in the DNA sequence itself but rather by epigenetic mechanisms such as DNA methylation, histone modifications, and microRNA regulation that alter gene expression patterns in gametes or during early development (Amrom and Schwartz, 2023). In addition, factors such as mitochondrial dysfunction, which is maternally inherited, placental adaptations, and microbial colonization patterns further mediate the intergenerational passage of metabolic traits (Basak et al., 2024).

Clinical and epidemiological evidence supports this paradigm. For instance, offspring of mothers who experienced famine during the Dutch Hunger Winter (1944–45) exhibited increased risks of obesity, insulin resistance, and cardiovascular disease in adulthood, decades after the initial insult (Veenendaal et al., 2013). Similarly, studies among Pima Indian populations, known for their high prevalence of obesity and T2DM, have shown that children born to mothers with diabetes during pregnancy face significantly higher risks of developing metabolic disorders themselves (Guan et al., 2023). These patterns have been reproduced in animal models, offering mechanistic insights and confirming causality.

The implications of these findings are far-reaching. They underscore the critical influence of prenatal and early postnatal nutrition, not only in determining an individual's lifelong metabolic trajectory but also in shaping the health of subsequent generations. The concept of developmental origins of health and disease (DOHaD) converges with that of metabolic memory, emphasizing that nutritional exposures during key developmental windows, such as

Metabolic Memory. https://doi.org/10.1016/B978-0-443-44591-0.00001-1

gametogenesis, embryogenesis, gestation, and infancy, program organ development, energy metabolism, hormonal regulation, and even appetite control (Hagemann et al., 2021).

This chapter delves into the biological mechanisms underlying intergenerational metabolic memory, with a particular focus on epigenetic regulation, mitochondrial inheritance, placental programming, and vertical microbiome transmission. We explore both human epidemiological studies and experimental animal models that offer compelling evidence for these processes. Furthermore, we examine the clinical and public health implications, emphasizing how maternal and early life nutrition can be harnessed as a preventative strategy to curb the rising incidence of metabolic diseases. Finally, we address key challenges in the field, such as the difficulty of conducting multigenerational human studies and the need for more detailed molecular mapping, and discuss promising future directions, including personalized nutrition, epigenetic therapeutics, and precision medicine approaches.

Understanding how metabolic states are passed across generations represents not just a scientific advancement but a public health imperative. It opens new avenues for intervention at the earliest stages of life, potentially altering disease risk before it begins, an opportunity to improve health not only for individuals but for entire lineages.

2. Conceptualizing metabolic memory

The concept of metabolic memory first gained prominence through diabetes research, particularly in studies examining the long-term effects of glycemic control on diabetic complications (Alqahtani et al., 2020). Clinical trials such as the Diabetes Control and Complications Trial (DCCT) and the follow-up Epidemiology of Diabetes Interventions and Complications (EDIC) study demonstrated that early intensive glycemic control in individuals with type 1 diabetes significantly reduced the risk of microvascular and macrovascular complications years later, even when glycemic control later became less stringent (Lachin and Nathan, 2021). This phenomenon indicated that the metabolic environment experienced during critical early periods could leave a lasting imprint on disease progression, a finding that led to the broader understanding of metabolic memory.

At its core, metabolic memory refers to the persistence of adverse metabolic effects long after an initial harmful exposure has ceased. This persistence is underpinned by molecular and cellular mechanisms that translate transient metabolic insults, such as hyperglycemia, oxidative stress, or nutrient imbalances, into durable changes within cells and tissues (González et al., 2023). Key among these are epigenetic modifications, including DNA methylation and histone modifications, which alter gene expression patterns without changing the underlying DNA sequence. These epigenetic changes can "lock in" maladaptive gene expression profiles that impair insulin signaling, glucose metabolism, and inflammatory responses (Scott et al., 2021).

Additionally, mitochondrial dysfunction plays a critical role in metabolic memory. Mitochondria, the energy powerhouses of the cell, are particularly susceptible to damage from metabolic stressors such as elevated glucose and free fatty acids. This damage leads to increased production of reactive oxygen species (ROS), which further exacerbate oxidative stress and impair cellular energy homeostasis. The resulting mitochondrial dysfunction can persist, contributing to chronic metabolic disturbances (Wang et al., 2018).

At the organ level, metabolic memory manifests as altered function in key metabolic tissues such as the pancreas, liver, and adipose tissue. In pancreatic β-cells, early metabolic insults can reduce insulin secretory capacity, while in the liver and adipose tissue, they can promote insulin resistance and dysregulated lipid metabolism (Newsholme et al., 2019; Cao et al., 2025). These functional impairments perpetuate a vicious cycle of metabolic imbalance. Ultimately, the persistent molecular and cellular alterations characteristic of metabolic memory contributes to the development and progression of chronic metabolic diseases, including type 2 diabetes, obesity, and cardiovascular disorders. Understanding metabolic memory has important implications for timing and targeting interventions to prevent or mitigate these diseases by addressing metabolic insults early and decisively.

3. Mechanisms underlying intergenerational transmission

Parental metabolic health plays a critical role in shaping the long-term metabolic outcomes of their offspring through nongenetic mechanisms (Fig. 9.1). Understanding these intergenerational pathways is essential for breaking the cycle of chronic metabolic diseases.

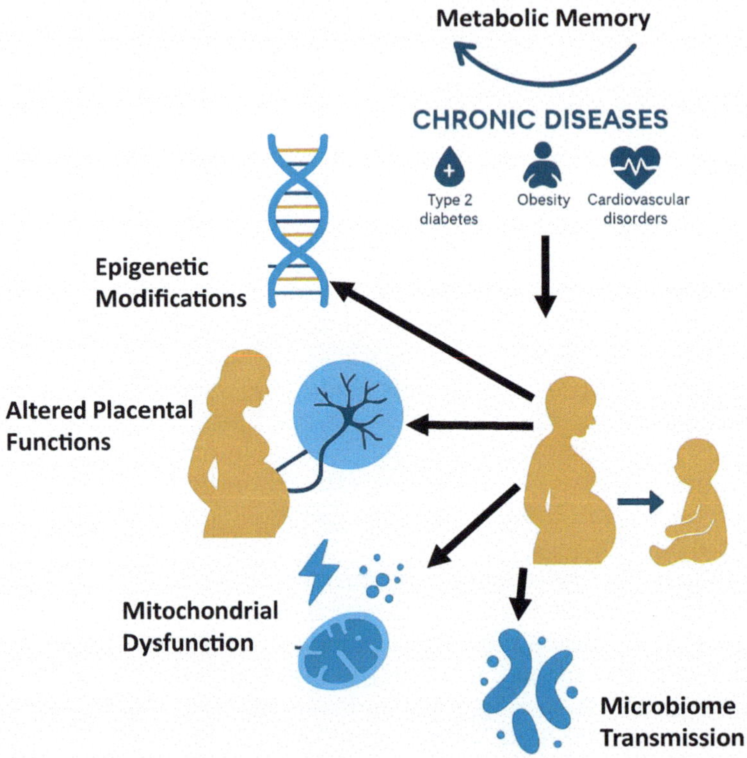

Figure 9.1 Mechanisms of intergenerational transmission of metabolic traits. Parental health influences offspring metabolism through epigenetic changes, mitochondrial dysfunction, placental alterations, and microbiome transmission. These pathways program metabolic risk even before birth, emphasizing early preventive strategies.

3.1 Epigenetic modifications

Epigenetic mechanisms serve as a molecular interface between environmental exposures and genome function, making them central to the concept of metabolic memory and its transmission across generations. During critical developmental windows, such as gametogenesis (the formation of sperm and eggs), embryogenesis (early development of the embryo), and the early postnatal period, environmental factors including maternal nutrition, stress, exposure to toxins, and metabolic status can induce stable epigenetic changes (Safi-Stibler and Gabory, 2020). These changes can persist throughout the lifespan and, importantly, be passed on to the next generation, thereby influencing offspring metabolic phenotypes.

One key mechanism is germline epigenetic inheritance, whereby epigenetic marks established in parental sperm or oocytes can be transmitted directly to the offspring (Zhu et al., 2022). For instance, if a parent experiences metabolic stress such as obesity or diabetes before conception, the epigenome of their germ cells can be altered, modifying the expression of genes involved in energy metabolism, insulin signaling, and inflammation in their children. This epigenetic "memory" enables the transmission of metabolic traits without changes in the DNA sequence itself.

Following fertilization, the early embryonic environment further shapes the epigenetic landscape in a process known as embryonic programming (Wilkinson et al., 2023). During this time, the developing embryo undergoes widespread epigenetic reprogramming, which is highly sensitive to environmental cues. Nutrient availability, oxygen levels, and hormonal signals can influence DNA methylation patterns and histone modifications, effectively programming the expression of genes that regulate metabolism, growth, and organ development. These programmed changes can persist into adulthood, predisposing the individual to metabolic dysfunction or resilience depending on the nature of the exposure (Safi-Stibler and Gabory, 2020).

In addition to DNA methylation and histone modifications, non-coding RNAs such as microRNAs and long non-coding RNAs are increasingly recognized as important regulators of gene expression that mediate epigenetic inheritance. These molecules can be packaged into sperm or oocytes and influence early embryonic gene regulation, further contributing to intergenerational transmission of metabolic states (Yuan et al., 2016).

Therefore, epigenetic modifications act as molecular conduits through which parental metabolic experiences influence the gene expression and metabolic health of subsequent generations. This epigenetic memory underscores the importance of optimizing parental health and environment well before conception and during early development to prevent the perpetuation of metabolic disease risk.

3.2 Mitochondrial dysfunction

Mitochondria are essential organelles responsible for producing the majority of cellular energy through oxidative phosphorylation. Because mitochondria carry their own DNA (mtDNA) and are maternally inherited, any mitochondrial damage or dysfunction in the mother can be transmitted directly to the offspring (Chiaratti et al., 2020). Maternal metabolic stressors, such as obesity, diabetes, or malnutrition, can induce oxidative damage and mutations in mtDNA or impair mitochondrial biogenesis and function. These alterations compromise the efficiency of ATP production and increase the generation of reactive oxygen species (ROS), which further exacerbate oxidative stress (Espinosa et al., 2023).

In the context of intergenerational transmission, dysfunctional maternal mitochondria can program offspring metabolism in several ways. Offspring may inherit mitochondria with compromised energy production capacity, which can affect tissues highly dependent on metabolic energy such as skeletal muscle, liver, and pancreatic β-cells (Wang et al., 2023). This can manifest as impaired glucose metabolism, reduced insulin secretion, and increased susceptibility to metabolic disorders like insulin resistance and type 2 diabetes.

Moreover, mitochondrial dysfunction in the mother can alter the intrauterine environment, leading to increased oxidative stress and inflammation during fetal development, which in turn programs the offspring's cellular metabolism and stress responses ("Obeagu, E. I., Muhimbura, E., & Obeagu, G. U. (2024). Hypoxia-Induced Oxidative Stress: Maternal and Fetal Implications. Elite Journal of Hematology, 2(8), 57–72.," no date). Given the pivotal role of mitochondria in energy homeostasis, inherited mitochondrial defects represent a critical mechanism linking maternal metabolic health to offspring disease risk.

3.3 Altered placental function

The placenta serves as the crucial biological interface that facilitates nutrient, gas, and waste exchange between mother and fetus, while also producing hormones that regulate fetal growth and development. Maternal metabolic conditions, such as obesity, gestational diabetes, or undernutrition, can detrimentally affect placental structure and function, thereby influencing fetal metabolic programming (Kelly et al., 2020).

In metabolic diseases, the placenta may exhibit altered expression of nutrient transporters, leading to either excessive or insufficient transfer of glucose, amino acids, and lipids to the fetus. For example, hyperglycemia in the mother can increase placental glucose transport, exposing the fetus to high glucose levels and promoting excessive fetal insulin production and adiposity, a process known as fetal overnutrition (Valent et al., 2021).

Additionally, impaired placental hormone production, including alterations in leptin, adiponectin, and insulin-like growth factors, can disrupt fetal energy regulation and organ development (Downs et al., 2024). Placental inflammation and oxidative stress, often seen in metabolic disorders, further impair placental function, resulting in fetal growth restriction or macrosomia (excessive growth), both of which are associated with later metabolic disease risk (Joo et al., 2021).

Thus, the placenta acts as a metabolic gatekeeper, translating maternal metabolic cues into fetal developmental signals, shaping the offspring's lifelong metabolic health.

3.4 Microbiome transmission

The human microbiome, particularly the gut microbiota, plays a vital role in regulating host metabolism, immune function, and energy balance. Increasingly, evidence shows that the maternal microbiome influences the initial colonization and subsequent development of the offspring's microbiota, thereby affecting their metabolic outcomes (Romano-Keeler and Weitkamp, 2015).

Vertical transmission of microbiota occurs during vaginal birth, breastfeeding, and close maternal contact in early life (Wang et al., 2020). Maternal metabolic diseases such as obesity and diabetes are associated with dysbiosis, an imbalance in microbial composition, that can be passed to the offspring. This dysbiotic microbiome is characterized by reduced microbial diversity and altered abundances of key bacterial taxa involved in energy harvest, short-chain fatty acid production, and inflammation regulation (Neri et al., 2021).

An altered microbiome in offspring can lead to increased gut permeability, systemic inflammation, and disrupted metabolic signaling pathways, predisposing children to obesity, insulin resistance, and other metabolic disorders. Moreover, early-life microbiome composition influences nutrient absorption and immune development, which are critical for long-term metabolic health (Sarkar et al., 2021).

Interventions aimed at restoring healthy maternal microbiota during pregnancy or modulating the infant's microbiome through probiotics, diet, or breastfeeding practices represent promising strategies to break the cycle of metabolic disease transmission (Moumne et al., 2021).

4. Evidence of intergenerational metabolic memory

Understanding the mechanisms of intergenerational metabolic memory requires evidence from both human populations and controlled animal experiments. This section explores key epidemiological studies that reveal the long-term metabolic consequences of prenatal exposures in humans, as well as animal model research that clarifies causal pathways and molecular mechanisms (Table 9.1).

4.1 Epidemiological studies

One of the most compelling human examples of intergenerational metabolic memory comes from the Dutch Hunger Winter during World War II (1944–45). During this period of severe famine, pregnant women experienced extreme nutritional deprivation. Follow-up studies decades later found that the children born to these mothers exhibited a significantly higher prevalence of metabolic diseases, including obesity, type 2 diabetes, and cardiovascular disorders, compared to those born before or after the famine (Veenendaal et al., 2013). Importantly, the timing of exposure during pregnancy was critical; famine during early gestation was associated with increased risk of cardiovascular disease and obesity, whereas mid-to late-gestation exposure more strongly affected glucose metabolism and insulin resistance (Conti et al., 2021). This historical natural experiment illustrates how transient prenatal nutritional insults can leave a persistent metabolic imprint, increasing susceptibility to chronic diseases in adulthood.

Another well-documented population is the Pima Indians of the southwestern United States, who exhibit some of the highest rates of obesity and type 2 diabetes worldwide. Studies in this population reveal that children born to mothers with obesity or diabetes have a markedly increased risk of developing metabolic disorders themselves ("Guan, Y., Tsai, C. J., & Zhang, S. (2023, October). Research on Diabetes Prediction Model of Pima Indian Females. In Proceedings of the 2023 fourth International Symposium on Artificial Intelligence for Medicine Science (pp. 294–303).," no date). This increased risk persists even after controlling for shared genetic and postnatal environmental factors, highlighting the powerful influence of the intrauterine metabolic environment on offspring health (Hsueh et al., 2018). The Pima studies underscore the concept that maternal metabolic status before and during pregnancy programs offspring metabolic pathways, contributing to the perpetuation of metabolic disease across generations.

Additional epidemiological evidence comes from diverse populations worldwide showing that maternal undernutrition, gestational diabetes, or obesity is associated with altered birth

Table 9.1 Summary of epidemiological and experimental evidence supporting intergenerational metabolic memory.

Study type	Key findings	Population/ Model	Mechanisms implicated	References
Epidemiological	Offspring exposed to famine in early gestation had increased risk of CVD and obesity; mid-late gestation linked to glucose/insulin issues.	Dutch Hunger Winter cohort	Timing-specific prenatal nutrient deprivation → lasting metabolic imprint	(Veenendaal et al., 2013; Conti et al., 2021)
Epidemiological	Maternal obesity/diabetes increases risk of metabolic disease in offspring, independent of genetics or shared postnatal environment.	Pima Indian population	Intrauterine metabolic environment programming	(Guan et al., 2023; Hsueh et al., 2018)
Epidemiological	Maternal undernutrition, obesity, and GDM linked to altered birth weight, insulin resistance, and adiposity in children.	Global diverse populations	Prenatal exposures affect fetal growth and metabolic outcomes	Carvalho et al. (2023)
Animal model (rodent)	Maternal high-fat/sugar diet leads to adiposity, insulin resistance, and glucose intolerance in offspring.	Rodents	Epigenetic changes, mitochondrial dysfunction, hypothalamic dysregulation	(Mishra et al., 2022; Harmancıoğlu and Kabaran, 2023)
Animal model (rodent)	Maternal undernutrition/protein restriction causes β-cell dysfunction and altered lipid metabolism in offspring.	Rodents	Reduced insulin production and impaired metabolic regulation	Calzada et al. (2016)
Animal model (primate)	High-fat maternal diet impairs insulin sensitivity, alters gene expression in liver and adipose tissue of offspring.	*Rhesus macaques*	Developmental programming of metabolism in liver/adipose	Thorn et al. (2014)
Animal model (rodent/ Primate)	Programmed defects transmitted to next generations; reversible with dietary interventions.	Rodents, primates	Inter/transgenerational inheritance, potential for intervention	(Fernandez-Twinn et al., 2015; Castro-Rodríguez et al., 2020)

outcomes (low or high birth weight), insulin resistance, and adiposity in offspring, further supporting the intergenerational transmission of metabolic memory (Carvahlo et al., 2023).

4.2 Animal models

While human studies provide crucial correlational data, controlled animal models have been indispensable for establishing causality and exploring underlying mechanisms. Rodent models, in particular, have been extensively used to investigate how maternal nutrition influences offspring metabolic programming.

In these studies, maternal overnutrition, typically modeled by feeding high-fat or high-sugar diets, leads to offspring with increased adiposity, insulin resistance, and altered glucose metabolism (Mishra et al., 2022). Molecular analyses reveal that these changes are mediated by epigenetic modifications in key metabolic genes, altered mitochondrial function, and disrupted hypothalamic regulation of appetite and energy expenditure (Harmancıoğlu and Kabaran, 2023). Similarly, maternal undernutrition or protein restriction during gestation results in offspring with impaired pancreatic β-cell development, glucose intolerance, and altered lipid metabolism, recapitulating findings from famine-exposed human cohorts (Calzada et al., 2016).

Primate studies provide further translational relevance. For example, rhesus macaques subjected to maternal high-fat diets produce offspring with impaired insulin sensitivity and altered gene expression in liver and adipose tissue (Thorn et al., 2014), confirming that maternal metabolic status directly programs offspring metabolism in species closer to humans.

These animal studies also demonstrate that many programmed effects can be transmitted beyond the first generation, indicating true intergenerational (and possibly transgenerational) inheritance of metabolic memory (Fernandez-Twinn et al., 2015). Interventions such as maternal dietary supplementation or postnatal nutritional modulation in offspring can sometimes reverse or mitigate these programmed metabolic defects, suggesting potential avenues for breaking the cycle of inherited metabolic disease (Castro-Rodríguez et al., 2020).

Together, epidemiological and animal research establish that intergenerational metabolic memory is a biologically plausible and clinically significant phenomenon. These findings emphasize the importance of maternal health and nutrition for preventing the propagation of metabolic disorders across generations.

5. Implications for prenatal and early life nutrition

The understanding that metabolic memory can be passed from one generation to the next has profound implications for how we approach nutrition and health during critical developmental periods. Interventions aimed at improving maternal and early-life nutrition can serve as powerful tools to prevent the onset of metabolic diseases in offspring and potentially reverse the trajectory of inherited metabolic dysfunction. Three key windows, preconception, gestation, and the early postnatal period, offer opportunities to mitigate the risks of metabolic memory transmission (Fig. 9.2).

5.1 Critical windows of development

The period before conception is increasingly recognized as a crucial window during which parental metabolic health, especially

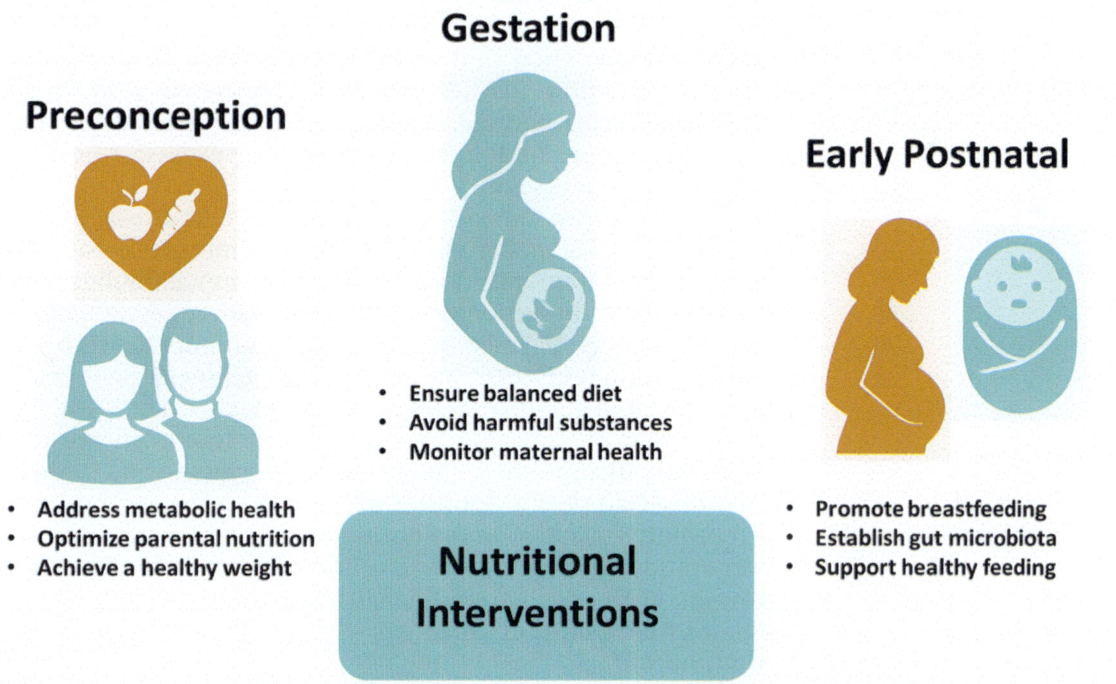

Figure 9.2 Implications of prenatal and early life nutrition on intergenerational transmission of metabolic diseases. This figure highlights the three critical windows-preconception, gestation, and early postnatal period, where targeted nutritional care can shape long-term metabolic health. Effective interventions during these stages can reduce intergenerational transmission of metabolic diseases.

that of the mother, but also of the father, can influence the quality and epigenetic integrity of gametes (Lucas and Watkins, 2017). For instance, obesity, insulin resistance, and micronutrient deficiencies in either parent have been shown to induce aberrant DNA methylation patterns in sperm and oocytes. These epigenetic changes can alter gene expression in the early embryo, impacting developmental trajectories and increasing the risk of obesity and type 2 diabetes in the offspring (Jahan-Mihan et al., 2024)+. Preconception care should, therefore, include not only reproductive health but also metabolic screening and intervention.

During gestation, the intrauterine environment exerts powerful programming effects on fetal development. The fetus is entirely dependent on maternal nutrient supply, and even subtle imbalances in maternal nutrition can affect the structure and function of key organs involved in metabolism, including the pancreas, liver, adipose tissue, and brain. For example, maternal hyperglycemia, whether due to gestational diabetes or pre-existing type 2 diabetes, can lead to fetal hyperinsulinemia, promoting increased fat deposition and larger birth weight (Vambergue and Fajardy, 2011). These infants are often at higher risk for developing insulin resistance and obesity later in life. Conversely, maternal undernutrition can result in intrauterine growth restriction (IUGR), which is associated with "thrifty phenotype" programming, predisposing individuals to metabolic syndrome under conditions of adequate or excessive postnatal nutrition (Bar et al., 2021).

The early postnatal period, including the first 2 years of life, is another pivotal stage for metabolic programming. Breastfeeding provides more than nutrition, it delivers immunoglobulins, oligosaccharides, and hormones like leptin and adiponectin that help regulate energy balance and support immune development. These components can influence appetite regulation, insulin sensitivity, and gut microbiota colonization (Du et al., 2015). Early introduction of unhealthy complementary foods, on the other hand, can disrupt these finely tuned processes and promote early-onset adiposity (Johnson et al., 2019). The establishment of a healthy gut microbiome during infancy is also shaped by delivery mode, antibiotic exposure, and maternal microbial transmission, all of which are influenced by maternal health and diet (Suárez-Martínez et al., 2023).

5.2 Nutritional interventions

Given the importance of these developmental windows, targeted nutritional strategies can play a transformative role in breaking the cycle of metabolic disease (Muhlhausler et al., 2013). Balanced macronutrient intake is fundamental, excessive consumption of saturated fats and refined sugars should be avoided, while diets should emphasize whole grains, lean proteins, healthy fats (such as omega-3 fatty acids), and fiber-rich fruits and vegetables. Both maternal undernutrition and overnutrition have been linked to negative programming effects, so achieving optimal energy balance is critical.

Micronutrient adequacy is another cornerstone of maternal and fetal health. Folate is vital for DNA methylation and neural tube development, and its deficiency can result in both structural anomalies and epigenetic dysregulation (Cao et al., 2022). Iron supports oxygen transport and brain development, while vitamin D is increasingly recognized for its role in immune regulation and insulin sensitivity (Backe et al., 2016; Szymczak-Pajor et al., 2020). Choline, zinc, iodine, and vitamin B12 are other essential nutrients that influence fetal development through both direct and epigenetic mechanisms. Supplementation programs that ensure adequate intake of these nutrients during pregnancy and lactation can significantly improve health outcomes (Razzaque and Wimalawansa, 2025).

It is also critical to avoid metabolic stressors such as ultra-processed foods, trans fats, high-fructose corn syrup, and environmental toxins (e.g., endocrine-disrupting chemicals like BPA). These substances can exacerbate oxidative stress and inflammation, disrupt hormonal balance, and interfere with placental function (Xanthakos et al., 2025). Behavioral interventions such as promoting physical activity, stress reduction, and smoking cessation should be integrated into maternal care to support a healthy metabolic environment.

5.3 Public health and policy

At the population level, the prevention of intergenerational metabolic disease requires systemic changes in public health infrastructure and policy (Zhang et al., 2023). Preconception and prenatal care should include metabolic health assessments, nutritional counseling, and supplementation where needed. These services must be accessible and affordable to reach the populations most at risk, especially in low-resource settings.

Government-led maternal nutrition programs, such as the provision of iron-folic acid tablets, fortified foods, and conditional cash transfers for pregnant women, can play a crucial role in improving maternal and neonatal outcomes (Aidoo, 2025). Education campaigns promoting healthy dietary habits, physical activity, and breastfeeding can empower women with the knowledge needed to support optimal fetal development.

Early childhood interventions should prioritize exclusive breastfeeding for the first 6 months and promote appropriate weaning practices to reduce childhood obesity and related conditions (Anderson et al., 2020). Public health guidelines must be updated to reflect the long-term impact of early nutrition on chronic disease risk (Saavedra et al., 2022). Additionally, policies addressing social determinants of health, including food security, poverty, education, and access to healthcare, are essential for creating environments that support healthy pregnancies and child development.

Collectively, these interventions offer a powerful strategy to reduce the prevalence of non-communicable diseases by interrupting the biological and social pathways that transmit metabolic risk from one generation to the next. Investing in maternal and early-life nutrition is not only a health imperative but a cornerstone of sustainable public health policy.

6. Challenges and future directions

Despite growing evidence supporting the concept of intergenerational metabolic memory, several scientific and practical challenges hinder its full understanding and clinical application. Addressing these challenges through innovative research and policy strategies will be crucial for translating current knowledge into effective interventions.

6.1 Complexity of human studies

One of the primary challenges in studying intergenerational metabolic memory is the complexity of human longitudinal research. Investigating how early life exposures influence health outcomes across generations requires tracking individuals over decades, often from preconception into adulthood and even into the next generation. These studies are logistically demanding, resource-intensive, and vulnerable to high attrition rates. Furthermore, it is difficult to isolate the effects of specific nutritional or metabolic insults from the myriad of environmental, behavioral, and socioeconomic factors that individuals are exposed to over their lifetimes. For instance, diet, physical activity, stress levels, healthcare access, and cultural practices all interact to influence health outcomes, making causal inferences challenging. Moreover, ethical constraints limit the extent to which certain experimental designs, such as controlled deprivation or overnutrition, can be implemented in human populations.

6.2 Molecular mechanism elucidation

Although associations between early-life exposures and later metabolic outcomes are well documented, the molecular mechanisms that mediate the intergenerational transmission of metabolic memory remain incompletely understood. While epigenetic mechanisms such as DNA methylation, histone modification, and non-coding RNA regulation are clearly involved, the specific genes, regulatory elements, and biochemical pathways responsible for transmitting these effects across generations require further elucidation. Advances in multi-omics technologies, like epigenomics, transcriptomics, proteomics, and metabolomics, offer promising tools to dissect these mechanisms at a systems level. However, translating the findings from animal models to human biology remains a major hurdle due to differences in developmental timing, placentation, and lifespan. Additionally, the reversible nature of these epigenetic marks, and how they may be modulated by targeted nutritional or pharmacological interventions, is still an area of active investigation.

6.3 Personalized medicine approaches

The future of managing intergenerational metabolic memory lies in the realm of personalized and precision medicine (Lonardo et al., 2021). Individual susceptibility to metabolic programming likely depends on a combination of genetic predisposition, epigenetic landscape, and environmental exposures. Understanding these individual-level differences could allow for the development of targeted interventions tailored to a person's unique biological and environmental profile. For example, genomic and epigenomic screening might 1 day be used to identify individuals at high risk of transmitting metabolic dysfunction to their offspring, thereby guiding preconception counseling and nutritional optimization. Nutrigenomics involving how diet interacts with genes and epigenetic markers, holds significant promise in designing precision nutrition strategies that are more effective than one-size-fits-all approaches. However, achieving this vision will require integrated data systems, bioinformatics infrastructure, and ethical frameworks to support personalized care while protecting individual privacy and preventing health disparities.

7. Conclusion

The transmission of metabolic traits across generations challenges the traditional boundaries of genetic inheritance and individual health responsibility. As evidence mounts linking parental metabolic status, particularly maternal nutrition and glycemic control, to long-term health risks in offspring, the concept of *intergenerational metabolic memory* has emerged as a critical determinant of public health outcomes. Mechanisms such as epigenetic modifications, mitochondrial dysfunction, placental adaptations, and microbiome inheritance play key roles in this process, offering potential targets for intervention.

Recognizing the importance of critical windows, preconception, gestation, and early infancy, opens new opportunities for preventive strategies that begin well before the onset of disease. Optimizing maternal and early life nutrition can attenuate or even reverse harmful metabolic programming, setting the foundation for healthier future generations. However, major challenges remain, including the complexity of long-term human studies, the need for clearer mechanistic understanding, and the development of equitable and effective precision medicine tools.

Moving forward, interdisciplinary collaboration between researchers, clinicians, and public health policymakers is essential. By shifting focus toward early-life and intergenerational interventions, we have the potential not only to reduce the prevalence of metabolic diseases but to fundamentally reshape our approach to health across the human lifespan.

References

Aidoo, E.M., 2025. Advancing precision medicine and health education for chronic disease prevention in vulnerable maternal and child populations. World J. Adv. Res. Rev. 25 (2), 2355–2376. https://doi.org/10.30574/wjarr.2025.25.2.0623.

Alqahtani, A.A., Alzidany, A.M., Alenazi, S.M., Dhifallah, T., Alotaibi, B.J.E.M., 2020. Long term complication of poor glycemic control in diabetic patients. EC Microbiol. 2, 1–7.

Amrom, D., Schwartz, S.S., 2023. Maternal metabolic health, lifestyle, and environment – understanding how epigenetics drives future offspring health. Curr. Diabetes Rev. 19 (2), 50–73. https://doi.org/10.2174/1573399818666220422085016.

Anderson, C.E., Whaley, S.E., Crespi, C.M., Wang, M.C., Chaparro, M.P., 2020. Every month matters: longitudinal associations between exclusive breastfeeding duration, child growth and obesity among WIC-participating children. J. Epidemiol. Commun. Health 74 (10), 785–791. https://doi.org/10.1136/jech-2019-213574.

Backe, M.B., Moen, I.W., Ellervik, C., Hansen, J.B., Mandrup-Poulsen, T., 2016. Iron regulation of pancreatic beta-cell functions and oxidative stress. Annu. Rev. Nutr. 36, 241–273. https://doi.org/10.1146/annurev-nutr-071715-050939.

Bar, J., Weiner, E., Levy, M., Gilboa, Y., 2021. The thrifty phenotype hypothesis: The association between ultrasound and Doppler studies in fetal growth restriction and the development of adult disease. Am. J. Obstet. Gynecol. MFM 3 (6), 100473. https://doi.org/10.1016/j.ajogmf.2021.100473.

Basak, S., Mallick, R., Navya Sree, B., Duttaroy, A., 2024. Placental epigenome impacts fetal development: Effects of maternal nutrients and gut microbiota. Nutrients 16 (12), 1860. https://doi.org/10.3390/nu16121860.

Calzada, L., Morales, A., Sosa-Larios, T.C., Reyes-Castro, L.A., Rodríguez-González, G.L., Rodríguez-Mata, V., Zambrano, E., Morimoto, S., 2016. Maternal protein restriction during gestation impairs female offspring pancreas development in the rat. Nutr. Res. 36 (8), 855–862. https://doi.org/10.1016/j.nutres.2016.03.007.

Cao, R., Xie, J., Zhang, L., 2022. Abnormal methylation caused by folic acid deficiency in neural tube defects. Open Life Sci. 17 (1), 1679–1688. https://doi.org/10.1515/biol-2022-0504.

Cao, X., Wang, N., Yang, M., Zhang, C., 2025. Lipid accumulation and insulin resistance: bridging metabolic dysfunction-associated fatty liver disease and chronic kidney disease. Int. J. Mol. Sci. 26 (14), 6962. https://doi.org/10.3390/ijms26146962.

Carvalho de, L.S., Oliveira de, A.A.D., Cristina Martins Grabovski, T., Christina Renzo, C., Silva, R.R.e, Hafemann Loz, S., Silva, J.C., 2023. Maternal prepregnancy obesity and gestational diabetes influence on adverse perinatal outcomes. Arch. Endocrinol. Metab. 67 (4). https://doi.org/10.20945/2359-3997000000605.

Castro-Rodríguez, D.C., Rodríguez-González, G.L., Menjivar, M., Zambrano, E., 2020. Maternal interventions to prevent adverse fetal programming outcomes due to maternal malnutrition: Evidence in animal models. Placenta 102, 49–54. https://doi.org/10.1016/j.placenta.2020.04.002.

Chiaratti, M.R., Macabelli, C.H., Neto, J.D.A., Grejo, M.P., Pandey, A.K., Perecin, F., Collado, M.D., 2020. Maternal transmission of mitochondrial diseases. Genet. Mol. Biol. 43 (1). https://doi.org/10.1590/1678-4685-GMB-2019-0095. http://www.scielo.br/pdf/gmb/v43n1s1/1415-4757-GMB-43-1-s1-20190095.pdf.

Conti, G., Poupakis, S., Ekamper, P., Bijwaard, G.E., Lumey, L.H., 2021. Severe prenatal shocks and adolescent health: Evidence from the Dutch Hunger Winter. medRxiv. https://doi.org/10.1101/2021.10.13.21264971. https://www.medrxiv.org/.

Downs, T., da Silva Costa, F., de Freitas Paganoti, C., Holland, O.J., Hryciw, D. H., 2024. Adiponectin and leptin during pregnancy: A systematic review of their association with pregnancy disorders, fetal growth and placental function. Endocrines 5 (3), 382–394. https://doi.org/10.3390/endocrines5030028.

Du, Q., Hosoda, H., Umekawa, T., Kinouchi, T., Ito, N., Miyazato, M., Kangawa, K., Ikeda, T., 2015. Postnatal weight gain induced by overfeeding pups and maternal high-fat diet during the lactation period modulates glucose metabolism and the production of pancreatic and gastrointestinal peptides. Peptides 70, 23–31. https://doi.org/10.1016/j.peptides.2015.05.003.

Espinosa, A., Casas, M., Jaimovich, E., 2023. Energy (and reactive oxygen species generation) saving distribution of mitochondria for the activation of ATP production in skeletal muscle. Antioxidants 12 (8), 1624. https://doi.org/10.3390/antiox12081624.

Fernandez-Twinn, D.S., Constância, M., Ozanne, S.E., 2015. Intergenerational epigenetic inheritance in models of developmental programming of adult disease. Semin. Cell Dev. Biol. 43, 85–95. https://doi.org/10.1016/j.semcdb.2015.06.006.

Godfrey, K.M., Gluckman, P.D., Hanson, M.A., 2010. Developmental origins of metabolic disease: Life course and intergenerational perspectives. Trends Endocrinol. Metabol. 21 (4), 199–205. https://doi.org/10.1016/j.tem.2009.12.008.

González, P., Lozano, P., Ros, G., Solano, F., 2023. Hyperglycemia and oxidative stress: An integral, updated and critical overview of their metabolic interconnections. Int. J. Mol. Sci. 24 (11), 9352. https://doi.org/10.3390/ijms24119352.

Guan, Y., Tsai, C.J., Zhang, S., October 2023. Research on diabetes prediction model of Pima Indian females. In: Proceedings of the 2023 4th International symposium on artificial intelligence for medicine science, pp. 294–303.

Hagemann, E., Silva, D.T., Davis, J.A., Gibson, L.Y., Prescott, S.L., 2021. Developmental Origins of health and disease (DOHaD): The importance of life-course and transgenerational approaches. Paediatr. Respir. Rev. 40, 3–9. https://doi.org/10.1016/j.prrv.2021.05.005.

Harmancıoğlu, B., Kabaran, S., 2023. Maternal high fat diets: Impacts on offspring obesity and epigenetic hypothalamic programming. Front. Genet. 14. https://doi.org/10.3389/fgene.2023.1158089.

Hsueh, W.C., Bennett, P.H., Esparza-Romero, J., Urquidez-Romero, R., Valencia, M.E., Ravussin, E., Williams, R.C., Knowler, W.C., Baier, L.J., Schulz, L.O., Hanson, R.L., 2018. Analysis of type 2 diabetes and obesity genetic variants in Mexican Pima Indians: Marked allelic differentiation among Amerindians at HLA. Ann. Hum. Genet. 82 (5), 287–299. https://doi.org/10.1111/ahg.12252. http://onlinelibrary.wiley.com/journal/10.1111/(ISSN)1469-1809.

Jahan-Mihan, A., Leftwich, J., Berg, K., Labyak, C., Nodarse, R.R., Allen, S., Griggs, J., 2024. The impact of parental preconception nutrition, body weight, and exercise habits on offspring health outcomes: A narrative review. Nutrients 16 (24), 4276. https://doi.org/10.3390/nu16244276.

Johnson, M.L., Jill Saffrey, M., Taylor, V.J., 2019. Gastrointestinal capacity, gut hormones and appetite change during rat pregnancy and lactation. Reproduction 157 (5), 431–443. https://doi.org/10.1530/REP-18-0414.

Joo, E.H., Kim, Y.R., Kim, N., Jung, J.E., Han, S.H., Cho, H.Y., 2021. Effect of endogenic and exogenic oxidative stress triggers on adverse pregnancy outcomes: Preeclampsia, fetal growth restriction, gestational diabetes mellitus and preterm birth. Int. J. Mol. Sci. 22 (18). https://doi.org/10.3390/ijms221810122. https://www.mdpi.com/1422-0067/22/18/10122/pdf.

Kelly, A.C., Powell, T.L., Jansson, T., 2020. Placental function in maternal obesity. Clin. Sci. 134 (8), 961–984. https://doi.org/10.1042/CS20190266.

Lachin, J.M., Nathan, D.M., 2021. Understanding metabolic memory: The prolonged influence of glycemia during the diabetes control and complications trial (dcct) on future risks of complications during the study of the epidemiology of diabetes interventions and complications (edic). Diabetes Care 44 (10), 2216–2224. https://doi.org/10.2337/dc20-3097.

Lonardo, A., Byrne, C.D., Targher, G., 2021. Precision medicine approaches in metabolic disorders and target organ damage: where are we now, and where are we going? Metabo. Target Organ Damage 1 (1). https://doi.org/

10.20517/mtod.2021.03. https://oaepublishstorage.blob.core.windows.net/98a97e5f-3801-42aa-996b-cd342ec808d0/4220.pdf.

Lucas, E.S., Watkins, A.J., 2017. The long-term effects of the periconceptional period on embryo epigenetic profile and phenotype; the paternal role and his contribution, and how males can affect offspring's phenotype/epigenetic profile. Adv. Exp. Med. Biol. 1014, 137–154. https://doi.org/10.1007/978-3-319-62414-3_8.

Mishra, A., Ruano, S.H., Saha, P.K., Pennington, K.A., 2022. A novel model of gestational diabetes: Acute high fat high sugar diet results in insulin resistance and beta cell dysfunction during pregnancy in mice. PLoS One 17 (12). https://doi.org/10.1371/journal.pone.0279041. https://journals.plos.org/plosone/article/file?id=10.1371/journal.pone.0279041&type=printable.

Moumne, O., Hampe, M.E., Montoya-Williams, D., Carson, T.L., Neu, J., Francois, M., Rhoton-Vlasak, A., Lemas, D.J., 2021. Implications of the vaginal microbiome and potential restorative strategies on maternal health: A narrative review. J. Perinat. Med. 49 (4), 402–411. https://doi.org/10.1515/jpm-2020-0367.

Muhlhausler, B.S., Gugusheff, J.R., Ong, Z.Y., Vithayathil, M.A., 2013. Nutritional approaches to breaking the intergenerational cycle of obesity. Can. J. Physiol. Pharmacol. 91 (6), 421–428. https://doi.org/10.1139/cjpp-2012-0353.

Neri, C., Serafino, E., Morlando, M., Familiari, A., Goebl, C.S., 2021. Microbiome and gestational diabetes: Interactions with pregnancy outcome and long-term infant health. J. Diabetes Res. 2021, 1–10. https://doi.org/10.1155/2021/9994734.

Newsholme, P., Keane, K.N., Carlessi, R., Cruzat, V., 2019. Oxidative stress pathways in pancreatic β-cells and insulin-sensitive cells and tissues: Importance to cell metabolism, function, and dysfunction. Am. J. Physiol. Cell Physiol. 317 (3), C420. https://doi.org/10.1152/ajpcell.00141.2019. https://www.physiology.org/doi/pdf/10.1152/ajpcell.00141.2019.

Obeagu, E.I., Muhimbura, E., Obeagu, G.U., 2024. Hypoxia-Induced oxidative stress: Maternal and fetal implications. Elite J. Haematol. 2 (8), 57–72.

Razzaque, M.S., Wimalawansa, S.J., 2025. Minerals and human health: From deficiency to toxicity. Nutrients 17 (3). https://doi.org/10.3390/nu17030454. http://www.mdpi.com/journal/nutrients/.

Romano-Keeler, J., Weitkamp, J.H., 2015. Maternal influences on fetal microbial colonization and immune development. Pediatr. Res. 77, 189–195. https://doi.org/10.1038/pr.2014.163.

Saavedra, J.M., Dattilo, A.M. (Eds.), 2022. Early nutrition and long-term health: mechanisms, consequences, and opportunities. Woodhead Publishing.

Safi-Stibler, S., Gabory, A., 2020. Epigenetics and the Developmental Origins of Health and Disease: Parental environment signalling to the epigenome, critical time windows and sculpting the adult phenotype. Semin. Cell Dev. Biol. 97, 172–180. https://doi.org/10.1016/j.semcdb.2019.09.008.

Sarkar, A., Yoo, J.Y., Dutra, S.V.O., Morgan, K.H., Groer, M., 2021. The association between early-life gut microbiota and long-term health and diseases. J. Clin. Med. 10 (3), 459. https://doi.org/10.3390/jcm10030459.

Scott, A.K., Casas, E., Schneider, S.E., Swearingen, A.R., Van Den Elzen, C.L., Seelbinder, B., Neu, C.P., 2021. Epigenetic remodeling during monolayer cell expansion reduces therapeutic potential. bioRxiv. https://doi.org/10.1101/2021.12.14.472696, 2021-12.

Suárez-Martínez, C., Santaella-Pascual, M., Yagüe-Guirao, G., Martínez-Graciá, C., 2023. Infant gut microbiota colonization: influence of prenatal and postnatal factors, focusing on diet. Front. Microbiol. 14. https://doi.org/10.3389/fmicb.2023.1236254.

Szymczak-Pajor, I., Drzewoski, J., Śliwińska, A., 2020. The molecular mechanisms by which vitamin D prevents insulin resistance and associated disorders. Int. J. Mol. Sci. 21 (18), 6644. https://doi.org/10.3390/ijms21186644.

Thorn, S.R., Baquero, K.C., Newsom, S.A., El Kasmi, K.C., Bergman, B.C., Shulman, G.I., Grove, K.L., Friedman, J.E., 2014. Early life exposure to maternal insulin resistance has persistent effects on hepatic NAFLD in juvenile nonhuman primates. Diabetes 63 (8), 2702–2713. https://doi.org/10.2337/db14-0276.

Valent, A.M., Choi, H., Kolahi, K.S., Thornburg, K.L., 2021. Hyperglycemia and gestational diabetes suppress placental glycolysis and mitochondrial function and alter lipid processing. FASEB (Fed. Am. Soc. Exp. Biol.) J. 35 (3). https://doi.org/10.1096/fj.202000326RR. https://onlinelibrary.wiley.com/journal/15306860.

Vambergue, A., Fajardy, I., 2011. Consequences of gestational and pregestational diabetes on placental function and birth weight. World J. Diabetes 2 (11), 196. https://doi.org/10.4239/wjd.v2.i11.196.

Veenendaal, M.V.E., Painter, R.C., De Rooij, S.R., Bossuyt, P.M.M., Van Der Post, J.A.M., Gluckman, P.D., Hanson, M.A., Roseboom, T.J., 2013. Transgenerational effects of prenatal exposure to the 1944-45 Dutch famine. BJOG Int. J. Obstet. Gynaecol. 120 (5), 548–554. https://doi.org/10.1111/1471-0528.12136. http://obgyn.onlinelibrary.wiley.com/hub/journal/10.1111/(ISSN)1471-0528/.

Wang, L., O'Kane, A.M., Zhang, Y., Ren, J., 2023. Maternal obesity and offspring health: Adapting metabolic changes through autophagy and mitophagy. Obes. Rev. 24 (7). https://doi.org/10.1111/obr.13567. http://onlinelibrary.wiley.com/journal/10.1111/(ISSN)1467-789X.

Wang, S., Ryan, C.A., Boyaval, P., Dempsey, E.M., Ross, R.P., Stanton, C., 2020. Maternal vertical transmission affecting early-life microbiota development. Trends Microbiol. 28 (1), 28–45. https://doi.org/10.1016/j.tim.2019.07.010.

Wang, Z., Zhao, H., Guan, W., Kang, X., Tai, X., Shen, Y., 2018. Metabolic memory in mitochondrial oxidative damage triggers diabetic retinopathy. BMC Ophthalmol. 18 (1). https://doi.org/10.1186/s12886-018-0921-0.

Wilkinson, A.L., Zorzan, I., Rugg-Gunn, P.J., 2023. Epigenetic regulation of early human embryo development. Cell Stem Cell 30 (12), 1569–1584. https://doi.org/10.1016/j.stem.2023.09.010.

Xanthakos, S.A., Ibrahim, S.H., Adams, K., Kohli, R., Sathya, P., Sundaram, S., Vos, M.B., Dhawan, A., Caprio, S., Behling, C.A., Schwimmer, J.B., 2025. AASLD Practice Statement on the evaluation and management of metabolic dysfunction–associated steatotic liver disease in children. Hepatology 82 (5), 1352–1394. https://doi.org/10.1097/HEP.0000000000001368.

Yuan, S., Schuster, A., Tang, C., Yu, T., Ortogero, N., Bao, J., Zheng, H., Yan, W., 2016. Sperm-borne miRNAs and endo-siRNAs are important for fertilization and preimplantation embryonic development. Development (Camb.) 143 (4), 635–647. https://doi.org/10.1242/dev.131755.

Zhang, K., Ma, Y., Luo, Y., Song, Y., Xiong, G., Ma, Y., Sun, X., Kan, C., 2023. Metabolic diseases and healthy aging: identifying environmental and behavioral risk factors and promoting public health. Front. Public Health 11. https://doi.org/10.3389/fpubh.2023.1253506.

Zhu, H., Cheng, Y., Huang, H., 2022. Diabetes predisposition inherited through maternal germline. Clin. Transl. Med. 12 (7). https://doi.org/10.1002/ctm2.969.

10

Personalized medicine and metabolic memory

1. Introduction

Personalized medicine (PM), also called precision medicine, groups patients based on their risk of disease or expected response to treatment. It is a major shift in healthcare because it focuses on tailoring medical care to each individual. This approach customizes medical decisions, procedures, interventions, and products according to the needs of each patient (Dolgopolov and Rykov, 2023). Personalized medicine works by considering differences in genetics, environment, and lifestyle, with the goal of giving the right treatment to the right patient at the right time (Sadee et al., 2023). Both personalized medicine and precision medicine aim to move away from the traditional "one-size-fits-all" approach. Precision medicine is often seen as a part of personalized medicine because it mainly uses genetic and molecular information to develop targeted therapies for specific patient subgroups (such as those with certain genetic mutations). In contrast, personalized medicine takes a broader view by including factors beyond biology, such as lifestyle and environmental influences (Elemento, 2020).

Rapid growth in genomics, transcriptomics, proteomics, metabolomics, and knowledge of disease mechanisms is now influencing routine clinical practice (Jacob et al., 2019). Doctors can increasingly use genetic, RNA, protein, and metabolic markers to guide treatment decisions, leading to more effective and individualized patient care. Since the completion of the Human Genome Project in 2003, progress in personalized medicine research, product development, and clinical use has accelerated (Huang et al., 2022). Over the past decade, the concept of personalized medicine has gained wide recognition in the scientific community, media, and the general public (Jørgensen, 2009). These advances support a more detailed understanding of patient profiles and enable more targeted therapies.

Metabolic Memory. https://doi.org/10.1016/B978-0-443-44591-0.00008-4

According to the European Parliamentary Research Service, personalized medicine is an evolving approach that applies genetic and molecular knowledge to guide disease prediction, prevention, diagnosis, and treatment (Causio et al., 2022). Similarly, the National Institutes of Health emphasize that personalized medicine aims to prevent, diagnose, and treat disease using information about each patient's genes, proteins, and environment (Di Sanzo et al., 2017).

The human genome and epigenome forms the foundation of personalized medicine and is considered central to next-generation diagnosis and treatment (Morganti et al., 2019). Advances such as SNP analysis, genotyping, and biochips have helped bring personalized medicine into clinical practice. Genetic variations, including SNPs, insertions, deletions, structural variants, and copy number variations, play important roles in diseases such as cancer, diabetes, cardiovascular disorders, and neurodegenerative diseases. The epigenome plays a key role in personalized medicine by capturing how genes are regulated by environment and lifestyle, enabling more precise prediction of disease risk and individualized treatment responses (Chen et al., 2023). Importantly, personalized medicine does not mean creating a unique drug for each individual. Instead, patients are grouped into subpopulations based on their disease risk or response to treatment. This allows treatments to be targeted to those most likely to benefit, while reducing unnecessary side effects and costs for others (Soni et al., 2020).

Big data links diverse datasets to reveal new disease pathways and correlations, allowing greater precision and customization than before (Schaefer et al., 2020). High-throughput technologies now enable cost-effective analysis of large health datasets. However, handling and integrating these data require advanced computing tools, such as powerful processors, improved algorithms, better sensors, and cloud computing. These developments can support future clinical decision-making (Verma and Barh, 2016).

Big data approaches have improved our ability to study normal and abnormal biological processes, but many precision strategies remain difficult to apply in routine practice. Major challenges include identifying which biological factors matter most for treatment selection, determining which patients will benefit, and choosing the best time for intervention. Although these challenges are significant, hypothesis-free, data-driven approaches offer promising solutions (Hulsen et al., 2019). In theory, treatments based on genetic profiles should be more effective and cause fewer side effects. In reality, personalized medicine can be costly, complex, and difficult to implement, and simpler options may sometimes work just as well. Challenges also include data privacy concerns, regulatory limitations, and the need for large clinical trials to prove safety and effectiveness. Despite these barriers, progress continues (Sigman, 2018).

In the future, personalized medicine may reduce drug development costs, treatment expenses, and time, leading to better healthcare outcomes (Goetz and Schork, 2018). For this approach to transform healthcare, patients, researchers, clinicians, industry, and regulators must work together to support innovation, new technologies, advanced diagnostics, and personalized care models (Antoñanzas et al., 2015). Pharmaceutical companies worldwide see precision medicine as a major opportunity, but many face scientific, regulatory, and commercial challenges. Although pharmacogenomics can help identify disease-related genes and new drug targets, concerns remain about developing therapies for small, genetically defined patient groups (Mathur and Sutton, 2017).

Mechanistically, metabolic memory is driven by epigenetic modifications (e.g., DNA methylation, histone acetylation), persistent oxidative stress, and inflammatory signaling that alter gene expression without changing DNA sequences (Reddy and Natarajan, 2011). For instance, hyperglycemia-induced methylation of promoters such as *TXNIP* or persistent activation of NF-κB signaling have been implicated in vascular and renal complications long after glucose levels are controlled (El-Osta et al., 2008; Keating et al., 2016).

The integration of metabolic memory into personalized medicine facilitates anticipatory care, enabling clinicians to identify high-risk individuals before overt disease manifests. This is particularly valuable in vulnerable populations such as offspring of mothers with gestational diabetes mellitus (GDM), who are at increased risk for obesity and type 2 diabetes due to adverse utero programming (Dabelea and Crume, 2011). Mechanistically, metabolic memory is driven by epigenetic modifications (e.g., DNA methylation, histone acetylation), persistent oxidative stress, and inflammatory signaling that alter gene expression without changing DNA sequences (Reddy and Natarajan, 2011). For instance, hyperglycemia-induced methylation of promoters such as *TXNIP* or persistent activation of NF-κB signaling have been implicated in vascular and renal complications long after glucose levels are controlled (El-Osta et al., 2008; Keating et al., 2016). Similarly, individuals exposed to early-life malnutrition, as seen in historical famines or socioeconomic deprivation, often exhibit altered epigenetic profiles linked to insulin resistance and metabolic syndrome later in life (Turnbaugh et al., 2006).

By merging the temporal lens of metabolic memory with individualized therapeutic strategies, personalized medicine offers a proactive model of care that addresses both present and latent metabolic risks. This chapter explores the biological foundations of metabolic memory, its interface with personalized medicine, and real-world applications which range from tailored diabetes management and microbiome-guided obesity therapy to epigenetic interventions in reproductive health.

2. The biology of metabolic memory in precision healthcare

2.1 Epigenetic profiling and predictive risk stratification

Metabolic memory is primarily driven by stable epigenetic modifications that are established during exposure to hyperglycemia, inflammation, oxidative stress, or nutrient excess, and these modifications can persist even after metabolic normalization. The three major classes of epigenetic alterations contributing to this phenomenon are DNA methylation, histone posttranslational modifications, and non-coding RNA regulation.

DNA methylation, particularly at CpG islands in promoter regions, leads to gene silencing by inhibiting the binding of transcription factors. For example, hypermethylation of the TXNIP (Thioredoxin-Interacting Protein) gene in response to chronic hyperglycemia contributes to persistent oxidative stress and β-cell dysfunction, which are hallmarks of metabolic memory (Zhuo et al., 2016). TXNIP inhibits thioredoxin, a key antioxidant, thereby increasing reactive oxygen species (ROS) levels and activating downstream inflammatory pathways such as NF-κB.

Histone modifications, including acetylation (e.g., H3K9ac) and methylation (e.g., H3K4me3 and H3K27me3), regulate chromatin accessibility. For instance, increased H3K9 acetylation at the promoters of pro-inflammatory genes like IL-6 and TNF-α has been observed in monocytes exposed to high glucose levels, maintaining their expression even after glucose normalization (El-Osta et al., 2008).

Non-coding RNAs, including microRNAs (e.g., miR-375, miR-29a) and long non-coding RNAs (lncRNAs), fine-tune gene expression posttranscriptionally. For instance, miR-29a, which targets insulin signaling and extracellular matrix genes, is upregulated by hyperglycemia and remains elevated, contributing to fibrosis and endothelial dysfunction (Zhuang et al., 2025).

In personalized medicine, these epigenetic changes are now detectable using high-throughput tools such as reduced representation bisulfite sequencing (RRBS) and epigenome-wide association studies (EWAS). Reduced Representation Bisulfite Sequencing (RRBS) is a cost-effective method to measure DNA methylation at single-base resolution, focusing on CpG-rich regions of the genome. It uses restriction enzyme digestion, bisulfite conversion, and next-generation sequencing to identify methylated versus unmethylated cytosines (Gu et al., 2021). Epigenome-Wide Association Studies (EWAS) investigate how variations in DNA methylation or other epigenetic marks across the genome are associated with specific traits or diseases. They scan thousands to millions of epigenetic sites to identify biomarkers and potential causal mechanisms (Xiong et al., 2022). These methods enable the construction of epigenetic risk scores (ERS) that complement genomic data. Individuals with unfavorable epigenetic profiles can be identified prior to phenotypic disease onset, allowing for targeted early interventions such as lifestyle modification, dietary epigenetic reprogramming, or early pharmacological therapy (Fig. 10.1).

2.2 Genomic and transcriptomic insights

Beyond epigenetic mechanisms, germline genetic variations modulate an individual's susceptibility to establishing and responding to metabolic memory. These include single nucleotide polymorphisms (SNPs) in genes involved in glucose metabolism, insulin signaling, mitochondrial function, and inflammation.

SNPs in TCF7L2 (rs7903146) significantly increase risk for type 2 diabetes by reducing insulin secretion and impairing β-cell function. This variant is also associated with incomplete reversal of hyperglycemia-induced gene expression, a hallmark of metabolic memory (Grant et al., 2006; Florez et al., 2006).

Variants in SLC30A8, encoding the zinc transporter ZnT8, affect insulin granule formation and β-cell resilience to oxidative stress. Individuals carrying the R325W variant are more prone to oxidative stress-induced epigenetic changes, reinforcing metabolic memory (Rutter and Chimienti, 2015).

Transcriptomic profiling using RNA-Seq has revealed persistent upregulation of pro-inflammatory genes (e.g., IL1B, TNFAIP3) and oxidative stress markers (e.g., NOX4, SOD2) in endothelial and immune cells from patients with previous

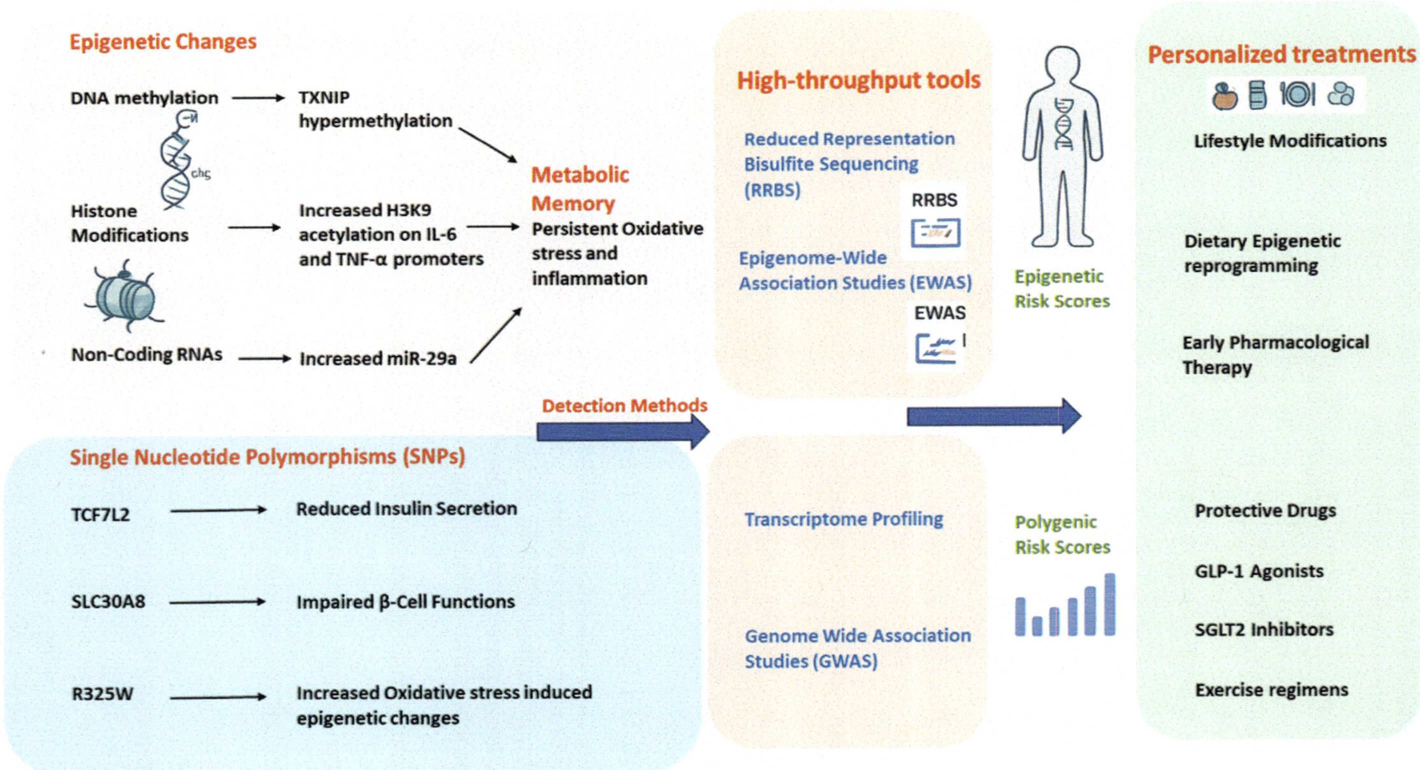

Figure 10.1 The biology of metabolic memory in precision healthcare. Epigenetic, genomic, and transcriptomic mechanisms drive the persistence of metabolic memory, influencing disease risk even after metabolic normalization. Integrating high throughput techniques, epigenetic risk scores and polygenic risk scores enables predictive stratification for personalized interventions.

episodes of poor glycemic control, even after glycemic normalization (Kato and Natarajan, 2019).

Polygenic Risk Scores (PRS) combine the effects of many genetic variants across the genome into a single score that estimates an individual's inherited risk for a disease. They are calculated using genome-wide association study (GWAS) data and weighted by each variant's effect size. PRS can now quantify cumulative risk based on thousands of SNPs. When combined with transcriptomic and epigenetic data, PRS can stratify patients not only by disease susceptibility but also by likely persistence of metabolic damage despite treatment (Fig. 10.1). This has powerful implications for personalized treatment algorithms, guiding early initiation of protective drugs (e.g., GLP-1 agonists, SGLT2 inhibitors), nutritional interventions, and exercise regimens tailored to genetic and molecular profiles (Holloszy, 2005).

3. Applications of personalized medicine in managing metabolic memory

3.1 Precision diabetes management

The Diabetes Control and Complications Trial (DCCT) and its long-term follow-up, the Epidemiology of Diabetes Interventions and Complications (EDIC) study, were landmark clinical trials that first highlighted the phenomenon of "legacy effects" or metabolic memory. These studies demonstrated that early intensive glycemic control in type 1 diabetes patients conferred long-lasting protective effects against microvascular and macrovascular complications, even years after glycemic control deteriorated (Diabetes Control and Complications Trial/Epidemiology of Diabetes Interventions and Complications (DCCT/EDIC) Study Research Group, 2005). Building on these insights, modern precision medicine approaches now optimize individualized diabetes management by integrating continuous glucose monitoring (CGM), metabolomics profiling, and machine learning algorithms. Such tools allow clinicians to dynamically assess glycemic variability, insulin sensitivity, and β-cell function to tailor therapies more precisely.

For example, metabolomics panels can detect subtle shifts in metabolic pathways that may predispose patients to sustained oxidative stress or inflammation, signaling a higher risk for persistent metabolic memory. Patients exhibiting these profiles are increasingly considered for early initiation of glucagon-like peptide-1 (GLP-1) receptor agonists or sodium-glucose co-transporter 2 (SGLT2) inhibitors. Beyond glucose lowering, these drug classes have demonstrated cardiovascular and renal protective effects, which are particularly valuable in mitigating the downstream impacts of metabolic memory (Zinman et al., 2015; Marso et al., 2016). Personalized medicine thus moves beyond a "one-size-fits-all" model by incorporating molecular markers and patient-specific metabolic phenotypes to optimize long-term outcomes.

3.2 Tailored nutrition and lifestyle plans

Nutrigenomics and nutrigenetics form the cornerstone of applying personalized nutrition to modulate metabolic memory. These disciplines study how individual genetic variants influence dietary responses, enabling customized nutritional plans that enhance metabolic health. For instance, the FTO (fat mass and obesity-associated) gene variant, strongly linked to obesity risk, affects how individuals metabolize and respond to high-fat diets (Frayling et al., 2007). Clinical trials have shown that individuals with risk alleles in FTO achieve more significant weight loss and better glycemic control when diet plans are tailored to their genetic makeup compared to standardized recommendations (Celis-Morales et al., 2017).

Furthermore, lifestyle interventions such as physical activity and targeted dietary changes have been shown to partially reverse deleterious epigenetic modifications associated with metabolic memory. Exercise induces beneficial epigenetic remodeling in skeletal muscle and adipose tissue, including altered DNA methylation and histone acetylation patterns that improve insulin sensitivity and mitochondrial function (Barres and Zierath, 2011). These findings emphasize the potential of integrating lifestyle medicine with genetic and epigenetic information to sustain metabolic health and counteract earlier metabolic insults.

3.3 Maternal and prenatal interventions

The intergenerational transmission of metabolic memory underscores the critical window of opportunity during preconception and pregnancy for personalized intervention. Emerging clinical programs combine genetic counseling, microbiome profiling, and nutritional assessment to optimize maternal and fetal health. For example, maternal folate status is closely linked to fetal DNA methylation patterns via the one-carbon metabolism pathway. Genetic polymorphisms in key enzymes such

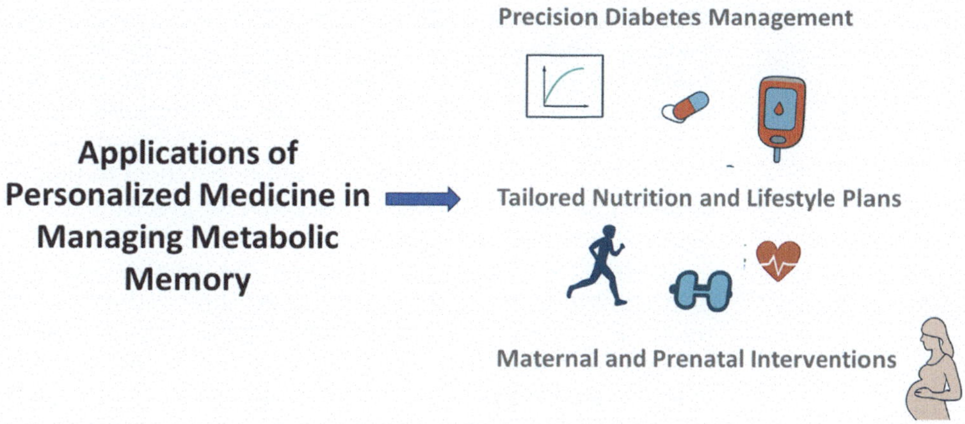

Figure 10.2 Applications of personalized medicine in metabolic memory. Precision therapies, tailored nutrition, and prenatal interventions help mitigate the long-term effects of metabolic memory. By integrating genetics, epigenetics, and lifestyle factors, personalized medicine optimizes health across generations.

as MTHFR (methylenetetrahydrofolate reductase) affect folate metabolism efficiency and consequently influence fetal epigenetic programming (Crider et al., 2012).

Tailoring folate supplementation and other micronutrients based on maternal genotype and nutritional status can reduce adverse metabolic programming in offspring, lowering their long-term risk for obesity, diabetes, and cardiovascular diseases. Additionally, modulation of the maternal microbiome during pregnancy through probiotics or diet adjustments is being investigated as a strategy to favorably shape fetal metabolic development and prevent transmission of dysbiotic microbial patterns linked to metabolic disorders (Koren et al., 2012). These personalized prenatal approaches have significant potential to disrupt the vicious cycle of metabolic memory across generations (Fig. 10.2).

4. Emerging technologies with transformative potential

Technological advances are dramatically expanding the possibilities for integrating metabolic memory into personalized medicine.

Single-cell multi-omics profiling now enables the simultaneous mapping of genomic, epigenomic, transcriptomic, proteomic, and even metabolomic changes within individual cells. This technology captures cellular heterogeneity and reveals early disease signatures that are often missed by bulk tissue analyses. For example, single-cell RNA sequencing of pancreatic islets from type 2 diabetes patients has identified discrete β-cell subpopulations with unique stress-response signatures and epigenetic marks linked to metabolic memory (Lawlor et al., 2017; Miragaia et al., 2019). Such approaches allow clinicians and researchers to pinpoint cell-specific pathways that could be targeted for precision interventions before irreversible damage occurs.

Artificial intelligence (AI)-driven risk prediction models are also revolutionizing metabolic disease prevention and management. By integrating large-scale clinical records, multi-omics profiles, and longitudinal lifestyle data, machine learning algorithms can predict the onset of diseases like type 2 diabetes or cardiovascular complications years before clinical symptoms appear (Liang et al., 2019; Krittanawong et al., 2019). These models can also run simulations of different therapeutic strategies, providing clinicians with evidence-based recommendations tailored to each patient's molecular and metabolic profile.

CRISPR-based epigenome editing is another groundbreaking avenue with transformative potential. Unlike conventional CRISPR-Cas9 gene editing, which alters DNA sequences, epigenome editing uses modified Cas proteins (e.g., dCas9 fused with DNA methyltransferases or histone acetyltransferases) to add, remove, or modify epigenetic marks (Liu et al., 2016). This makes it possible to reverse maladaptive DNA methylation or histone modifications associated with metabolic memory, potentially restoring normal gene expression without changing the underlying genetic code (Horlbeck et al., 2016). For instance, targeted demethylation of promoters involved in insulin sensitivity or oxidative stress regulation could mitigate long-term complications in individuals with a history of poor glycemic control.

Together, these emerging technologies, when integrated into a personalized medicine framework, hold the promise of identifying, predicting, and actively reversing the molecular imprints of metabolic memory, fundamentally changing how chronic metabolic diseases are prevented and treated.

5. Main challenges of personalized medicine

Personalized medicine offers major healthcare benefits but faces technical, ethical, regulatory, and economic challenges that limit its widespread adoption. Implementing it requires collaboration among genomics, bioinformatics, clinical medicine, and data science, which is often difficult due to differences in terminology, methods, and work cultures (Horgan et al., 2014). Overcoming these barriers needs coordinated efforts from researchers, clinicians, policymakers, and other stakeholders to ensure effective and equitable implementation (Wells, 2020).

5.1 Data privacy and security

Personalized medicine relies heavily on genetic and sensitive health data, making privacy and security critical. Unauthorized access to genetic data can cause privacy breaches, discrimination, and social stigma (Laschinger et al., 2008). Data sharing among healthcare providers, researchers, and third parties increases risks due to varying security standards and the challenges of securely storing large genomic datasets (Raisaro, 2018).

To minimize risks, strong encryption, regular security audits, strict access control, secure cloud practices, and clear policies on data retention and disposal are essential (Jin et al., 2019). Ethical use of data requires informed consent, compliance with GDPR and HIPAA, anonymization during data sharing, and ethical review of all research involving personal data (Gymrek et al., 2013; Vayena and Blasimme, 2018).

5.2 Ethical and social issues

Personalized medicine raises ethical and social concerns, including genetic discrimination, informed consent, psychological impact of knowing genetic risks, and cultural differences in perceptions of genetic testing (Brothers and Rothstein, 2015; Garrison, 2013). Unequal access between high- and low-income regions and underrepresentation of diverse populations in genomic research can reduce treatment accuracy and fairness. Ethical, inclusive, and socially responsible implementation is essential to ensure equitable benefits of personalized medicine (Sharrer, 2017).

5.3 Regulatory hurdles

Regulatory systems are not fully adapted to personalized medicine, which requires validation of genetically targeted diagnostics and therapies (Zhang et al., 2013; Knowles et al., 2017). Traditional clinical trial models are not suitable for small, genetically defined patient groups, especially for gene therapies. Adaptive regulatory pathways, conditional approvals, accelerated reviews, interdisciplinary advisory boards, and international regulatory harmonization can help overcome these challenges (Beccia et al., 2022a,b).

5.4 Economic barriers

High costs of sequencing technologies, bioinformatics tools, genetic testing, and targeted therapies limit access to personalized medicine (Shabaruddin et al., 2015). Insurance coverage is inconsistent, and high research and trial costs increase treatment prices (Trosman et al., 2011). Addressing economic barriers requires policy reforms, funding support, innovative pricing models, and equity-focused strategies to ensure affordability and sustainability (Davis et al., 2009).

5.5 Integration into clinical practice

Integrating personalized medicine into routine care requires upgrading healthcare infrastructure, updating clinical guidelines, training professionals, and strengthening data management systems (Hamburg and Collins, 2010). Medical education must include genomics, genetic counseling, test interpretation, and ethical considerations. Interdisciplinary collaboration and standardized protocols are essential for reliable implementation, supported by secure and efficient data systems (Daack-Hirsch et al., 2013; Bowdin et al., 2016).

5.6 Interdisciplinary collaboration

Effective personalized medicine depends on collaboration among genomic scientists, bioinformaticians, clinicians, and pharmacologists. Genomic data must be integrated into clinical decision-making systems, while pharmacologists optimize drug choice and dosing based on genetic variation (Beccia et al., 2022a,b; Mirnezami et al., 2012). This interdisciplinary approach improves precision, innovation, ethical practice, and patient-centered care (Branco and Choupina, 2021; Bashraheel et al., 2020).

5.7 Scientific challenges

Personalized medicine is challenged by complex gene-environment-lifestyle interactions, polygenic diseases, variable phenotypes, and the integration of multi-omics data (Agarwal et al., 2021; Collins and Varmus, 2015). Large-scale data analysis requires advanced computational tools, while understanding interactions with environmental factors and the microbiome remains incomplete (Kaur et al., 2024). Biomarker discovery, sequencing accuracy, reproducibility, and cost-effectiveness are ongoing challenges (Arifuzzaman et al., 2024). Addressing these issues through multidisciplinary collaboration will enable personalized medicine to achieve its full potential in improving healthcare outcomes (Stanojevic et al., 2022).

6. Future directions

Despite the transformative potential of personalized medicine in managing metabolic memory, several challenges hinder its widespread implementation in routine clinical care. A major obstacle lies in the interpretation and accessibility of high-throughput omics data, including genomics, epigenomics, metabolomics, and microbiome profiles. These complex datasets require specialized bioinformatics expertise and advanced computational tools, which remain limited in many clinical settings (Vitorino, 2024). Furthermore, the integration of multi-omics data for comprehensive patient stratification demands standardized protocols and interoperable data platforms that are not yet fully developed (Chahal et al., 2025).

Ethical and equity considerations also pose significant challenges. Personalized medicine risks exacerbating health disparities if access is restricted to populations with greater resources or if genetic information leads to discrimination in insurance and employment (Tawfik et al., 2023). Ensuring equitable distribution of these advanced healthcare modalities is essential to avoid widening existing social and health inequities. Moreover, patient consent, data privacy, and the responsible use of genetic information require robust regulatory frameworks to protect individual rights (Balagurunathan and Sethuraman, 2024).

Another critical gap is the paucity of long-term longitudinal studies validating the clinical utility and cost-effectiveness of personalized interventions. While many small-scale trials demonstrate promise, large cohort studies and randomized controlled trials are needed to confirm sustained benefits, optimal timing of interventions, and potential unintended consequences (Greene, 2015). Without such evidence, clinical guidelines and reimbursement policies remain cautious.

Looking forward, the development of novel epigenetic editing technologies, such as CRISPR-based targeted DNA methylation or histone modification tools, may enable precise reversal of adverse metabolic programming, offering potential curative strategies beyond symptom management (McCutcheon et al., 2024). Artificial intelligence (AI) and machine learning algorithms are poised to enhance clinical decision-making by integrating complex omics and clinical data to generate personalized risk scores and treatment recommendations in real time (Ali, 2023). Furthermore, population-wide screening platforms utilizing blood-based epigenetic biomarkers could facilitate early identification of at-risk individuals, allowing timely preventive interventions before clinical disease onset (Caraballo et al., 2024).

Together, addressing these challenges and leveraging emerging technologies will be critical to realizing the full potential of personalized medicine in breaking the cycle of metabolic memory and improving metabolic health outcomes across diverse populations.

7. Conclusion

Metabolic memory is a powerful concept that redefines our understanding of chronic disease progression and risk. Personalized medicine offers the tools to decode this memory and respond with precision interventions tailored to each individual's genetic, epigenetic, metabolic, and environmental context. From preventing diabetes to interrupting the intergenerational cycle of obesity, personalized approaches are proving to be not just more effective but also more sustainable in the long run. As technology advances, the integration of metabolic memory into personalized healthcare will enable a new standard of care, one that is proactive, predictive, and profoundly personal.

References

Agarwal, A., Pritchard, D., Gullett, L., Amanti, K.G., Gustavsen, G., 2021. A quantitative framework for measuring personalized medicine integration into us healthcare delivery organizations. J. Personalized Med. 11 (3). https://doi.org/10.3390/jpm11030196. https://www.mdpi.com/2075-4426/11/3/196/pdf.

Ali, H., 2023. Artificial intelligence in multi-omics data integration: Advancing precision medicine, biomarker discovery and genomic-driven disease interventions. Int. J. Sci. Res. Arch. 8 (1), 1012–1030. https://doi.org/10.30574/ijsra.2023.8.1.0189.

Antoñanzas, F., Juárez-Castelló, C.A., Rodríguez-Ibeas, R., 2015. Some economics on personalized and predictive medicine. Eur. J. Health Econ. 16 (9), 985–994. https://doi.org/10.1007/s10198-014-0647-8.

Arifuzzaman, M., Collins, N., Guo, C.J., Artis, D., 2024. Nutritional regulation of microbiota-derived metabolites: Implications for immunity and inflammation. Immunity 57 (1), 14–27. https://doi.org/10.1016/j.immuni.2023.12.009.

Balagurunathan, Y., Sethuraman, R.R., 2024. An analysis of ethics-based foundation and regulatory issues for genomic data privacy. J. Inst. Eng.: Ser. Bibliogr. 105 (4), 1097–1107. https://doi.org/10.1007/s40031-024-01058-3.

Barres, R., Zierath, J.R., 2011. DNA methylation in metabolic disorders. Am. J. Clin. Nutr. 93 (4), 897S. https://doi.org/10.3945/ajcn.110.001933.
Bashraheel, S.S., Domling, A., Goda, S.K., 2020. Update on targeted cancer therapies, single or in combination, and their fine tuning for precision medicine. Biomed. Pharmacother. 125. https://doi.org/10.1016/j.biopha.2020.110009. https://www.journals.elsevier.com/biomedicine-and-pharmacotherapy.
Beccia, F., Causio, F., Farina, S., Savoia, C., Osti, T., Di Marcantonio, M., Morsella, A., Cadeddu, C., Ricciardi, W., Boccia, S., 2022a. Personalised medicine in shaping sustainable healthcare: A Delphi survey within the IC2PerMed project. Eur. J. Publ. Health 32 (Suppl. 3). https://doi.org/10.1093/eurpub/ckac129.429 ckac129.429.
Beccia, F., Hoxhaj, I., Castagna, C., Strohäker, T., Cadeddu, C., Ricciardi, W., Boccia, S., 2022b. An overview of personalized medicine landscape and policies in the European Union. Eur. J. Publ. Health 32, 844–851. https://doi.org/10.1093/eurpub/ckac103.
Bowdin, S.C., Hayeems, R.Z., Monfared, N., Cohn, R.D., Meyn, M.S., 2016. The SickKids Genome Clinic: developing and evaluating a pediatric model for individualized genomic medicine. Clin. Genet. 89 (1), 10–19. https://doi.org/10.1111/cge.12579.
Branco, I., Choupina, A., 2021. Bioinformatics: new tools and applications in life science and personalized medicine. Appl. Microbiol. Biotechnol. 105 (3), 937–951. https://doi.org/10.1007/s00253-020-11056-2.
Brothers, K.B., Rothstein, M.A., 2015. Ethical, legal and social implications of incorporating personalized medicine into healthcare. Pers. Med. 12 (1), 43–51. https://doi.org/10.2217/pme.14.65.
Caraballo, E.V., Centeno-Girona, H., Torres-Velásquez, B.C., Martir-Ocasio, M. M., González-Pons, M., López-Acevedo, S.N., Cruz-Correa, M., 2024. Diagnostic accuracy of a blood-based biomarker panel for colorectal cancer detection: a pilot study. Cancers 16 (24). https://doi.org/10.3390/cancers16244176. http://www.mdpi.com/journal/cancers/.
Causio, F.A., Hoxhaj, I., Beccia, F., Marcantonio, M.D., Strohäker, T., Cadeddu, C., Boccia, S., 2022. Big data and ICT solutions in the European Union and in China: a comparative analysis of policies in personalized medicine. Digit. Health 8, 20552076221129060.
Celis-Morales, C., Livingstone, K.M., Marsaux, C.F.M., Macready, A.L., Fallaize, R., O'Donovan, C.B., Woolhead, C., Forster, H., Walsh, M.C., Navas-Carretero, S., San-Cristobal, R., Tsirigoti, L., Lambrinou, C.P., Mavrogianni, C., Moschonis, G., Kolossa, S., Hallmann, J., Godlewska, M., Surwiłło, A., Traczyk, I., Drevon, C.A., Bouwman, J., Van Ommen, B., Grimaldi, K., Parnell, L.D., Matthews, J.N.S., Manios, Y., Daniel, H., Martinez, J.A., Lovegrove, J.A., Gibney, E.R., Brennan, L., Saris, W.H.M., Gibney, M., Mathers, J.C., 2017. Effect of personalized nutrition on health-related behaviour change: Evidence from the Food4Me European randomized controlled trial. Int. J. Epidemiol. 46 (2), 578–588. https://doi.org/10.1093/ije/dyw186.
Chahal, A.A.C., Alahdab, F., Asatryan, B., Addison, D., Aung, N., Chung, M.K., Denaxas, S., Dunn, J., Hall, J.L., Pamir, N., Slotwiner, D.J., Vargas, J.D., Armoundas, A.A., 2025. Data interoperability and harmonization in cardiovascular genomic and precision medicine. Circulation: Genomic and Precision Medicine 18 (3). https://doi.org/10.1161/CIRCGEN.124.004624. https://www.ahajournals.org/journal/circgen.

Chen, M., Liu, X., Liu, Q., Shi, D., Li, H., 2023. 3D genomics and its applications in precision medicine. Cellul. Mol. Biol. Lett. 28 (1), 19.

Collins, F.S., Varmus, H., 2015. A new initiative on precision medicine. N. Engl. J. Med. 372 (9), 793–795. https://doi.org/10.1056/NEJMp1500523.

Crider, K.S., Yang, T.P., Berry, R.J., Bailey, L.B., 2012. Folate and DNA methylation: A review of molecular mechanisms and the evidence for Folate's role. Adv. Nutr. 3 (1), 21–38. https://doi.org/10.3945/an.111.000992.

Daack-Hirsch, S., Jackson, B., Belchez, C.A., Elder, B., Hurley, R., Kerr, P., Nissen, M.K., 2013. Integrating genetics and genomics into nursing curricula. You can do it too. Nurs. Clin. 48 (4), 661–669. https://doi.org/10.1016/j.cnur.2013.08.005.

Dabelea, D., Crume, T., 2011. Maternal environment and the transgenerational cycle of obesity and diabetes. Diabetes 60 (7), 1849–1855. https://doi.org/10.2337/db11-0400.

Davis, J.C., Furstenthal, L., Desai, A.A., Norris, T., Sutaria, S., Fleming, E., Ma, P., 2009. The microeconomics of personalized medicine: today's challenge and tomorrow's promise. Nat. Rev. Drug Discov. 8 (4), 279–286. https://doi.org/10.1038/nrd2825.

Di Sanzo, M., Cipolloni, L., Borro, M., La Russa, R., Santurro, A., Scopetti, M., Frati, P., 2017. Clinical applications of personalized medicine: a new paradigm and challenge. Curr. Pharmaceut. Biotechnol. 18 (3), 194–203.

Diabetes Control and Complications Trial/Epidemiology of Diabetes Interventions and Complications (DCCT/EDIC) Study Research Group, 2005. Intensive diabetes treatment and cardiovascular disease in patients with type 1 diabetes. N. Engl. J. Med. 353 (25), 2643–2653.

Dolgopolov, I.S., Rykov, M.Y., 2023. Medicine of the future: personalized, stratified or precision? (literature review). Health Care Russian Feder. 67 (3), 259–266.

Elemento, O., 2020. The future of precision medicine: towards a more predictive personalized medicine. Emerg. Topic. Life Sci. 4 (2), 175–177.

El-Osta, A., Brasacchio, D., Yao, D., Pocai, A., Jones, P.L., Roeder, R.G., Cooper, M.E., Brownlee, M., 2008. Transient high glucose causes persistent epigenetic changes and altered gene expression during subsequent normoglycemia. J. Exp. Med. 205 (10), 2409–2417. https://doi.org/10.1084/jem.20081188Australia.

Florez, J.C., Jablonski, K.A., Bayley, N., Pollin, T.I., De Bakker, P.I.W., Shuldiner, A.R., Knowler, W.C., Nathan, D.M., Altshuler, D., 2006. TCF7L2 polymorphisms and progression to diabetes in the Diabetes Prevention Program. N. Engl. J. Med. 355 (3), 241–250. https://doi.org/10.1056/NEJMoa062418.

Frayling, T.M., Timpson, N.J., Weedon, M.N., Zeggini, E., Freathy, R.M., Lindgren, C.M., Perry, J.R.B., Elliott, K.S., Lango, H., Rayner, N.W., Shields, B., Harries, L.W., Barrett, J.C., Ellard, S., Groves, C.J., Knight, B., Patch, A.M., Ness, A.R., Ebrahim, S., Lawlor, D.A., Ring, S.M., Ben-Shlomo, Y., Jarvelin, M. R., Sovio, U., Bennett, A.J., Melzer, D., Ferrucci, L., Loos, R.J.F., Barroso, I., Wareham, N.J., Karpe, F., Owen, K.R., Cardon, L.R., Walker, M., Hitman, G.A., Palmer, C.N.A., Doney, A.S.F., Morris, A.D., Smith, G.D., Hattersley, A.T., McCarthy, M.I., 2007. A common variant in the FTO gene is associated with body mass index and predisposes to childhood and adult obesity. Science 316 (5826), 889–894. https://doi.org/10.1126/science.1141634.

Garrison, N.A., 2013. Genomic justice for native Americans: Impact of the havasupai case on genetic research. Sci. Technol. Hum. Val. 38 (2), 201–223. https://doi.org/10.1177/0162243912470009.

Goetz, L.H., Schork, N.J., 2018. Personalized medicine: motivation, challenges, and progress. Fertil. Steril. 109 (6), 952–963.

Grant, S.F.A., Thorleifsson, G., Reynisdottir, I., Benediktsson, R., Manolescu, A., Sainz, J., Helgason, A., Stefansson, H., Emilsson, V., Helgadottir, A., Styrkarsdottir, U., Magnusson, K.P., Walters, G.B., Palsdottir, E., Jonsdottir, T., Gudmundsdottir, T., Gylfason, A., Saemundsdottir, J., Wilensky, R.L., Reilly, M.P., Rader, D.J., Bagger, Y., Christiansen, C., Gudnason, V., Sigurdsson, G., Thorsteinsdottir, U., Gulcher, J.R., Kong, A., Stefansson, K., 2006. Variant of transcription factor 7-like 2 (TCF7L2) gene confers risk of type 2 diabetes. Nat. Genet. 38 (3), 320–323. https://doi.org/10.1038/ng1732.

Greene, T., 2015. Randomized controlled trials 5: determining the sample size and power for clinical trials and cohort studies. In: Clinical Epidemiology: Practice and Methods. Springer New York, New York, NY, pp. 225–247.

Gu, H., Raman, A.T., Wang, X., Gaiti, F., Chaligne, R., Mohammad, A.W., Arczewska, A., Smith, Z.D., Landau, D.A., Aryee, M.J., Meissner, A., Gnirke, A., 2021. Smart-RRBS for single-cell methylome and transcriptome analysis. Nat. Protoc. 16 (8), 4004–4030. http://www.natureprotocols.com/. doi: 10.1038/s41596-021-00571-9.

Gymrek, M., McGuire, A.L., Golan, D., Halperin, E., Erlich, Y., 2013. Identifying personal genomes by surname inference. Science 339 (6117), 321–324. https://doi.org/10.1126/science.1229566.

Hamburg, M.A., Collins, F.S., 2010. The path to personalized medicine. N. Engl. J. Med. 363 (4), 301–304. https://doi.org/10.1056/NEJMp1006304.

Holloszy, J.O., 2005. Exercise-induced increase in muscle insulin sensitivity. J. Appl. Physiol. 99 (1), 338–343. https://doi.org/10.1152/japplphysiol.00123.2005.

Horgan, D., Jansen, M., Leyens, L., Lal, J.A., Sudbrak, R., Hackenitz, E., Bußhoff, U., Ballensiefen, W., Brand, A., 2014. An index of barriers for the implementation of personalised medicine and pharmacogenomics in Europe. Public Health Genom. 17, 287–298. https://doi.org/10.1159/000368034.

Horlbeck, M.A., Witkowsky, L.B., Guglielmi, B., Replogle, J.M., Gilbert, L.A., Villalta, J.E., Torigoe, S.E., Tjian, R., Weissman, J.S., 2016. Nucleosomes impede cas9 access to DNA in vivo and in vitro. eLife 5. https://doi.org/10.7554/eLife.12677. https://elifesciences.org/content/5/e12677-download.pdf.

Huang, X., Chen, Z., Xiang, X., Liu, Y., Long, X., Li, K., Liu, J., 2022. Comprehensive multi-omics analysis of the m7G in pan-cancer from the perspective of predictive, preventive, and personalized medicine. EPMA J. 13 (4), 671–697.

Hulsen, T., Jamuar, S.S., Moody, A.R., Karnes, J.H., Varga, O., Hedensted, S., McKinney, E.F., 2019. From big data to precision medicine. Front. Med. 6, 34.

Jacob, M., Lopata, A.L., Dasouki, M., Abdel Rahman, A.M., 2019. Metabolomics toward personalized medicine. Mass Spectrometry Rev. 38 (3), 221–238.

Jin, H., Luo, Y., Li, P., Mathew, J., 2019. A review of secure and privacy-preserving medical data sharing. IEEE Access 7, 61656–61669. https://doi.org/10.1109/access.2019.2916503.

Jørgensen, J.T., 2009. New era of personalized medicine: a 10-year anniversary. Oncologist 14 (5), 557–558.

Kato, M., Natarajan, R., 2019. Epigenetics and epigenomics in diabetic kidney disease and metabolic memory. Nat. Rev. Nephrol. 15 (6), 327–345. https://doi.org/10.1038/s41581-019-0135-6.

Kaur, R., Mandal, D., Potdar, V., Gosavi, M.S., Kumar, A., 2024. Multi-omics and its clinical application. In: Multi-omics analysis of the human microbiome: From technology to clinical applications. Springer Nature, India, pp. 295–319. https://doi.org/10.1007/978-981-97-1844-3_14. https://link.springer.com/book/10.1007/978-981-97-1844-3.

Keating, S.T., Plutzky, J., El-Osta, A., 2016. Epigenetic changes in diabetes and cardiovascular risk. Circ. Res. 118 (11), 1706–1722. https://doi.org/10.1161/CIRCRESAHA.116.306819.

Knowles, L., Luth, W., Bubela, T., 2017. Paving the road to personalized medicine: recommendations on regulatory, intellectual property and reimbursement challenges. J. Law Biosci. 4 (3), 453–506. https://doi.org/10.1093/jlb/lsx030.

Koren, O., Goodrich, J.K., Cullender, T.C., Spor, A., Laitinen, K., Kling Bäckhed, H., Gonzalez, A., Werner, J.J., Angenent, L.T., Knight, R., Bäckhed, F., Isolauri, E., Salminen, S., Ley, R.E., 2012. Host remodeling of the gut microbiome and metabolic changes during pregnancy. Cell 150 (3), 470–480. https://doi.org/10.1016/j.cell.2012.07.008.

Krittanawong, C., Johnson, K.W., Rosenson, R.S., Wang, Z., Aydar, M., Baber, U., Min, J.K., Tang, W.H.W., Halperin, J.L., Narayan, S.M., 2019. Deep learning for cardiovascular medicine: a practical primer. Eur. Heart J. 40 (25), 2058–2073. https://doi.org/10.1093/eurheartj/ehz056.

Laschinger, S., Medves, J., Pulling, C., McGraw, R., Waytuck, B., Harrison, M.B., Gambeta, K., 2008. Effectiveness of simulation on health profession students' knowledge, skills, confidence and satisfaction. Int. J. Evid. Base. Healthc. 6 (3), 278–302. https://doi.org/10.1111/j.1744-1609.2008.00108.x. http://onlinelibrary.wiley.com/store/10.1111/j.1744-1609.2008.00108.x/asset/j.1744-1609.2008.00108.x.pdf?v=1&t=hztaer97&s=7291390a4f6172208ffee472f4a6374f96a9b93d.

Lawlor, N., George, J., Bolisetty, M., Kursawe, R., Sun, L., Sivakamasundari, V., Kycia, I., Robson, P., Stitzel, M.L., 2017. Single-cell transcriptomes identify human islet cell signatures and reveal cell-type-specific expression changes in type 2 diabetes. Genome Res. 27 (2), 208–222. https://doi.org/10.1101/gr.212720.116.

Liang, H., Tsui, B.Y., Ni, H., Valentim, C.C.S., Baxter, S.L., Liu, G., Cai, W., Kermany, D.S., Sun, X., Chen, J., He, L., Zhu, J., Tian, P., Shao, H., Zheng, L., Hou, R., Hewett, S., Li, G., Liang, P., Zang, X., Zhang, Z., Pan, L., Cai, H., Ling, R., Li, S., Cui, Y., Tang, S., Ye, H., Huang, X., He, W., Liang, W., Zhang, Q., Jiang, J., Yu, W., Gao, J., Ou, W., Deng, Y., Hou, Q., Wang, B., Yao, C., Liang, Y., Zhang, S., Duan, Y., Zhang, R., Gibson, S., Zhang, C.L., Li, O., Zhang, E.D., Karin, G., Nguyen, N., Wu, X., Wen, C., Xu, J., Xu, W., Wang, B., Wang, W., Li, J., Pizzato, B., Bao, C., Xiang, D., He, W., He, S., Zhou, Y., Haw, W., Goldbaum, M., Tremoulet, A., Hsu, C.N., Carter, H., Zhu, L., Zhang, K., Xia, H., 2019. Evaluation and accurate diagnoses of pediatric diseases using artificial intelligence. Nat. Med. 25 (3), 433–438. https://doi.org/10.1038/s41591-018-0335-9.

Liu, X.S., Wu, H., Ji, X., Stelzer, Y., Wu, X., Czauderna, S., Shu, J., Dadon, D., Young, R.A., Jaenisch, R., 2016. Editing DNA methylation in the mammalian genome. Cell 167 (1), 233. https://doi.org/10.1016/j.cell.2016.08.056.

Marso, S.P., Daniels, G.H., Frandsen, K.B., Kristensen, P., Mann, J.F.E., Nauck, M.A., Nissen, S.E., Pocock, S., Poulter, N.R., Ravn, L.S., Steinberg, W. M., Stockner, M., Zinman, B., Bergenstal, R.M., Buse, J.B., 2016. Liraglutide and cardiovascular outcomes in type 2 diabetes. N. Engl. J. Med. 375 (4), 311–322. https://doi.org/10.1056/NEJMoa1603827.

Mathur, S., Sutton, J., 2017. Personalized medicine could transform healthcare. Biomed. Rep. 7 (1), 3–5. https://doi.org/10.3892/br.2017.922.

McCutcheon, S.R., Rohm, D., Iglesias, N., Gersbach, C.A., 2024. Epigenome editing technologies for discovery and medicine. Nat. Biotechnol. 42 (8), 1199–1217. https://doi.org/10.1038/s41587-024-02320-1.

Miragaia, R.J., Zhang, X., Gomes, T., Svensson, V., Ilicic, T., Henriksson, J., Teichmann, S.A., 2019. Single-cell transcriptomics of regulatory T cells reveals trajectories of tissue adaptation. Immunity 50 (2), 493–504.e7.

Mirnezami, R., Nicholson, J., Darzi, A., 2012. Preparing for precision medicine. N. Engl. J. Med. 366 (6), 489–491. https://doi.org/10.1056/NEJMp1114866.

Morganti, S., Tarantino, P., Ferraro, E., D'Amico, P., Duso, B.A., Curigliano, G., 2019. Next generation sequencing (NGS): a revolutionary technology in pharmacogenomics and personalized medicine in cancer. Transl. Res. Onco-omics Appl. Era Cancer Personal Genom. 9–30.

Raisaro, J.L., 2018. Privacy-enhancing technologies for medical and genomic data: From theory to practice. Swiss Federal Institute of Technology Lausanne. Doctoral dissertation.

Reddy, M.A., Natarajan, R., 2011. Epigenetics in diabetic kidney disease. J. Am. Soc. Nephrol. 22 (12), 2182–2185. https://doi.org/10.1681/ASN.2011060629.

Rutter, G.A., Chimienti, F., 2015. SLC30A8 mutations in type 2 diabetes. Diabetologia 58 (1), 31–36. https://doi.org/10.1007/s00125-014-3405-7.

Sadee, W., Wang, D., Hartmann, K., Toland, A.E., 2023. Pharmacogenomics: driving personalized medicine. Pharmacol. Rev. 75 (4), 789–814.

Schaefer, G.O., Tai, E.S., Sun, S.H.L., 2020. Navigating conflicts of justice in the use of race and ethnicity in precision medicine. Bioethics 34 (8), 849–856.

Shabaruddin, F.H., Fleeman, N.D., Payne, K., 2015. Economic evaluations of personalized medicine: Existing challenges and current developments. Pharmacogenomics Personalized Med. 8, 115–126. https://doi.org/10.2147/PGPM.S35063.

Sharrer, G.T., 2017. Personalized medicine: Ethical aspects. In: Molecular profiling: Methods and protocols. Humana Press, pp. 37–50. https://doi.org/10.1007/978-1-4939-6990-6_3.

Sigman, M., 2018. Introduction: Personalized medicine: what is it and what are the challenges? Fertil. Steril. 109 (6), 944–945.

Soni, N., Soni, N., Maheshwari, R., Thakkar, S., Sharma, D., Tekade, R.K., Tekade, M., 2020. Pharmacogenomics and pharmacoepigenomics: Impact on therapeutic strategies. In: *The Future of Pharmaceutical Product Development and Research*. Academic Press, pp. 413–446.

Stanojevic, S., Li, Y., Ristivojevic, A., Garmire, L.X., 2022. Computational Methods for single-cell multi-omics integration and alignment. Genom. Proteom. Bioinform. 20 (5), 836–849. https://doi.org/10.1016/j.gpb.2022.11.013.

Tawfik, S.M., Elhosseiny, A.A., Galal, A.A., William, M.B., Qansuwa, E., Elbaz, R. M., Salama, M., 2023. Health inequity in genomic personalized medicine in underrepresented populations: a look at the current evidence. Funct. Integr. Genomics 23 (1). https://doi.org/10.1007/s10142-023-00979-4. https://www.springer.com/journal/10142.

Trosman, J.R., Van Bebber, S.L., Phillips, K.A., 2011. Health technology assessment and private payers' coverage of personalized medicine. J. Oncol. Pract. 7 (3). https://doi.org/10.1200/JOP.2011.000300(. http://jop.ascopubs.org/content/7/3S/18s.full.pdf+html. United States).

Turnbaugh, P.J., Ley, R.E., Mahowald, M.A., Magrini, V., Mardis, E.R., Gordon, J. I., 2006. An obesity-associated gut microbiome with increased capacity for energy harvest. Nature 444 (7122), 1027–1031. https://doi.org/10.1038/nature05414.

Vayena, E., Blasimme, A., 2018. Health research with big data: Time for systemic oversight. J. Law Med. Ethics 46 (1), 119–129. https://doi.org/10.1177/1073110518766026.

Verma, M., Barh, D. (Eds.), 2016. Progress and Challenges in Precision Medicine.

Vitorino, R., 2024. Transforming clinical research: The power of high-throughput omics integration. Proteomes 12 (3), 25. https://doi.org/10.3390/proteomes12030025.

Wells, C.J., 2020. A consensus on collaboration: reviewing the 15th annual personalized medicine conference at harvard medical school. Pers. Med. 17 (2), 79–81. https://doi.org/10.2217/pme-2020-0001.

Xiong, Z., Yang, F., Li, M., Ma, Y., Zhao, W., Wang, G., Li, Z., Zheng, X., Zou, D., Zong, W., Kang, H., Jia, Y., Li, R., Zhang, Z., Bao, Y., 2022. EWAS Open Platform: integrated data, knowledge and toolkit for epigenome-wide association study. Nucleic Acids Res. 50 (D1), D1004. https://doi.org/10.1093/nar/gkab972.

Zhang, B., Gaiteri, C., Bodea, L.G., Wang, Z., McElwee, J., Podtelezhnikov, A.A., Zhang, C., Xie, T., Tran, L., Dobrin, R., Fluder, E., Clurman, B., Melquist, S., Narayanan, M., Suver, C., Shah, H., Mahajan, M., Gillis, T., Mysore, J., MacDonald, M.E., Lamb, J.R., Bennett, D.A., Molony, C., Stone, D.J., Gudnason, V., Myers, A.J., Schadt, E.E., Neumann, H., Zhu, J., Emilsson, V., 2013. Integrated systems approach identifies genetic nodes and networks in late-onset Alzheimer's disease. Cell 153 (3), 707–720. https://doi.org/10.1016/j.cell.2013.03.030.

Zhuang, S., Liu, S., Li, R., Duan, H., 2025. Electroacupuncture alleviates insulin resistance and impacts the hypothalamic IRS-1/PI3K/AKT pathway and miRNA-29a-3p in a rat model of type 2 diabetes. Acupunct. Med. 43 (2), 104–113. https://doi.org/10.1177/09645284251327205.

Zhuo, C., Feng, M., Andrew, D.P., John, M.L., Lingxiao, Z., Dustin, E.S., Xiwei, W., Jinhui, W., Joshua, D.T., Saul, G., Barbara, H.B., Arthur, D.R., Rama, N., 2016. Epigenomic profiling reveals an association between persistence of DNA methylation and metabolic memory in the DCCT/EDIC type 1 diabetes cohort. Proc. Natl. Acad. Sci. U. S. A 113 (21), E3002. https://doi.org/10.1073/pnas.1603712113.

Zinman, B., Wanner, C., Lachin, J.M., Fitchett, D., Bluhmki, E., Hantel, S., Mattheus, M., Devins, T., Johansen, O.E., Woerle, H.J., Broedl, U.C., Inzucchi, S.E., 2015. Empagliflozin, cardiovascular outcomes, and mortality in type 2 diabetes. N. Engl. J. Med. 373 (22), 2117–2128. https://doi.org/10.1056/NEJMoa1504720. http://www.nejm.org/doi/pdf/10.1056/NEJMoa1504720.

11

Metabolic memory: Future outlook

1. Introduction

Metabolic diseases, particularly diabetes and obesity, represent a growing global health burden, with complications often persisting or emerging even after clinical parameters such as blood glucose levels are brought under control. This paradox has led to the conceptualization of metabolic memory, a phenomenon wherein early metabolic insults, such as hyperglycemia, oxidative stress, and chronic inflammation, induce long-lasting molecular changes that continue to influence disease progression long after the inciting stimuli have been mitigated (Brownlee, 2005; Hurrle and Hsu, 2017).

The evidence for metabolic memory was first established in seminal clinical trials like the Diabetes Control and Complications Trial (DCCT) and its follow-up, the Epidemiology of Diabetes Interventions and Complications (EDIC) study. These studies revealed that early intensive glycemic control in patients with type 1 diabetes significantly reduced the risk of long-term complications such as nephropathy and retinopathy, even when glycemic control in both study groups later converged (Nathan, 2014). These findings suggested that the biological consequences of early hyperglycemia could become ingrained in cellular function, exerting long-term pathogenic effects.

At the molecular level, epigenetic modifications, including DNA methylation, histone modifications, and non-coding RNA regulation, have emerged as key mediators of metabolic memory (El-Osta et al., 2008). These changes can persist long after normalization of metabolic parameters, influencing gene expression profiles associated with inflammation, vascular damage, and insulin resistance. Furthermore, oxidative stress, mitochondrial dysfunction, and pro-inflammatory signaling pathways such as NF-κB and p38 MAPK are deeply implicated in the persistence of these effects, creating a self-sustaining cycle of cellular damage (Brownlee, 2005; Hurrle and Hsu, 2017).

Metabolic Memory. https://doi.org/10.1016/B978-0-443-44591-0.00009-6

Importantly, recent research has expanded the scope of metabolic memory to include intergenerational transmission. Maternal metabolic conditions, such as obesity, undernutrition, or gestational diabetes, can epigenetically program the offspring's susceptibility to metabolic diseases later in life, mediated through changes in placental function, fetal gene expression, and the developing microbiome (Aiken and Ozanne, 2014; Godfrey et al., 2016). This growing understanding underscores the critical importance of early-life interventions and preconception health.

Given its profound clinical implications, metabolic memory is becoming a focal point in efforts to transition from reactive to predictive and preventive medicine. By integrating tools such as DNA methylation profiling, transcriptomics, and metabolomics, researchers and clinicians are beginning to identify at-risk individuals even before clinical symptoms manifest (Rehman, 2024). Moreover, novel therapeutic avenues, ranging from epigenetic-modifying agents and microbiome-targeted interventions to precision public health strategies, offer the potential to interrupt or even reverse the long-term imprint of metabolic insults.

This chapter provides a comprehensive overview of the foundational concepts, biological mechanisms, clinical evidence, and translational implications of metabolic memory, setting the stage for future innovations in personalized healthcare and chronic disease prevention (Fig. 11.1).

1.1 Future outlook on research and clinical practice

The future of metabolic memory research lies in translating epigenetic and molecular discoveries into practical clinical tools that can inform diagnosis, prognosis, and intervention strategies. A growing body of research suggests that epigenetic biomarkers, such as specific DNA methylation patterns and histone modification signatures, have immense potential for identifying individuals at elevated risk of chronic metabolic diseases, especially those who appear clinically normal but have a history of early-life metabolic insults (Rehman, 2024; Ling and Rönn, 2019). These biomarkers could enable the identification of latent molecular risk long before overt symptoms emerge, allowing for preventive, rather than reactive, care.

Emerging technologies such as longitudinal epigenomic profiling which involves repeated tracking of genome-wide epigenetic changes in the same individuals over time to study

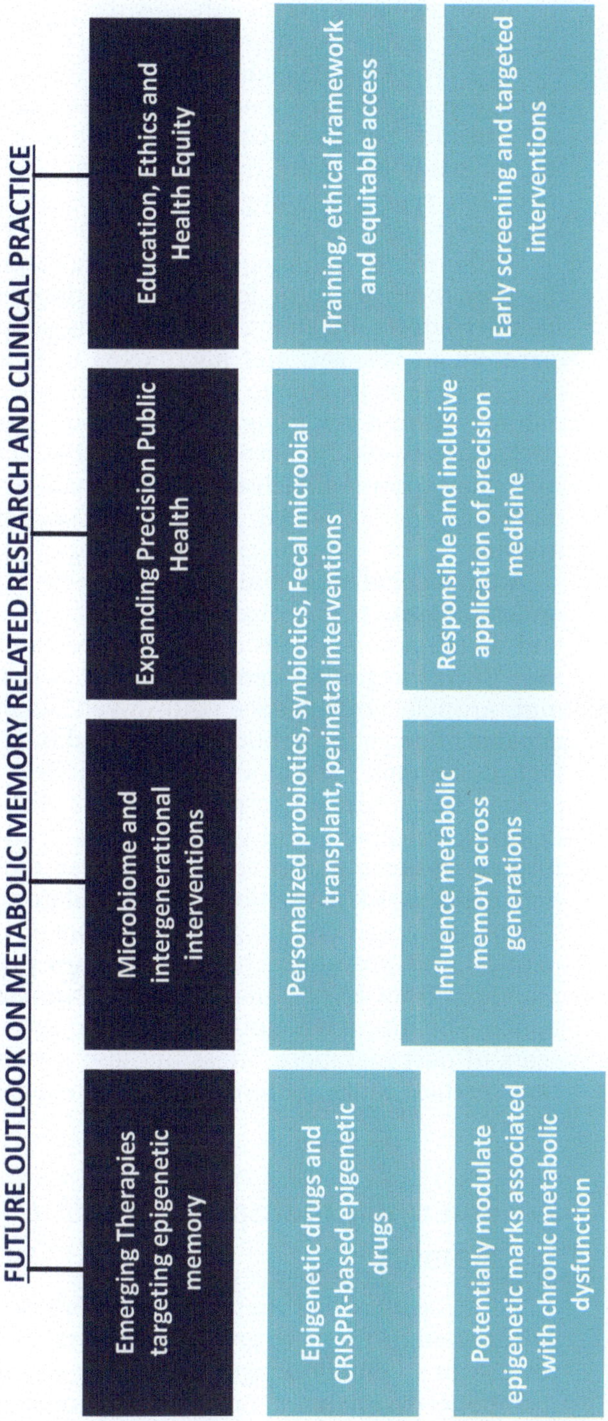

Figure 11.1 Future outlook on research and clinical practice. Paradigm shift from reactive to proactive interventions, ensuring equity and inclusivity.

dynamic regulation in health and disease, could revolutionize our ability to monitor disease trajectories and treatment responsiveness. Tracking epigenetic changes over time in response to therapy may provide a sensitive and dynamic window into metabolic health. For instance, demethylation of certain inflammatory or oxidative stress-related gene loci could signal effective metabolic reprogramming following a lifestyle or pharmacological intervention (El-Osta et al., 2008; Dayeh et al., 2014).

Furthermore, minimally invasive platforms, including liquid biopsies, hold promise for assessing tissue-specific metabolic memory effects. By analyzing circulating cell-free DNA (cfDNA), extracellular vesicles, and microRNAs in blood or saliva, clinicians may soon be able to monitor organ-specific epigenetic signatures without requiring invasive tissue sampling (Wan et al., 2017). This would be particularly valuable in populations where early-life exposures, such as maternal malnutrition or gestational diabetes, are suspected to have left a persistent molecular imprint.

A major challenge and opportunity lie in integrating multi-omics datasets (e.g., epigenomics, transcriptomics, proteomics, and metabolomics) with clinical records and lifestyle information. Such integration demands robust bioinformatics pipelines and artificial intelligence (AI)-driven analytical frameworks capable of detecting subtle, multilayered interactions across biological systems. Machine learning models, for example, are already being trained to predict type 2 diabetes risk based on complex epigenetic and genetic inputs (Zou et al., 2019). With further refinement and validation, these tools could transform personalized risk prediction into a standard part of routine care.

The convergence of omics technologies, personalized therapeutics, and preventive health strategies promises to shift the paradigm from disease management to proactive health maintenance. The future will not only focus on reversing the molecular scars of past metabolic stress but also on intercepting them at their earliest stage, before they are etched into the biological record.

2. Emerging therapies targeting epigenetic memory

As the concept of metabolic memory becomes increasingly substantiated, there is growing interest in therapies that can reverse or modulate epigenetic marks associated with chronic metabolic dysfunction. Epigenetic modifications such as DNA methylation and histone modifications are not necessarily permanent and may be therapeutically altered to restore gene expression patterns associated with metabolic homeostasis.

Histone deacetylase (HDAC) inhibitors and DNA methyltransferase (DNMT) inhibitors are among the most studied epigenetic drugs. Originally developed and approved for use in certain cancers, these agents are now being repurposed and investigated for their effects on metabolic and cardiovascular diseases. For example, HDAC inhibitors like valproic acid and trichostatin A have shown promise in preclinical models of diabetes and cardiac hypertrophy by enhancing insulin sensitivity and reducing inflammatory gene expression (Rafehi et al., 2014; Huang et al., 2021).

Dietary and naturally occurring compounds that modulate the epigenome are also being explored as safer and more accessible therapeutic agents. Compounds such as resveratrol, a polyphenol found in grapes, and butyrate, a short-chain fatty acid produced by gut microbiota, are known to inhibit HDACs and improve metabolic function in animal models (Tennen et al., 2010; Gao et al., 2009). Similarly, folate and other one-carbon donors play crucial roles in methylation reactions and have been shown to influence epigenetic regulation of metabolic genes, especially during early development and pregnancy (Waterland and Jirtle, 2003).

Perhaps the most cutting-edge approach involves CRISPR/dCas9-based epigenetic editing, which allows for precise, locus-specific reprogramming of gene expression without altering the underlying DNA sequence. By fusing the catalytically inactive Cas9 (dCas9) protein to epigenetic modifiers such as DNA demethylases or histone acetyltransferases, researchers can selectively target and reverse aberrant epigenetic silencing of protective metabolic genes (Liu et al., 2016; Nuñez et al., 2021). While still in its experimental stages, this approach holds transformative potential for long-term reprogramming of metabolic pathways.

Despite these advances, several challenges remain, including off-target effects, delivery efficiency, and the ethical implications of modifying the human epigenome. Rigorous long-term studies and ethical guidelines will be essential as these novel therapies transition from bench to bedside.

3. Microbiome and intergenerational interventions

Given the pivotal role of the gut microbiome in regulating host metabolism, inflammation, and immune responses, the field of microbiome-modulating therapy is gaining traction as a promising avenue for mitigating metabolic memory. The human gut harbors trillions of microorganisms that influence nutrient absorption, insulin sensitivity, bile acid metabolism, and systemic inflammation, processes closely linked to obesity, type 2 diabetes, and cardiovascular diseases (Tilg et al., 2020).

3.1 Personalized probiotics and synbiotics

Emerging approaches emphasize individualized probiotic and synbiotic formulations designed to address a person's specific dysbiosis profile. Traditional probiotics often follow a one-size-fits-all model, but advancements in metagenomic sequencing and machine learning algorithms now allow precise identification of microbial imbalances in individuals. For example, patients with a high Firmicutes-to-Bacteroidetes ratio, associated with obesity and insulin resistance, may benefit from strains like *Akkermansia muciniphila* or *Bifidobacterium animalis,* which promote mucosal barrier integrity and antiinflammatory signaling (Depommier et al., 2019). Synbiotics, combinations of probiotics and prebiotic substrates, can be tailored to support the engraftment and activity of beneficial taxa.

3.2 Fecal microbiota transplantation (FMT)

Fecal microbiota transplantation (FMT), involving the transfer of stool from healthy donors to recipients, is being explored not only for treating recurrent *Clostridioides difficile* infection but also for resetting microbiome-metabolome interactions in metabolic disease. In a landmark study, obese patients receiving FMT from lean donors exhibited increased insulin sensitivity within weeks, correlating with shifts in microbial taxa such as *Roseburia* and *Eubacterium hallii,* known producers of short-chain fatty acids like butyrate (Vrieze et al., 2012). These findings underscore the potential of FMT as a therapeutic reset for persistent dysbiosis-driven metabolic programming.

3.3 Perinatal and early-life microbiome interventions

The early-life microbiome is critical for metabolic and immune development, making pregnancy and infancy strategic windows for intervention. Maternal diet, antibiotic exposure, and delivery mode can shape the infant gut microbiome in ways that influence long-term metabolic risk. Interventions targeting maternal microbiota, such as supplementation with specific probiotics or prebiotics during pregnancy, have been shown to modulate offspring gut microbiota and reduce the risk of obesity and allergic disease (Kalliomäki et al., 2003). Furthermore, breast milk-derived human milk oligosaccharides (HMOs) act as natural prebiotics that selectively enrich protective bacteria like *Bifidobacterium*, reinforcing mucosal immunity and metabolic resilience (Zivkovic et al., 2011).

Collectively, these strategies represent a paradigm shift in how clinicians may intervene not just in overt disease states but at the microbial and metabolic level to influence long-term health trajectories.

4. Expanding precision public health

Future clinical practice is expected to witness a strategic convergence between precision medicine and public health, giving rise to a new interdisciplinary model known as precision public health. This approach emphasizes the integration of genomic, epigenomic, and environmental data at the population level, not merely for treatment, but for anticipatory prevention of chronic metabolic diseases rooted in early-life exposures.

4.1 Maternal-child health and early screening

One of the most promising domains of precision public health is maternal-child health, where programs increasingly incorporate epigenetic and metabolic screening during preconception, pregnancy, and infancy. For example, early identification of DNA methylation patterns in placental or cord blood DNA associated with insulin resistance or adiposity can guide prenatal nutrition and lifestyle interventions (Lillycrop and Burdge, 2011). In addition, maternal genomic profiling, including polymorphisms in folate and one-carbon metabolism pathways, can inform targeted supplementation strategies to mitigate epigenetic imprinting in the fetus (Steegers-Theunissen et al., 2013).

4.2 Population-level genomic and epigenomic risk profiling

Advancements in population-scale omics, including polygenic risk scores (PRS) and epigenome-wide association studies (EWAS), enable stratification of individuals based on their inherited or acquired risk of metabolic disease. Tools such as epigenetic clocks and biological age estimators are emerging as predictors of long-term health and disease burden (Horvath and Raj, 2018). These tools hold promise for incorporation into public health screening programs, facilitating early identification and intervention among high-risk populations, even in the absence of clinical symptoms.

4.3 Policy and environmental interventions

Metabolic memory is not shaped by biology alone but is deeply influenced by social determinants of health, including dietary patterns, air pollution, socioeconomic status, and early-life stress. Therefore, future directions in policy must address these upstream drivers. Reforms in food systems, such as restricting ultra-processed food marketing, improving maternal nutrition programs, and supporting breastfeeding, can reduce early metabolic insults. Similarly, policies to curb air pollution have been linked to decreased incidence of childhood obesity and metabolic dysfunction through mechanisms involving inflammation and oxidative stress (Thiering and Heinrich, 2015).

4.4 Disrupting the cycle of metabolic memory

Ultimately, precision public health aims to break the intergenerational cycle of metabolic memory by targeting the earliest stages of life, from gametogenesis and embryonic development to early childhood. This preventive framework redefines health promotion by integrating multi-omics data, environmental risk mapping, and social policy, offering a proactive, rather than reactive, approach to chronic disease prevention.

5. Education, ethics, and health equity

As precision medicine becomes increasingly integrated into clinical care, healthcare education, bioethics, and equity frameworks must evolve accordingly to ensure responsible and inclusive application, especially in managing metabolic memory.

5.1 Education and clinical readiness

The education of healthcare professionals is foundational for successful translation of personalized medicine into practice. Clinicians will require fluency in systems biology, genomics, epigenetics, bioinformatics, and data interpretation to make informed decisions from multi-omics data and integrate them into individual patient care. Training programs must emphasize how epigenetic modifications, microbiome interactions, and metabolic phenotyping contribute to chronic disease risk and treatment response (Feero et al., 2010). Interdisciplinary curricula incorporating genomic literacy, machine learning applications, and ethical decision-making will prepare providers for the complexity of precision healthcare.

5.2 Evolving ethical frameworks

The application of personalized strategies also raises novel ethical challenges, especially in the context of metabolic memory, which can span generations. Issues of genetic privacy, data security, and informed consent must be addressed, particularly when intergenerational health decisions are at play, for example, in preconception screening or early-life interventions. Additionally, there is a growing need to consider non-maleficence and autonomy when dealing with predictive risk profiling in asymptomatic individuals (Kass, 2001). Ethical frameworks must evolve to handle longitudinal data use, AI-driven decision support, and biological determinism in clinical counseling.

5.3 Ensuring health equity

Perhaps the most critical challenge lies in ensuring equitable access to personalized healthcare. Historically marginalized populations, such as those from lower socioeconomic backgrounds or underrepresented ethnic groups, bear a disproportionate burden of metabolic diseases such as diabetes and obesity. Without intentional action, precision medicine may risk widening existing health disparities, as access to omics testing, personalized therapies, and expert interpretation remains limited in many settings (Manrai et al., 2016). Equity-driven models must include subsidized access, community-based implementation strategies, and policies that prevent discrimination based on genetic or epigenetic risk profiles.

Efforts such as community genomic literacy programs, inclusive research participation, and public-private partnerships can support equitable adoption. Moreover, regulatory oversight should ensure that new technologies undergo diverse population validation to avoid biases in predictive algorithms and treatment responses.

6. Conclusion

Metabolic memory provides a compelling biological explanation for the persistence of disease risk despite apparent clinical resolution. As the fields of epigenetics, genomics, and systems medicine continue to advance, integrating metabolic memory into clinical practice offers a unique opportunity to transform healthcare from reactive to proactive, and from generalized to personalized. Future efforts must prioritize the development of scalable, accessible, and ethically sound interventions that target both individual risk and intergenerational transmission. Through a combined lens of molecular insight and public health strategy, we can envision a future in which chronic metabolic diseases are not merely managed, but prevented at their molecular roots.

References

Aiken, C.E., Ozanne, S.E., 2014. Transgenerational developmental programming. Hum. Reprod. Update 20 (1), 63–75. https://doi.org/10.1093/humupd/dmt043.

Brownlee, M., 2005. The pathobiology of diabetic complications: a unifying mechanism. Diabetes 54 (6), 1615–1625. https://doi.org/10.2337/diabetes.54.6.1615.

Dayeh, T., Volkov, P., Salö, S., Hall, E., Nilsson, E., Olsson, A.H., Kirkpatrick, C. L., Wollheim, C.B., Eliasson, L., Rönn, T., Bacos, K., Ling, C., 2014. Genome-wide DNA methylation analysis of human pancreatic islets from type 2 diabetic and non-diabetic donors identifies candidate genes that influence insulin secretion. PLoS Genet. 10 (3). https://doi.org/10.1371/journal.pgen.1004160.

Depommier, C., Everard, A., Druart, C., Plovier, H., Van Hul, M., Vieira-Silva, S., Falony, G., Raes, J., Maiter, D., Delzenne, N.M., de Barsy, M., Loumaye, A., Hermans, M.P., Thissen, J.P., de Vos, W.M., Cani, P.D., 2019. Supplementation with Akkermansia muciniphila in overweight and obese human volunteers: a proof-of-concept exploratory study. Nat. Med. 25 (7), 1096–1103. https://doi.org/10.1038/s41591-019-0495-2.

El-Osta, A., Brasacchio, D., Yao, D., Pocai, A., Jones, P.L., Roeder, R.G., Cooper, M.E., Brownlee, M., 2008. Transient high glucose causes persistent epigenetic changes and altered gene expression during subsequent normoglycemia. J. Exp. Med. 205 (10), 2409–2417. https://doi.org/10.1084/jem.20081188Australia.

Feero, W.G., Guttmacher, A.E., Collins, F.S., 2010. Genomic medicine—an updated primer. N. Engl. J. Med. 362 (21), 2001–2011. https://doi.org/10.1056/NEJMra0907175.

Gao, Z., Yin, J., Zhang, J., Ward, R.E., Martin, R.J., Lefevre, M., Cefalu, W.T., Ye, J., 2009. Butyrate improves insulin sensitivity and increases energy expenditure in mice. Diabetes 58 (7), 1509–1517. https://doi.org/10.2337/db08-1637.

Godfrey, K.M., Costello, P.M., Lillycrop, K.A., 2016. Development, epigenetics and metabolic programming. Nestle Nutr. Inst. Workshop Ser. 85, 71–80. https://doi.org/10.1159/000439488.

Horvath, S., Raj, K., 2018. DNA methylation-based biomarkers and the epigenetic clock theory of ageing. Nat. Rev. Genet. 19 (6), 371–384. https://doi.org/10.1038/s41576-018-0004-3.

Huang, S., Chen, G., Sun, J., Chen, Y., Wang, N., Dong, Y., Shen, E., Hu, Z., Gong, W., Jin, L., Cong, W., 2021. Histone deacetylase 3 inhibition alleviates type 2 diabetes mellitus-induced endothelial dysfunction via Nrf2. Cell Commun. Signal. 19 (1). https://doi.org/10.1186/s12964-020-00681-z.

Hurrle, S., Hsu, W.H., 2017. The etiology of oxidative stress in insulin resistance. Biomed. J. 40 (5), 257–262. https://doi.org/10.1016/j.bj.2017.06.007.

Kalliomäki, M., Salminen, S., Poussa, T., Arvilommi, H., Isolauri, E., 2003. Probiotics and prevention of atopic disease: 4-year follow-up of a randomised placebo-controlled trial. Lancet 361 (9372), 1869–1871. https://doi.org/10.1016/s0140-6736(03)13490-3.

Kass, N.E., 2001. An ethics framework for public health. Am. J. Public Health 91 (11), 1776–1782. https://doi.org/10.2105/AJPH.91.11.1776.

Lillycrop, K.A., Burdge, G.C., 2011. Epigenetic changes in early life and future risk of obesity. Int. J. Obes. 35 (1), 72–83. https://doi.org/10.1038/ijo.2010.122.

Ling, C., Rönn, T., 2019. Epigenetics in human obesity and type 2 diabetes. Cell Metab. 29 (5), 1028–1044. https://doi.org/10.1016/j.cmet.2019.03.009.

Liu, X.S., Wu, H., Ji, X., Stelzer, Y., Wu, X., Czauderna, S., Shu, J., Dadon, D., Young, R.A., Jaenisch, R., 2016. Editing DNA methylation in the mammalian genome. Cell 167 (1), 233. https://doi.org/10.1016/j.cell.2016.08.056.

Manrai, A.K., Funke, B.H., Rehm, H.L., Olesen, M.S., Maron, B.A., Szolovits, P., Margulies, D.M., Loscalzo, J., Kohane, I.S., 2016. Genetic misdiagnoses and the potential for health disparities. N. Engl. J. Med. 375 (7), 655–665. https://doi.org/10.1056/NEJMsa1507092.

Nathan, D.M., 2014. The diabetes control and complications trial/epidemiology of diabetes interventions and complications study at 30 years: overview. Diabetes Care 37 (1), 9–16. https://doi.org/10.2337/dc13-2112.

Nuñez, J.K., Chen, J., Pommier, G.C., Cogan, J.Z., Replogle, J.M., Adriaens, C., Ramadoss, G.N., Shi, Q., Hung, K.L., Samelson, A.J., Pogson, A.N., Kim, J.Y. S., Chung, A., Leonetti, M.D., Chang, H.Y., Kampmann, M., Bernstein, B.E., Hovestadt, V., Gilbert, L.A., Weissman, J.S., 2021. Genome-wide programmable transcriptional memory by CRISPR-based epigenome editing. Cell 184 (9), 2503. https://doi.org/10.1016/j.cell.2021.03.025.

Rafehi, H., Balcerczyk, A., Lunke, S., Kaspi, A., Ziemann, M., Harikrishnan, K.N., Jun, O., Khurana, I., Ooi, J., Khan, A.W., Jun Du, X., Chang, L., Haviv, I., Keating, S.T., Karagiannis, T.C., El-Osta, A., 2014. Vascular histone deacetylation by pharmacological HDAC inhibition. Genome Res. 24 (8), 1271–1284. https://doi.org/10.1101/gr.168781.113.

Rehman, A., 2024. Advances in precision medicine for type 2 diabetes: integrating genomic, epigenetic, and metabolomic data for personalized therapeutic strategies. Life Sci. Perspect. 1 (1), 1–9.

Steegers-Theunissen, R.P.M., Twigt, J., Pestinger, V., Sinclair, K.D., 2013. The periconceptional period, reproduction and long-term health of offspring: the importance of one-carbon metabolism. Hum. Reprod. Update 19 (6), 640–655. https://doi.org/10.1093/humupd/dmt041.

Tennen, R.I., Berber, E., Chua, K.F., 2010. Functional dissection of SIRT6: identification of domains that regulate histone deacetylase activity and chromatin localization. Mech. Ageing Dev. 131 (3), 185–192. https://doi.org/10.1016/j.mad.2010.01.006.

Thiering, E., Heinrich, J., 2015. Epidemiology of air pollution and diabetes. Trends Endocrinol Metab 26 (7), 384–394. https://doi.org/10.1016/j.tem.2015.05.002.

Tilg, H., Zmora, N., Adolph, T.E., Elinav, E., 2020. The intestinal microbiota fuelling metabolic inflammation. Nat. Rev. Immunol. 20 (1), 40–54. https://doi.org/10.1038/s41577-019-0198-4.

Vrieze, A., Van Nood, E., Holleman, F., Salojärvi, J., Kootte, R.S., Bartelsman, J.F. W.M., Dallinga-Thie, G.M., Ackermans, M.T., Serlie, M.J., Oozeer, R., Derrien, M., Druesne, A., Van Hylckama Vlieg, J.E.T., Bloks, V.W., Groen, A. K., Heilig, H.G.H.J., Zoetendal, E.G., Stroes, E.S., De Vos, W.M., Hoekstra, J. B.L., Nieuwdorp, M., 2012. Transfer of intestinal microbiota from lean donors increases insulin sensitivity in individuals with metabolic syndrome. Gastroenterology 143 (4), 913. https://doi.org/10.1053/j.gastro.2012.06.031.

Wan, J.C.M., Massie, C., Garcia-Corbacho, J., Mouliere, F., Brenton, J.D., Caldas, C., Pacey, S., Baird, R., Rosenfeld, N., 2017. Liquid biopsies come of age: towards implementation of circulating tumour DNA. Nat. Rev. Cancer 17 (4), 223–238. https://doi.org/10.1038/nrc.2017.7.

Waterland, R.A., Jirtle, R.L., 2003. Transposable elements: targets for early nutritional effects on epigenetic gene regulation. Mol. Cell Biol. 23 (15), 5293–5300. https://doi.org/10.1128/MCB.23.15.5293-5300.2003.

Zivkovic, A.M., Bruce German, J., Lebrilla, C.B., Mills, D.A., 2011. Human milk glycobiome and its impact on the infant gastrointestinal microbiota. Proc. Natl. Acad. Sci. 108 (Suppl. 1), 4653–4658. https://doi.org/10.1073/pnas.1000083107.

Zou, J., Huss, M., Abid, A., Mohammadi, P., Ali, T., Telenti, A., 2019. A primer on deep learning in genomics. Nat. Genet. 51 (1), 12–18. https://doi.org/10.1038/s41588-018-0295-5.

Index

Note: 'Page numbers followed by "f" indicate figures, "t" indicate tables.'

Printed and bound by CPI Group (UK) Ltd, Croydon, CR0 4YY
25/07/2026
02176697-0002